Research for Advanced Practice Nurses

Magdalena A. Mateo, PhD, RN, FAAN, died of Parkinson's Disease on June 13, 2013 in Phoenix, Arizona, while in the care of Hospice of the Valley. She was 67 years old. She received her BSN and MN degrees in the Philippines and her PhD from The Ohio State University. While working in clinical and academic settings as a clinical nurse specialist, and director of nursing and faculty in the Philippines, Canada, and the United States, she conducted studies and used results of studies to improve patient care. Her primary areas of research included research development and dissemination in the clinical arena, workforce diversity, and neuroscience (mild traumatic brain injury).

She was the director of research for the Department of Nursing at The Ohio State University Hospital and later at Mayo Clinics. She had recently retired from Northeastern University School of Nursing in Boston where she taught research courses. *Research for Advanced Practice Nurses* was based on a research manual she developed for her staff at Ohio State, to improve patient care. The book twice received the *American Journal of Nursing* Book of the Year Award for the research category, and she was working on the fourth edition when her health failed. She was elected a Fellow of the American Academy of Nursing in 1992.

Marquis D. Foreman, PhD, RN, FAAN, is professor and executive associate dean, Rush University College of Nursing. He has actively sought to improve the care of hospitalized older people for more than 30 years. Foreman is known best for his research on delirium in hospitalized older people. He is a Fellow of the American Academy of Nursing, and the Institute of Medicine of Chicago, and has received numerous awards, including the Mary Opal Wolanin Award for Excellence in Gerontological Clinical Nursing Research, the Harriet H. Werley New Investigator Award, and the Mosby-Cameo Nursing Research Award, all for his work on delirium in hospitalized older people.

Research for Advanced Practice Nurses

From Evidence to Practice

Second Edition

Magdalena A. Mateo, PhD, RN, FAAN
Marquis D. Foreman, PhD, RN, FAAN

Editors

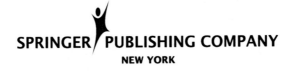

SPRINGER PUBLISHING COMPANY
NEW YORK

Springer Publishing Company, LLC
11 West 42nd Street
New York, NY10036
www.springerpub.com

Acquisitions Editor: Joseph Morita
Composition: Exeter Premedia Services Private Ltd.

ISBN: 978-0-8261-3725-8
e-book ISBN: 978-0-8261-3726-5

13 14 15 16 17/ 5 4 3 2 1

The author and the publisher of this Work have made every effort to use sources believed to be reliable to provide information that is accurate and compatible with the standards generally accepted at the time of publication. The author and publisher shall not be liable for any special, consequential, or exemplary damages resulting, in whole or in part, from the readers' use of, or reliance on, the information contained in this book. The publisher has no responsibility for the persistence or accuracy of URLs for external or third-party Internet websites referred to in this publication and does not guarantee that any content on such websites is, or will remain, accurate or appropriate.

Library of Congress Cataloging-in-Publication Data
Research for advanced practice nurses : from evidence to practice / [edited by] Magdalena Mateo, Marquis Foreman. — 2nd edition.
    p. ; cm.
  Includes bibliographical references and index.
  ISBN 978-0-8261-3725-8—ISBN 978-0-8261-3726-5 (e-book)
  I. Mateo, Magdalena A., editor of compilation. II. Foreman, Marquis D., editor of compilation.
  [DNLM: 1. Clinical Nursing Research. 2. Evidence-Based Practice. 3. Research Design. WY 20.5]
  RT81.5
  610′.73072—dc23

                                                            2013033785

Printed in the United States of America by Gasch Printing.

*This book is dedicated to my friend and colleague,
Magdalena A. Mateo.*

Contents

PART III. USING AVAILABLE EVIDENCE

PART IV. EVALUATING THE IMPACT OF EBP AND COMMUNICATING RESULTS

Contributors

Susan Adams, PhD, RN   Associate Director, Research Translation and Dissemination Core, Gerontological Nursing Interventions Research Center, College of Nursing, University of Iowa, Iowa City, Iowa

Mary D. Bondmass, PhD, RN, CNE   Associate Professor, Director of Distance Education, Georgetown University School of Nursing & Health Studies, Washington, DC

Elizabeth A. Carlson, RN, PhD   Associate Professor and Acting Chairperson, Department of Adult Health & Gerontological Nursing; Coordinator, Systems Leadership DNP, College of Nursing, Rush University Medical Center, Chicago, Illinois

Norma G. Cuellar, DSN, RN, FAAN   Professor, Capstone College of Nursing, University of Alabama, Tuscaloosa, Alabama

Ulrike Dieterle, MA, MLS   Senior Academic Librarian Emerita, Ebling Library for the Health Sciences, University of Wisconsin-Madison, Madison, Wisconsin

Marquis D. Foreman, PhD, RN, FAAN   Professor and Executive Associate Dean, Rush University College of Nursing

Susan K. Frazier, RN, PhD, FAHA   Associate Professor, College of Nursing, University of Kentucky, Lexington, Kentucky

Carol Glod, RN, PhD, FAAN   Lecturer, Harvard Medical School; Psychiatric Clinical Nurse Specialist, McLean Hospital; Dean, School of Graduate Studies, Salem State University, Salem, Massachusetts

Christopher Hooper-Lane, MA   Senior Academic Librarian, Ebling Library for the Health Sciences, University of Wisconsin—Madison, Madison, Wisconsin

Margaret Irwin, PhD, MN, RN, BA   Research Associate, Oncology Nursing Society, Pittsburgh, Pennsylvania

Briana J. Jegier, PhD   Assistant Professor, Department of Women, Children and Family Nursing, College of Nursing, Department of Health Systems Management, College of Health Sciences, Rush University Medical Center, Chicago, Illinois

Mary E. Johnson, RN, PhD, PMHCNS-BC, FAAN   Assistant Dean of Academic Affairs and Director of Specialty Programs, Community Systems and Mental Health Nursing, Rush University Medical Center, College of Nursing, Chicago, Illinois

Tricia J. Johnson, PhD   Associate Professor, Department of Health Systems Management, College of Health Sciences, Rush University Medical Center, Chicago, Illinois

Lea Ann Matura, PhD, RN, NP-C, CCRN   Assistant Professor, University of Pennsylvania School of Nursing, Philadelphia, Pennsylvania

Vivian Nowazek, PhD, MSN, RN-BC, CNS-CC, CCRN   Assistant Professor, University of Houston—Victoria at Sugar Land, Sugar Land, Texas

Marcia Phillips, RN, PhD   Assistant Professor, Department of Adult Health and Gerontological Nursing, College of Nursing, Rush University Medical Center, Chicago, Illinois

Beth Rodgers, PhD, RN, FAAN   Professor, College of Nursing, University of New Mexico, Albuquerque, New Mexico

Karen J. Saewert, RN, PhD, CPHQ, CNE, ANEF   Clinical Associate Professor, Arizona State University, College of Nursing & Health Innovation, Phoenix, Arizona

Mary Schira, PhD, RN, ACNP-BC   Associate Dean, Chair, Advanced Practice Nursing/ACNP Program, School of Nursing, The University of Texas at Arlington, Arlington, Texas

Leah L. Shever, PhD, RN   Director of Nursing Research, Quality, and Innovation, University of Michigan Health System, Ann Arbor, Michigan

Beth A. Staffileno, RN, PhD, FAHA   Associate Professor, Department of Adult Health and Gerontological Nursing, College of Nursing, Rush University Medical Center, Chicago, Illinois

Kathleen R. Stevens, RN, EdD, FANE, FAAN   Professor and Director, Academic Center for Evidence-Based, Practice, The University of Texas Health Science Center, San Antonio, Texas

Diane L. Stuenkel, EdD, RN   Professor, Assistant Director, Curriculum Coordinator, The Valley Foundation School of Nursing at San Jose State University, San Jose, California

Marita G. Titler, PhD, RN, FAAN   Associate Dean for Practice and Clinical Scholarship, Rhetaugh Dumas Endowed Chair, University of Michigan School of Nursing and University of Michigan Health System, Ann Arbor, Michigan

Julie Johnson Zerwic, PhD, RN, FAHA, FAAN   Professor and Executive Associate Dean, College of Nursing, University of Illinois at Chicago, Chicago, Illinois

Preface

The increasing focus on evidence needed for practice decisions propels us to integrate how we teach graduate students about research. The use of research summaries and the need for evidence-based quality and safety practices and for clarifying the conduct of research are all requirements for nurses functioning professionally in practice. We hope that this book meets all those needs in a single introductory volume that includes evaluation of single research reports along with summaries and guidelines that may be of use when establishing evidence-based practice (EBP). When using results from an individual report, one must have a working knowledge of the research conducted if one is to evaluate the scientific merit and relevance of a single study.

Evidence-based practice concepts related to patient care are integrated throughout the chapters, with important points highlighted in exhibits. Clinically relevant examples present ways students and staff nurses can apply knowledge to daily clinical practice. We have also expanded, from the previous edition of this book, the information on EBP and examples of clinical protocols.

Part I: Evidence-Based Practice. Chapters focus on an overview of EBP: the definitions of EBP that have evolved over time, types of evidence, and models of EBP. Ways of finding evidence are presented to guide the reader to respond to the mandate for EBP. This information on EBP is vital to graduate students who are developing skills that will prepare them to assume their advanced practice role in health care.

Part II: Building Blocks for Evidence. The section starts with appraising a single research article; a building block for evidence. Components of the research process are presented from a reviewer's perspective of using the article as supporting evidence for practice in subsequent chapters. One of the documented barriers to research utilization is that practitioners feel inadequate reading and interpreting research findings. Gaining knowledge about the research process is crucial for clinicians who must read, interpret, and determine the relevance of research findings (evidence) to practice and to consider those findings that may be used in developing practice guidelines. It also allows practitioners to advocate for patients who are considering whether to participate in research.

Part III: Using Available Evidence. Meta-analyses, systematic reviews, and practice guidelines from various sources, such as professional organizations and government websites, are other types of evidence that may be used in establishing EBP. Appraising information from these sources is suggested in this section. Program evaluation provides an opportunity for use of evidence. Considerations when planning and implementing EBP activities are also included in this section: identifying the focus of EBP activities (unit or organizational) and developing an EBP protocol.

Part IV: Evaluating the Impact of EBP and Communicating Results. Cost, outcomes, and ethical aspects are essential aspects of EBP. Communicating ideas through oral and written avenues is valuable in making EBP a reality. Techniques for acquiring oral and written methods for presenting ideas are included; such techniques are helpful in writing protocols and reporting outcomes of EBP activities.

Although graduate students are the primary audience for this book—a textbook for a graduate course in nursing research or an interdisciplinary health care course—nurses in clinical settings also will find the book helpful in fulfilling their research role toward achieving hospital Magnet Status. Our hope is that the information provided in this book can be used to provide optimal cost-efficient care to patients, which will increase their quality of life.

Magdalena A. Mateo, PhD, RN, FAAN

Marquis D. Foreman, PhD, RN, FAAN

A Tribute

Magdalena Mateo was a determined person whose impact was much larger than her small frame. As director of research at Ohio State University Hospital, she had a dream to help nurses use research, and she developed a research manual that was placed on every unit. When she invited me to speak to her staff, she proudly showed me the manual, which she intended to publish. I asked a few questions about it, and before long I found myself lined up as a co-editor of the project, with assigned chapters and responsibilities. That work led to publication of the first edition of this book. Magda said she would handle all the negotiations, communication with authors, and the business part of doing an edited book. She really knew how to make things happen. This made the process easy and smooth for me. She was born and raised in the Philippines, and received her education there, until she received her PhD at Ohio State. I found that the chapters I wrote came back to me with her helpful editing. She was a master at English, even though it was not her native language.

Our first edition focused solely on staff nurses, but we found that a number of baccalaureate programs were using it as a research textbook. For the second edition we tried to be more comprehensive to fit the textbook role.

Our many get-togethers were always fun, with food, laughter, and good times. Sometimes work on the book was a part of the plan. She was always the consummate hostess, preparing meals ahead of time and lining up things to do. She taught me to cook Asian food (stir fry and oriental barbecued ribs) and how to bake bread.

The subsequent edition was written for advanced practice nurses, with Springer Publishing Company. She always followed through with her responsibilities despite any health or work limitations. She was working on the latest edition of the advanced practice book when her life was cut short by Parkinson's disease. Her husband had died less than 3 months earlier, but she handled those arrangements with bravery and grace, despite her declining health. The hardest part for me was to watch her struggle to the podium after the service to express her thanks to those who had come.

Magda was my friend and I am better for that relationship.

Karin T. Kirchhoff, PhD, RN
Professor Emerita
University of Wisconsin School of Nursing

PART I

Evidence-Based Practice

1

Overview of Evidence-Based Practice

Mary D. Bondmass

For well over a decade, discussion and debate related to evidence-based practice (EBP) have ensued. Early data from the Institute of Medicine (IOM) suggested that health care in the United States is not as safe as it should and could be (IOM, 2000). In 2001, the IOM called for efforts to redesign health systems, including the mantra that decision making in health care be *evidence-based* opining that "Patients should receive care based on the best available scientific knowledge. Care should not vary illogically from clinician to clinician or from place to place" (IOM, 2001, p. 4). Core needs were identified and included in IOM's 2001 report in that health care should be *safe, effective, patient-centered, timely, efficient,* and *equitable.* A few years later (IOM, 2003), five core competencies were recommended for health care education curriculum with a focus on EBP. During the past two decades, we have seen debate and discussion in the health care literature about multiple issues, including EBP nomenclature ("evidence-based medicine" versus "evidence-based nursing," versus "evidence-based practice"), educational preparation and requirements (who, what, where, when, and how), and even some discussion of the very need for EBP (AACN, 1995, 2011; Burke et al., 2005; Estabrooks,1998,1999; IOM, 2001, 2003, 2008, 2010; Kleiber & Titler, 1998; Melnyk & Fineout-Overholt, 2005; National League for Nursing [NLN], 2005; O'Neil & The Pew Health Professions Commission, 1998; Stetler, 1994; Stetler et al., 1998; Stevens, 2002, 2004, 2009; Titler et al., 1994).

Today, as the latest edition of this text is prepared for publication, EBP and EBP curriculum in health care education changes are no longer optional or up for debate. Data are clear and compelling that health care education must change to meet the needs of EBP (IOM, 2010). In the advent of implementation of the 2010 legislation of the Health Care and Education Reconciliation Act (HCERA) and the Affordable Care Act (ACA), nursing is at the forefront to lead this change in both education and practice. *The Future of Nursing: Leading Change, Advancing Health* report from the IOM and Robert Wood Johnson Foundation (RWJF) (2010) and the *Quality and Safety Education for Nurses* (QSEN) initiative from the University of North Carolina and the American Association of Colleges of Nursing (AACN, 2011) are two examples of exciting initiatives available to advise and guide nursing on leading change in education and EBP (IOM, 2010; QSEN Institute, 2012).

Although the *Future of Nursing* report plots a course to position nurses for advanced practice, the QSEN competencies provide specific *skill, knowledge,* and *attitude* that are quite similar to, and no doubt developed from, the original five core competencies proposed by the IOM in 2003 to ensure quality in patient care. Of note, *The Essentials of Master's Education in Nursing* (AACN, 2011) was developed also using data and recommendations from the IOM 2003 report.

Comparisons of the core competencies proposed by the IOM in 2003 and the 2012 QSEN competency categories are displayed in Exhibit 1.1. The graduate level QSEN competencies for EBP are listed in Exhibit 1.2.

Exhibit 1.1
Comparisons of the Core Competencies Proposed by the IOM in 2003 and the 2012 QSEN Competency Categories

Institute of Medicine, 2003	QSEN: Skill, Knowledge and Attitude, 2012
• Patient-centered care	• Patient-centered care
• Interdisciplinary skills	• Teamwork and collaboration
• Quality improvement skills	• Quality improvement
• Information technology	• Informatics
• Evidence-based practice	• Evidence-based practice
	• Safety

DEFINITION OF EVIDENCE-BASED PRACTICE

Multiple definitions of EBP have been proposed and have evolved over the past decades. One of the most common definitions of EBP in use today was derived from an initial proposal for evidence-based medicine by Sackett, Straus, Richardson, Rosenberg, and Haynes

Exhibit 1.2
Graduate-Level QSEN Competencies for EBP

Knowledge	Skills	Attitudes
Demonstrate knowledge of health research methods and processes	Use health research methods and processes, alone or in partnership with scientists, to generate new knowledge for practice	Appreciate strengths and weaknesses of scientific bases for practice
Describe evidence-based practice (EBP) to include the components of research evidence, clinical expertise, and patient/family/community values	Role model clinical decision making based on evidence, clinical expertise, and patient/family/community preferences	Value all components of EBP
Identify efficient and effective search strategies to locate reliable sources of evidence	Employ efficient and effective search strategies to answer focused clinical or health system practices	Value development of search skills for locating evidence for best practice
Identify principles that comprise the critical appraisal of research evidence	Critically appraise original research and evidence summaries related to area of practice	Value knowing the evidence base for one's practice specialty area
Summarize current evidence regarding major diagnostic and treatment actions within the practice specialty and health care delivery system	Exhibit contemporary knowledge of best evidence related to practice and health care systems	Value cutting-edge knowledge of current practice
Determine evidence gaps within the practice specialty and health care delivery system	Promote a research agenda for evidence that is needed in practice specialty and health care system	Value working in an interactive manner with the Institutional Review Board

Data in the above table were retrieved from www.qsen.org. Terms and conditions from the QSEN Institute indicate "use of the graduate-level competencies is freely available for educational purposes" (Cronenwett et al., 2009).

(2000). This definition was later refined in 2005 to be more inclusive (Straus, Richardson, Glasziou, & Haynes, 2005). Over time, many texts and publications have agreed on the definition of EBP to be *"the integration of best research evidence with clinical expertise and patient values and circumstances"* (Straus et al., 2005, p. 1). Although many other excellent definitions are used in the literature, most would agree that the above definition is inclusive enough for universal use.

ORIGINS OF EVIDENCE-BASED PRACTICE

Many credit Archibald Leman Cochrane as one of the first proponents of EBP. In the 1970s, Cochrane began a series of studies on the health population studies, which pioneered the use of randomized controlled trials (RCTs). Through Cochrane's experiences in the Spanish Civil War and later in World War II, he developed the belief that much of the medical community did not have sufficient evidence to justify its practice. In his landmark monograph *Effectiveness and Efficiency: Random Reflections on Health Services* (Higgins & Green, 1972) he advocated RCTs as evidence for practice. Cochrane's initial work is credited to the eventual development of the Cochrane Library database of systematic reviews, and the establishment of the UK Cochrane Center in Oxford and the international Cochrane Collaboration.

In looking at the origins of EBP, it should be noted that Cochrane was not the only one advocating the use of research findings in practice. Well in advance of Cochrane's observations and publications, Nightingale (1858, 1859, 1863a, 1863b), wrote extensively about the use of evidence for practice. More recently, the concept of research utilization (RU) reappeared in the nursing literature in the 1970s. Some nurse leaders called it the translation of scientific evidence into practice and expressed the need for nurses to use scientific evidence from research studies to improve the quality of care in practice (Abdellah, 1970; Lindeman, 1975). By the mid-1970s, large RU projects developed several EBP models in the United States. In particular, three models for RU are considered the foundations for the initial understanding of EBP in nursing.

The Conduct and Utilization of Research in Nursing (CURN) project developed and tested a model for using research-based knowledge in clinical practice settings. The RU process is organizational with planned changes integrated throughout. System change is essential to establishing research-based practice on a large scale (Haller, Reynolds, & Horsley, 1979; Horsley, Crane, & Bingle, 1978; Horsley, Crane, Crabtree, & Wood, 1983).

The Stetler Model of Research Utilization applied research findings at the individual practitioner level. The model has six phases and emphasizes critical thinking and decision making (Stetler, 1983, 1985, 1994; Stetler & Marram, 1976).

The Iowa Model for Research in Practice consists of research integrated into practice to improve the quality of care (Titler et al., 1994), and is an outgrowth of the Quality Assurance Model Using Research (QAMUR; Watson, Bulecheck, & McCloskey, 1987). Research utilization is an organizational process, with planned change principles integrating research and practice using a multidisciplinary team approach (Kleiber & Titler, 1998).

Both the Stetler and Iowa models have continued to evolve over the past few decades and have become more consistent with the EBP versus the more limited RU paradigm (Stetler, 2001a; Titler & Everett, 2001; Titler et al., 2001). Both models still provide guidance for evidence-based clinical decision making, including change requirements at both the organizational/system and individual levels. An in-depth discussion of the pros and cons of all available models, although beyond the scope of this chapter, is encouraged prior to the implementation of an EBP model at any institution or within any practice.

TRANSITION FROM RESEARCH UTILIZATION TO EVIDENCE-BASED PRACTICE

Oftentimes in the literature and in practice conversation, the terms "EBP" and "RU" are often used interchangeably; although they are similar, they are not synonymous (Estabrooks, 1999). Kirchhoff (2009) made the case that the primary differences between EBP and RU are the processes (steps) used and the level of evidence being appraised for practice. Whereas summary evidence (systematic reviews) is considered the "heart" of EBP, the singular primary research article is the basic unit of analysis relied on in RU (Stevens, 2001).

ONE MODEL FOR EVIDENCE-BASED PRACTICE

ACE Star Model of Knowledge Transformation

Many models are available for learning and implementing EBP; one such model, more specific to learning and understanding EBP, is briefly presented here in this overview chapter. The ACE Star Model was selected to be presented here because it simply and parsimoniously "organizes both old and new concepts of improving care into a whole and provides a framework with which to organize EBP processes and approaches" (Stevens, 2004). The ACE Star Model of Knowledge Transformation depicts the cyclic stages that knowledge or evidence must pass through to be transformed into a smaller, more user-friendly form for health care decision making. Stevens conceptualized that the current volume was too large and the packaging or form of the tremendous health care knowledge base was just not usable. Stevens developed the model, as a simple five-point star with each star point representing knowledge in a form to be transformed: *Discovery, Evidence Summary, Translation, Integration,* and *Evaluation* (Stevens, 2004).

The first star point, *Discovery,* represents the stage wherein new knowledge is generated. The knowledge is in the form of individual or primary research reports and in this form can be found in research journals, abstracts and/or conference proceedings. Kirchhoff (2009) referred to knowledge from a single or individual research study as a "brick" that when added to other "bricks" (e.g., other single studies) will be transformed into a wall of evidence.

Evidence summary is the second star point, wherein the individual studies, that is, knowledge in the discovery form, are transformed through evidence synthesis and/or meta-analysis into a meaningful statement. This knowledge transformation is conducted by experts in their respective fields and the statements produced are often packaged as a systematic review. Few would argue that the most rigorous systematic reviews can be found within the Cochrane Collaboration. The rigorous steps involved in a Cochrane systematic review can be found in the *Cochrane Handbook* (Cochrane Collaboration, 2009).

Translation is the third star point, wherein the synthesized knowledge of multiple systematic reviews is transformed in an evidence-based clinical practice guideline (CPG). In this stage of the model, our knowledge is transformed into a very user-friendly form for practice. Evidence-base CPG generally contains an evidence rating for each intervention listed. The most comprehensive set of open access CPGs, most of which are evidence-based, can be found via the National Guideline Clearinghouse, under the auspices of the Agency for Healthcare Research and Quality (AHRQ) of the U.S. Department of Health and Human Services. Advanced practice nurses generally need to develop the skills required to critically appraise CPGs as this function is not done by AHRQ; it is the user's responsibility to determine value through evidence rating scales (Bondmass, 2009).

The fourth star point is *Integration,* wherein our knowledge has been transformed to the point at which it is usable by all clinicians and disseminated throughout our institutions. Frequently, systemwide change in practice is difficult, even change based on the best evidence and in the best possible form is difficult. Efforts to overcome barriers to EBP continue to be the focus of many outcomes by researchers.

The last star point is *Evaluation,* wherein knowledge in the form we are using is evaluated from the perspective of its impact on outcomes. Possible EBP outcomes at this stage include patient satisfaction, safety, efficacy, efficiency, and health status of whole populations. Evaluation knowledge directs further issues to be researched in *Discovery,* and the cycle continues as knowledge is transformed into usable evidence at each star point.

The ACE Star Model, although less specific about the implementation of EBP at the "bedside," has been found to be particularly useful for research related to the teaching and learning of EBP for nurses (Bondmass, 2011, in press; Bondmass, Kesten, & Dennison, 2012). It is important to note that the conceptual EBP knowledge obtained from the use of this model may be useful in preparing nurses and other health care providers for their roles in fulfilling the IOM's EBP recommendations (2003).

EBP COMPETENCIES

Essential Competencies for Evidence-Based Practice in Nursing (ECEBP) were developed by Stevens in 2005 (Stevens, 2005) and revised in 2009 to include all levels of education, associate through doctoral. The ECEBP are aligned with the ACE Star Model of Knowledge Transformation with specific competencies addressing each respective star point; the ECEBP are also divided by educational preparation per star point. Although the QSEN competencies are directed toward the education of nurses in the academic setting, the ECEBP are used by practicing nurses and set as an expectation for practice. Prior to the advent of the QSEN, researchers used the ECEBP in academic settings to evaluate the teaching and learning of EBP in both undergraduate and graduate nursing education (Bondmass, 2011, in press; Bondmass et al., 2012). Additional information about the ACE Star model and EBP competencies can be found at the website for the Academic Center for Evidence-Based Practice (http://www.acestar.uthscsa.edu).

SUMMARY

In the past 20 years, EBP has emerged as a global movement. This movement includes more than RU, and many relevant EBP models have been developed to promote scientific and other evidence sources to improve the quality of care (Burrow & McLeish, 1995; Camiah, 1997; Davies, 2002; Estabrooks, 1999; Goode, Lovett, Hayes, & Butcher, 1987; International Council of Nurses [ICN], 1990; Kitson, Ahmed, Harvey, Seers, & Thompson, 1996; Kitson, Harvey, & McCormack, 1998; Olade, 1990, 2001; Redfern & Christian, 2003; Rolfe, 1999; Rosswurm & Larrabee, 1999; Stetler, 2001a, 2001b, 2003; Stevens, 2004; Titler et al., 1994). In the new millennium, EBP is an umbrella term for many sources of evidence, including, but not limited to, meta-analysis, systematic reviews, consensus recommendations by experts, and clinical guidelines (Bondmass, 2009; IOM, 2003, 2010; Jenning & Loan, 2001; Kirchhoff, 2009; Melnyk & Fineout-Overholt, 2005; QSEN, 2012; Roberts, 1998; Rolfe, 1999; Stetler et al., 1998; Stevens, 2001).

This chapter intends to give a brief overview of EBP for the advanced practice nurse. Origins, definitions, EBP models, and academic and clinical EBP competencies were presented as a snapshot of the challenges and expectations of advanced practice nurses in an interprofessional EBP environment. In the various proceeding chapters of this text, in-depth and specific material will be presented with the intent to prepare advanced practice nurses for their leadership role in health care related to research and EBP.

SUGGESTED ACTIVITIES

1. Select a clinical topic and conduct a literature search to find evidence in the various stages of the knowledge transformation on that topic: *Discovery, Evidence Summary, Translation, Integration,* and *Evaluation.*
2. Gather a group of colleagues, either in your clinical or classroom setting, and conduct a self-assessment using the QSEN and/or the ECEBP. Compare your results.

REFERENCES

Abdellah, F. G. (1970). Overview of nursing research 1955–1968. *Nursing Research, 19*(3), 239–252.

American Association of Colleges of Nursing (AACN). (1995). *The essentials of baccalaureate education for professional nursing practice.* Available from http://www.aacn.nche.edu/education/bacessn.htm

American Association of Colleges of Nursing (AACN). (2011). *The essentials of master's education in nursing.* Washington, DC: Author. Available from http://www.aacn.nche.edu/education-resources/MastersEssentials11.pdf

Bondmass, M. (2009, July). Finding and appraising clinical practice guidelines. In M. Mateo, & K. Kirchhoff (Eds.), *Research for advanced practice nurses: From evidence to practice* (pp. 267–285). New York, NY: Springer Publishing Company.

Bondmass, M. (2011, July). *Application of the ACE Star Model© and essential competencies in a DNP program* [Abstract]. University of Texas Health Science Center, San Antonio: Summer Institute at the Academic Center for Evidence Based Practice.

Bondmass, M. (in press). The effects of teaching/learning evidence-based practice in a baccalaureate nursing program. *Nursing Education Perspectives.*

Bondmass, M., Kesten, K., & Dennison, R. (2012, July). *Application of the ACE Star Model© and essential competencies in an MS program* [Abstract]. University of Texas Health Science Center, San Antonio: Summer Institute at the Academic Center for Evidence Based Practice.

Burke, L. E., Schlenk, E. A., Sereika, S. M., Cohen, S. M., Happ, M. B., & Dorman, J. S. (2005). Developing research competence to support evidence-based practice. *Journal of Professional Nursing, 21*(6), 358–363.

Burrows, D. E., & McLeish, K. (1995). A model for research-based practice. *Journal of Clinical Nursing, 4*(4), 243–247.

Camiah, S. (1997). Utilization of nursing research in practice and application strategies to raise research awareness amongst nurse practitioners: A model for success. *Journal of Advanced Nursing, 26*(6), 1193–1202.

Cochrane, A. L. (1972). *Effectiveness and efficiency: Random reflections on health services.* London: Nuffield Provincial Hospitals Trust (reprinted in 1989 in association with the *BMJ* and reprinted in 1999 for Nuffield Trust by the Royal Society of Medicine Press, London).

Cronenwett, L., Sherwood, G., Pohl, J., Barnsteiner, J., Moore, S., Sullivan, D., Ward, D., & Warren, J. (2009). Quality and safety education for advanced nursing practice. *Nursing Outlook, 57*(6), 338–348. doi:10.1016/j.outlook.2009.07.00

Davies, B. L. (2002). Sources and models for moving research evidence into clinical practice. *Journal of Obstetric & Gynecologic Neonatal Nursing, 31*(5), 558–562.

Estabrooks, C. A. (1998). Will evidence-based nursing practice make practice perfect? *Canadian Journal of Nursing Research, 30*(1), 15–36.

Estabrooks, C. A. (1999). Modeling the individual determinants of research utilization. *Western Journal of Nursing Research, 21*(6), 758–772.

Goode, C. J., Lovett, M. K., Hayes, J. E., & Butcher, L. A. (1987). Use of research based knowledge in clinical practice. *Journal of Nursing Administration, 17*(12), 11–18.

Haller, K. B., Reynolds, M. A., & Horsley, J. A. (1979). Developing research-based innovation protocols: Process, criteria and issues. *Research in Nursing and Health, 2,* 45–51.

Higgins, J. P. T., & Green, S. (2009). *Cochrane handbook for systematic reviews of interventions.* In J. P. T. Higgins & S. Green (Eds.), Version 5.0.2. Available from http://www.cochrane-handbook.org

Horsley, J. A., Crane, J., & Bingle, J. D. (1978, July). Research utilization as an organizational process. *Journal of Nursing Administration, 8*(7), 4–6.

Horsley, J. A., Crane, J., Crabtree, M. K., & Wood, D. J. (1983). *Using research to improve practice.* Orlando, FL: Grune & Stratton.

Institute of Medicine (IOM). (2000). *To err is human: Building a safer health system.* Washington, DC: National Academies Press.

Institute of Medicine (IOM). (2001). *Crossing the quality chasm: A new health system for the 21st Century.* Committee on Quality of Health Care in America, Institute of Medicine. Washington, DC: National Academies Press.

Institute of Medicine (IOM). (2003). *Health professions education: A bridge to quality.* Washington, DC: National Academies Press.

Institute of Medicine (IOM). (2010). *The future of nursing: Leading change, advancing health.* Washington, DC: National Academies Press.

International Council of Nurses (ICN). (1990). *Nursing research worldwide: Current dimensions and future directions.* Geneva, Switzerland: Author.

Jennings, B. M., & Loan, L. A. (2001). Misconceptions among nurses about evidence-based practice. *Journal of Nursing Scholarship, 33*(2), 121–127.

Kirchhoff, K. T. (2009, July). Overview of evidence-based practice. In M. Mateo, & K. Kirchoff (Eds.), *Research for advanced practice nurses from evidence to practice* (pp. 155–166). New York, NY: Springer Publishing Company.

Kitson, A., Ahmed, L. B., Harvey, G., Seers, K., & Thompson, D. R. (1996). From research to practice: One organizational model for promoting research-based practice. *Journal of Advance Nursing, 23*(3), 430–440.

Kitson, A., Harvey, G., & McCormack, B. (1998). Enabling the implementation of evidence based practice: A conceptual framework. *Quality in Health Care, 7*(3), 149–158.

Kleiber, C., & Titler, M. G. (1998). *Evidence based practice and the revised Iowa Model.* Fifth international research utilization conference (April 23–24). Iowa City, IA: University of Iowa Hospitals and Clinics.

Lindeman, C. A. (1975). Priorities in clinical nursing research. *Nursing Outlook, 23*(11), 693–698.

Melnyk, B. M., & Fineout-Overholt, E. (2005). Making the case for evidence-based practice. In B. M. Melnyk, & E. Fineout-Overholt (Eds.), *Evidence-based practice in nursing & healthcare: A guide to best practice* (pp. 3–24). Philadelphia, PA: Lippincott Williams & Wilkins.

National League for Nursing (NLN) Position Statement. (2005, May 9). *Transforming nursing education.* New York, NY: Author.

Nightingale, F. (1858). *Notes on matters affecting the health, efficiency, and hospital administration of the British Army.* London: Harrison & Sons.

Nightingale, F. (1859). *A contribution to the sanitary history of the British Army during the late war with Russia.* London: John W. Parker & Sons.

Nightingale, F. (1863a). *Observation on the evidence contained in the statistical reports submitted by her to the Royal Commission on the sanitary state of the Army in India.* London: Edward Stanford.

Nightingale, F. (1863b). *Notes on hospitals.* London: Longman, Green, Roberts & Green.

Olade, R. A. (1990). A survey of nursing research in Nigeria. *International Nursing Review, 37*(4), 299–302.

Olade, R. A. (2001). *Correlates of nurses' attitudes to research and the desire for evidence-based practice.* Paper presented at the Hawaii nursing research conference: Searching for evidence & finding the answers, Honolulu, HI.

O'Neil, E. H., & The Pew Health Professions Commission. (1998). *Recreating health professional practice for a new century.* San Francisco, TX: Pew Health Professions Commission.

QSEN Institute. (2012). *Quality and safety education for nurses (QSEN) project.* Available from http://qsen.org

Redfern, S., & Christian, S. (2003). Achieving change in health care practice. *Journal of Advanced Nursing, 31*(3), 599–606.

Roberts, K. L. (1998). Evidence-based practice: An idea whose time has come. *Collegian, 4*(3), 24–27.

Rolfe, G. (1999). Insufficient evidence: The problems of evidence-based nursing. *Nurse Education Today, 19*(6), 433–442.

Rosswurm, M. A., & Larrabee, J. H. (1999). A model for change to evidence-based practice. *Image: Journal of Nursing Scholarship, 31*(4), 317–322.

Sackett, D. L., Straus, S. E., Richardson, W. S., Rosenberg, W., & Haynes, R. B. (Eds.) (2000). *Evidence-based medicine: How to practice and teach EBM.* Edinburgh, UK: Churchill Livingstone.

Stetler, C. B. (1983). Nurses and research responsibility and involvement. *Journal of the National Intravenous Therapy Association, 6*, 207–212.

Stetler, C. B. (1985). Research utilization: Defining the concept. *Image: The Journal of Nursing Scholarship XVII*(2), 40–44.

Stetler, C. B. (1994). Refinement of the Stetler/Marram model for application of research findings to practice. *Nursing Outlook, 42*(1), 15–25.

Stetler, C. B. (2001a). Updating the Stetler model of research utilization to facilitate evidence-based practice. *Nursing Outlook, 49,* 272–279. doi: 10.1067/mno.2001.120517

Stetler, C. B. (2001b). Evidence-based nursing: What it is and what it isn't. *Nursing Outlook, 49*(6), 286.

Stetler, C. B. (2003). Role of the organization in translating research into evidence-based practice. *Outcomes Management, 7*(3), 97–103.

Stetler, C. B., Brunnell, M., Guiliano, K. K., Morsi, D., Prince, L., & Newell-Stokes, V. (1998). Evidence-based practice and the role of nursing leadership. *Journal of Nursing Administration, 28*(7–8), 45–53.

Stetler, C. B., & Marram, G. (1976). Evaluating research findings for applicability in practice. *Nursing Outlook, 24*(9), 559–563.

Stevens, K. R. (2001). Systematic reviews: The heart of evidence-based nursing. *AACN Clinical Issues, 12*(4), 529–538.

Stevens, K. R. (2002). Evidence-based practice in advanced practice nursing. In K. Crabtree, & R. Pruitt (Eds.), *Building curriculum for quality nurse practitioner education.* Washington, DC: National Organization of Nurse Practitioner Faculties.

Stevens, K. R. (2004). *ACE star model of EBP: The cycle of knowledge transformation.* Available from http://www.acestar.uthscsa.edu/acestar-model.asp

Stevens, K. R. (2005). *Essential competencies for evidence-based practice in nursing* (1st ed.). The University of Texas Health Science Center at San Antonio: Academic Center for Evidence-Based Practice.

Stevens, K. R. (2009). *Essential competencies for evidence-based practice in nursing* (2nd ed.). The University of Texas Health Science Center at San Antonio: Academic Center for Evidence-Based Practice.

Straus, S. E., Richardson, W. S., Glasziou, P., & Haynes, R. B. (2005). *Evidence-based medicine* (3rd ed.). New York, NY: Churchill Livingstone.

Titler, M. G., & Everett, L. Q. (2001). Translating research into practice: Considerations for critical care investigators. *Critical Care Nursing Clinics of North America, 13*(4), 587–604.

Titler, M., Kleiber, C., Steelman, V., Goode, C., Rakel, B., & Barry-Walker, J., ... Buckwalter, K. (1994). Infusing research into practice to promote quality care. *Nursing Research, 43*(5), 307–313.

Titler, M., Kleiber, C., Steelman, V., Rakel, B., Budreau, G., & Everett, L., ... Goode, C. (2001). The Iowa model of evidence-based practice to promote quality care. *Critical Care Clinics of North America, 13*(4), 497–509.

Watson, C. A., Bulecheck, G. M., & McCloskey, J. C. (1987). QAMUR: A quality assurance model using nursing research. *Journal of Nursing Quality Assurance, 2*(1), 21–27.

General Searching: Finding Research Reports

Ulrike Dieterle and Christopher Hooper-Lane

Conducting a literature review in the 21st century poses numerous challenges for the researcher. The emphasis on evidence-based decision making in health care, the exponential increase in the volume of scientific literature, and the growing dependence on ever-changing computer technologies result in a more complicated research environment. The changing shape of information, and how it is retrieved and evaluated have profound effects at every level of the research process. Although the core concepts of research have remained relatively consistent, new tools, new technologies, and new information destinations continue to evolve and multiply. This chapter discusses the search for evidence as a systematic process consisting of four distinct phases that include preparation and planning, searching the literature, going beyond the literature, and pulling it all together.

A brief review of significant information trends related to the health sciences illustrates the impact on the advanced practice nurse's (APN's) search for evidence to support practice. One of the most dramatic changes in the past 10 years affecting all types of information gathering has been the shift from print to electronic resources. It is estimated that original information is increasing at a rate of approximately 30% a year, and most of this new information appears for the first time in digital formats (Lyman & Varian, 2003). Action verbs used 15 years ago for information gathering activities—scanning, browsing, and retrieving—conjure up very different mental pictures today. As research tools continue to develop, APNs find it difficult to refresh computer skills and to keep up to date in their fields. Staying current as information resources evolve, takes time, appropriate skill sets, and attention (Skiba, 2005). Researchers now find themselves spending the bulk of their research hours with computers and virtual research partners, often performing searches alone and developing their final papers in digital spaces. And, while the information explosion continues, the skills to navigate through denser, more crowded information landscapes seldom keep pace (Tanner, Pierce, & Pravikoff, 2004).

Another trend is the appearance of new information destinations. One variant of this is the open-access movement, which was spurred on by the library community and influential research-granting institutions such as the National Institutes of Health. This movement promises to dramatically increase public access to full-text scientific articles. A significant milestone was reached on December 26, 2007, when the FY 2008 appropriations process (Consolidated Appropriations Act of 2007 [H.R. 2764]) included wording to make articles reporting publicly funded research freely available to the world. As vendor providers find their inventories disappearing from behind their proprietary firewalls, even more information destinations will arise, adding to the existing "information diasporas." With additional places to look, it will become increasingly important to chart the research course in more detail in advance, identify resources more precisely, and evaluate the right skill sets early in the process.

The heightened focus, in recent years, on improving clinical outcomes through support of scientific knowledge has resulted in a greater emphasis on the integration of evidence-based practices (EBPs) at all levels of health care (Brancato, 2006). As nursing students and health care professionals learn to incorporate EBP into their clinical workflow, they must learn to identify evidence-based information resources and construct related information-seeking strategies. Practitioners now have mandates to adopt effective EBP recommendations. Effective EBPs are increasingly important in saving clinicians time, energy, and, ultimately, in achieving improved clinical outcomes (Polit & Beck, 2008).

PHASES IN THE SEARCH FOR EVIDENCE

Phase I—Preparation and Planning

Although much attention is traditionally paid to the process of formulating search statements and selecting appropriate search terminology, databases, and strategies, a literature review consists of more than this. It is, in a very real sense, a project waiting to be managed. Thinking about and identifying its many parts before beginning is time well spent. It will benefit the searcher and instill order in what may seem to be a string of chaotic activities. The preliminary literature review preparation phase, that is, Phase I, is discussed first.

A real-world, kitchen-table analogy may work here. Everyone has been challenged by the prospect of preparing a new recipe. It is best to first read the entire recipe from beginning to end before assembling the ingredients for the dish. One then gathers appropriate ingredients and needed utensils. After preparing the same recipe a number of times, one finds that the preparation is much easier. It becomes second nature. As the cook gains more assurance, more certainty in the procedure, a pattern begins to develop. As patterns develop, variations are incorporated with ease, and confidence increases over time.

Research is much the same. If searching a database is a rare occurrence, it will continue to be a slow and laborious process. Once evidence-based research is fully integrated into clinical cultures and professional workflow, it will become second nature.

Ask Questions

Before diving headfirst into database searching, it is important to ask a few questions to guide subsequent actions. Presearch preparation will tease out existing strengths and weaknesses. It will define the skills needed and pinpoint knowledge gaps. Asking the right questions *before* beginning a project is a valuable exercise in charting the most effective and efficient research course. Questioning the purpose of the literature review will determine the intent and the appropriate intensity, depth, and scope of the search(es).

A literature review may be undertaken for a variety of reasons.

1. To answer a clinical question
2. To prepare for a thesis, conduct a topical survey, and ready scholarly research for publication
3. To conduct a systematic review, respond to a professional curiosity, or some variation on these

An inclusive search for all relevant literature, such as demanded by systematic reviews and meta-analyses, requires more time and involves more databases than a selective review of limited scope. Which resources are best for the research question? It is advisable to identify the best information resources for the topic before constructing search strategies. Good preparation prevents distracting detours and lost time, resolves confusion, and serves to sequence the order in which databases are searched. In Phase I, exploratory searches are important for discovery and to determine the viability of the research topic.

MEDLINE (PubMed), for example, is an ideal choice for initial exploratory searches because it is the largest biomedical database available. It provides article citations at all levels of the evidence hierarchy, from the "gold standard" of systematic reviews to the most casual, subjective opinions.

What are the best search strategies? Because databases have their own "personalities," it is best to understand not only the basic features common to all but also the unique characteristics of each selected database before initiating the search process. Researchers who make repetitive use of a database will develop degrees of comfort and form patterns of recognition useful in attaining precision. Expert searching is an acquired skill developed over time with practice. Even seasoned researchers can benefit from added search acuity. Exhibit 2.1 lists factors to consider when searching relevant literature.

Exhibit 2.1
Questions to Ask During Phase I

- *What is the purpose of the literature review?*
- *Which resources are best for the research question?*
- *How are the resources best searched?*
- *Where can help be obtained?*
- *What resources are available?*
- *Is time a limiting factor?*
- *Which bibliographic management tools will be used?*
- *How is the information evaluated?*

Most online databases provide tutorials or help manuals that give at least rudimentary point-of-need assistance. MEDLINE (PubMed) has an extensive series of tutorials available from the PubMed home page, presented in well-defined learning increments. Medical librarians at academic health sciences libraries, hospitals, and clinics are also available to provide database suggestions, search guidance, and training opportunities.

What other resources are available? Is time a limiting factor in this project? Which bibliographic management tools will be used, if any? How does the researcher evaluate the information? Self-assessment questions similar to these will help to make necessary components transparent to the researcher and allow time to prepare. Conducting a literature review involves many intersecting, nonlinear processes, including planning, discovery, preparation, contemplation, search skills, and evaluation.

These phases do not always progress in a strict linear fashion from point A to point B. In fact, research is much like lining up the colors on a Rubik's cube, more a process of moving forward, pushing back, sliding sideways, re-evaluating, and refining. It is more a series of overlapping loops that propel momentum forward (Mellon, 1984). Through repeated checks, evaluations, confirmations, and reflections along the way, the APN avoids unplanned detours down a foggy path. Finding oneself in a research fog of uncertainty is not unusual but can be minimized by planning and preparation. The uncertainties faced by novice researchers are often inadvertently magnified, setting up needless hurdles. The aid of a multipart schematic for research success is a helpful tool.

Define Search Goal

Defining the scope of the planned research is an important element in moving forward. Assessing the intended outcome of the search provides clarity of purpose and direction. Is the impending literature review a class assignment with specific guidelines, requirements, and deadlines? Is it generated by unanswered health care questions that need immediate attention? Is it part of a team project leading to the creation of evidence-based guidelines in the clinical setting? Is the literature review part of a long-term research project to be published? Answers to these questions may drive the momentum of the literature review down slightly different search paths. Decisions made at this juncture will also impact the choice of databases and resources consulted. One size does not fit all. A small-sized research goal does not warrant an extensive research approach. Each literature review is the sum of its unique parts.

Gather Background Information

One important preliminary step is to understand how the research topic fits into its related field of knowledge. The APN must attain some degree of comfort with the nomenclature, and the topic in general, before moving into serious search phases. Background builds an information foundation that will support increased awareness of vocabulary (important when searching) and related issues. Background information can be found in many places, including textbooks, on trusted websites, reference resources, and review articles. If the topic is interdisciplinary, as many nursing topics are, the information destinations will be broader in scope, more numerous and, often, be less familiar. Reaching across disciplines can be a stretch, especially for the less experienced searcher. During the gathering of background information, it is advisable to clearly list and expand related terminology to aid in search strategy construction later.

Construct a Searchable Question

Formulating a searchable or answerable question is a technique that focuses on the most basic elements of the research topic. By focusing on only the core elements of a complex health care scenario, the researcher clarifies the central question and achieves a more precise definition of the subject. Precision and focus are also enhanced by the use of the PICO method. The PICO mnemonic (P = patient, population, problem, I = intervention, C = comparison, O = outcome) provides a useful instrument in peeling away the outer layers of the research question and directs the focus to only the most essential components. This concentrated effort removes other "noisy" narrative that may prove distracting when constructing search strategies. Not every query will fit neatly into the PICO format, but the approach of deconstructing the parts to their meaningful essence, clarifies the purpose and helps develop more effective search strategies.

Eliminate Search Barriers

Nursing literature is replete with documentation of potential barriers to the integration of evidence-based methods into practice. Identified barriers include following familiar practices that may be outdated, the perceived lack of value of EBP in practice, time constraints, lack of access to computers and databases at the point of need, limited database searching skills, and continued underutilization of evidence-based information in health care environments. Even trusted online resources are not as accessible or viewed as useful as consultation with a colleague (Dee & Stanley, 2005; Melnyk et al., 2009; Pravikoff, Tanner, & Pierce, 2005).

An overestimation of difficulties related to the research process can cause uncertainty, which, in turn, may lead the APN to avoid research or even the onset of research rigor mortis (Downs, 1969). Uncertainties surrounding the research process can inhibit forward momentum. It is important to identify and manage research uncertainties early and throughout the process. According to Klein (2003), there are five basic sources of uncertainty. These sources are as follows: missing or inaccessible information; unreliable or untrustworthy information; information that is inconsistent or conflicting; information that is confusing and that clouds decision making; and "noisy" or distracting information, which can result in time wasted sifting through unrelated resources.

Researchers are advised to follow a basic prescription when contemplating literature reviews: (1) spend presearch time on discovery, planning, and reflection; then (2) choose the appropriate information destinations and execute well-formulated searches; (3) critically evaluate and expand search parameters; and (4) sort, store, and organize gathered information throughout the process. Using a checklist, such as the one in Exhibit 2.2, will promote effective search habits.

Exhibit 2.2
Checklist—Phase I

Research Topic	☐
Due Date	☐
Background Information	☐
Information Management Tool	☐
PICO	☐
Searchable Question	☐
Major Database(s)	☐
Knowledge Gaps	☐

Phase II—Mining the Literature Databases

Choose the Best Resources

When a well-formulated question is created, researchers and practitioners must look for the best evidence to answer the question. In order to succeed in this venture, an understanding of the EBP hierarchy, adequate searching skills, and accessing and access to appropriate resources are all required. There is a remarkable amount of health research now published. With 75 trials and 11 systematic reviews published each day and over 2 million research papers on biomedical topics published annually, it is essential that a researcher have a solid grasp of the resources to find the proper evidence to answer clinical questions (Bastian, Glasziou, & Chalmers, 2010; Mulrow, 1994).

Start With Reviews

From an evidence-based perspective, the best bet is to start by using resources containing the secondary literature—articles that review or summarize peer-reviewed research on a topic. Keep in mind that there are several types of reviews. A *literature review* (also known as *narrative review*) tends to be a body of text that discusses the current knowledge on a topic from a wide variety of text sources. A *systematic review*, on the other hand, focuses on a specific clinical topic or question, includes a thorough literature search, appraises individual studies, and offers a conclusion on that topic or an answer to the clinical question. A *meta-analysis* is a type of systematic review that applies statistical methods to combine the evidence from individual trials. Some also place *practice guidelines* into the review category. This is true only if their statements are developed using rigorous scientific evidence (i.e., systematic reviews and randomized controlled trials).

Search the Primary Literature

Although the amount (and value) of review literature has seen phenomenal growth in the last decade, much of the evidence, particularly in nursing and allied health fields, still resides within the *primary literature*—individual reports of findings. These single studies are the building blocks from which the systematic reviews, meta-analyses, and evidence-based guidelines are built. As one might guess, studies are not created equal and there is a great range of publication types found in the journal literature. All levels of the evidence hierarchy from double-blind randomized controlled trials, to cohort studies, to case studies, to qualitative and descriptive studies are found in journals. Researchers and clinicians should initiate a search in the review literature and turn to primary literature to fill in the gaps (both in content and currency).

Select Resources to Search

There are thousands of electronic and print resources that cover the scholarly output of the health sciences. Some are freely available on the Internet through government agencies, health organizations, or even commercial enterprises; others are restricted to individuals and/ or institutions with, at times costly, subscriptions. The highest quality health research is normally found in the scholarly, peer-reviewed, journals and literature databases that cover them. Literature databases are indices of journal articles. The majority of these databases contain citations and abstracts of articles from journals covering specific topics. Some also provide either the full articles or links to providers of the articles.

It is in the best interest of the health researcher or clinician to commence with searches in the core health databases. The two literature databases considered essential are MEDLINE (PubMed) and CINAHL (Cumulative Index to Nursing and Allied Health Literature). These databases are the best starting point for both clinical and research topics in the health sciences. For a list of core database descriptions and features see Table 2.1.

There are, of course, other databases with unique content that might be useful, if not integral, to the searcher. For instance, Embase, a large international health database, contains unique global literature particularly in drug-related fields; ERIC (Education Resources Information Center) can be tapped for articles, reports, and other publications concerning education; and PsycINFO, as its name implies, covers the mental health literature. Table 2.2 lists peripheral databases of interest to researchers and clinicians in nursing.

Speak the Database Language

Nurses have identified a lack of searching skills as a barrier to EBP (Melnyk et al., 2004; Pravikoff et al., 2005). It is therefore essential for database users to develop a skill set to gain confidence and search efficiently. This chapter will proceed with a discussion of some of the basic search concepts and tools that all searchers should understand and employ. Keep in mind that attending a continuing education (CE) session provided by a health library or institution, a consultation with a librarian, or even a few moments reviewing a resource-specific guide or tutorial will often pay great dividends.

The search terms (words or phrases) entered into a literature database search box will have a significant bearing on the quality of the results. The terminology in the health literature is replete with synonyms (different words, same definition) and homonyms (same word, different definition). For example, the concept *cancer* can be entered in a database as *cancer, tumor, malignancy, neoplasm*, and so on. Therefore, challenging decisions need to be made regarding the selection of appropriate terms.

TABLE 2.1 Selected Core Literature Databases

	COVERAGE	PUBLICATION TYPES	FEATURES	FINDING REVIEWS
CINAHL http://www.ebscohost .com/cinahl	Comprehensive source for nursing and allied health journals, providing coverage of 5,000 journals along with 80 other document types.	Systematic Reviews guidelines Primary literature dissertations Books, book chapters Audiovisual Pamphlets, etc.	Controlled Vocabulary Advanced Search EBM Filters Explode Major Concept Allows Boolean Limits Includes Exclude MEDLINE option	Use the Systematic Reviews publication type limit or the Evidence-Based Practice Special Interest filter
Cochrane Database of Systematic Reviews (Systematic Reviews) http://www.cochrane .org	Includes ~7,500 reviews and protocols involving therapy and prevention in all areas of health care. Recently added reviews of diagnostic tools.	Systematic Reviews protocols (detailed plan to create a systematic review)	Controlled Vocabulary Allows Boolean Limits (Systematic Review or Protocol)	If available, use reviews limit
Database of Abstracts of Reviews of Effects (DARE) http://www.crd.york .ac.uk/crdweb	Includes ~20,000 reviews of systematic reviews found in the journal literature. Covers health-related interventions and diagnostic tests, public health, pharmacology, surgery, psychology, etc. Complements the Cochrane Database by including reviews on topics not completed by the Cochrane Collaboration.	Abstracts/Reviews of Systematic Reviews	Controlled Vocabulary Allows Boolean	All contents are reviews
MEDLINE (PubMed) http://www.pubmed .gov	Largest health database covering over 5,000 journals and some other publication types in all areas of the health sciences.	Systematic Reviews guidelines Primary literature	Controlled Vocabulary Explode Major Topic Allows Boolean Limits Filters (Clinical Queries)	Use Clinical Queries: Systematic Reviews filter or the Systematic Reviews article type filter

TABLE 2.2 Selected Peripheral Literature Databases

DATABASES	COVERAGE
AMED—the Allied and Complementary Medicine Database www.ebscohost.com/biomedical-libraries/AMED-The-Allied-and-Complementary-Medicine-Database	AMED covers references to articles from 600 journals, in three separate subject areas: professions allied to medicine, complementary medicine, and palliative care. The scope of coverage is mainly European.
British Nursing Index http://www.bniplus.co.uk	BNI is a UK nursing and midwifery database, covering over 270 UK journals and other English language titles, including international nursing and midwifery journals, and selected content from medical, allied health, and management titles.
Cochrane Central Register of Controlled Trials (CENTRAL) http://www.cochrane.org	CENTRAL includes citations and summaries of over 600,000 trials culled from literature databases and other published and unpublished sources used to create *Cochrane Reviews*.
Embase http://www.embase.com	Embase is a large international biomedical and pharmacological database containing over 25 million records from 7,600 biomedical journals, including more than 2,000 titles not covered in MEDLINE. Embase has a broad biomedical scope, with in-depth coverage of pharmacology, pharmaceutical science, and clinical research. Embase also includes over 600,000 conference abstracts from over 2,000 conferences.
ERIC http://www.eric.ed.gov	Sponsored by the U.S. Department of Education, ERIC provides free access to more than 1.4 million records of journal articles from 600+ journals and other education-related materials (books, research syntheses, conference papers, tech reports, policy papers, etc.) and, if available, includes links to full text.
HealthSource: Nursing/Academic Edition http://www.ebscohost.com/academic/health-source-nursing-academic-edition	This EBSCO database provides coverage of nursing and allied health topics and includes citation/abstracts from 820 journals and the full text of nearly 550 scholarly journals.
MIDRIS Reference Database http://www.midirs.org	MIDRIS contains over 186,000 references with abstracts to journal articles from over 500 international English-language journals, books, and grey literature relating to the midwifery profession, pregnancy, labor, birth, postnatal care, neonatal care, and the first year of an infant's life.
PsycINFO http://www.apa.org/pubs/databases/psycinfo	Produced by the American Psychological Association, PsycINFO is a large behavioral science and mental health database with more than 3 million records from 2,500 journals, books, book chapters, and dissertations.

In some cases, using common or everyday language is effective and appropriate. This is called *free-text* or *keyword* searching. However, searching with terms offered from a database-specific thesaurus, often referred to as a *controlled vocabulary*, will often prove the best way to improve the breadth and accuracy of the retrieval set.

Search Using Keywords

Keyword (free-text, natural language, and common language) searches are commonly used in search boxes on the Internet (e.g., Google) and all literature databases allow searchers to create search queries with keywords. Keyword searches are by nature fairly restrictive, as records retrieved by the database must have the exact term(s) entered in the search box. For example, if an author of an article uses the term *ascorbic acid* and the searcher enters *vitamin C*, the searcher would not necessarily retrieve that specific potentially relevant article.

Keyword searches can be used to find good information on a topic and are appropriate in certain circumstances. Expert searchers will often begin the process of searching a database by entering a few important keywords to obtain a quick and dirty initial retrieval set. This set is then scrutinized to uncover any appropriate additional search terms to refine and focus the query.

Although the use of natural language may not be the best way to search a given resource (see "Search Using a Controlled Vocabulary"), there are techniques to improve the results of your search query. *Truncation*, also called stemming, allows searching for various word endings and spellings of a keyword term simultaneously. Databases that allow truncation will designate database-specific characters, or wildcards, to initiate the truncation feature. The asterisk (*) and question mark (?) are commonly used wildcards. For example, a search in MEDLINE (PubMed) using the keyword *communit** will retrieve records with the terms: community, communities, communitarian, communitarians, etc. Some resources also allow for internal (wom?n) or beginning truncation ($natal). *Phrase searching* is a good way to search for specific phrases or words that are unusually formed. Many resources will allow a searcher to surround a phrase with brackets, parentheses, or quotes (depending on the resource) to retrieve only results including these specific phrases within the database record. This modification can reduce irrelevant results by requiring that the component words appear consecutively and in the order specified. For example, a search for "community acquired pneumonia" will find only results containing that particular string of words.

Search Using a Controlled Vocabulary

A *controlled vocabulary* is a carefully selected standardized list of terms, or thesaurus, that indexers (generally librarians who review individual articles before inclusion into a database) use to determine the main and minor topics discussed in the article. These standardized terms may or may not be the same words that the author uses in his or her writings, but are embedded within the database record. Therefore, a searcher using a standardized or controlled term will retrieve articles on a topic, regardless of the ambiguity of terms. Many studies have shown that utilizing a controlled term will improve searches in both size and accuracy. Be aware that not all health databases use a controlled vocabulary system, and even in databases that do, many concepts do not have precise matches within the system. Also, it takes databases time to incorporate new concepts/terms into its thesaurus. For example, the term *AIDS* was coined in 1981, but it took years before it was introduced into MEDLINE's Medical Subject Heading (MeSH) thesaurus. In these cases, a searcher must resort to a keyword search.

There are many examples of a controlled vocabulary in the health literature and most are database specific:

- MeSH (*Me*dical *S*ubject *H*eadings) is the National Library of Medicine's controlled vocabulary for MEDLINE. MeSH is presented as a hierarchy of over 26,000 descriptive terms covering virtually all medical concepts.
- The CINAHL database uses a different controlled vocabulary, named CINAHL Subject Headings. Although CINAHL Subject Headings follow the structure of MeSH, the vocabulary reflects the terminology used by nursing and allied health professionals.

Some databases have addressed the problems associated with keyword searches by developing a built-in term-mapping system where free-text terms are matched against a controlled vocabulary translation table. For example, although MEDLINE's MeSH list includes 26,000 terms, yet another 200,000 synonyms are included in the translation table. So a search query with term *vitamin C* will be matched and searched (behind the scenes) with the proper MeSH term *ascorbic acid*. Although this is reliable for many common health terms, not all have such straightforward and successful mapping.

Explode and Focus Terms

The subject headings of a controlled vocabulary are often presented in a hierarchical structure. For example, MEDLINE's MeSH thesaurus presents the term *depressive disorder* within broader and narrower terms:

Mood Disorders
    Affective Disorders, Psychotic
        Depressive Disorder
            Depression, Postpartum
            Depressive Disorder, Major
            Dysthymic Disorder
            Seasonal Affective Disorder

Many databases allow searchers to *explode* a subject heading, which instructs the database to retrieve records with the requested subject heading as well as any more specific/narrower terms that are related to the topic. In MEDLINE, a search query with the exploded MeSH term *depressive disorder* will not only search the MeSH term *depressive disorder*, but also the terms *depression, postpartum; depressive disorder, major; dysthymic disorder,* and *seasonal affective disorder.*

The *focus* (major concepts, etc.) command instructs the database to retrieve only those articles in which the subject term selected is considered to be the primary focus of the article. This command narrows your search by eliminating articles that peripherally discuss the topic of the subject heading.

Combine Concepts (Boolean Operators)
Boolean logic defines the relationship among terms in a search. There are three Boolean operators: AND, OR, and NOT. Database searchers can apply operators to create broader or narrower searches:

- *AND* combines search terms so that the retrieval set contains all of the terms. The *AND* operator is generally placed between different concepts. For example, the search *St John's wort AND depression* will retrieve results containing *both* terms.
- *OR* combines search terms so that the retrieval set contains at least one of the terms. The *OR* operator is generally placed between synonyms of the same concept. For example, *St John's wort OR hypericum* will retrieve results containing *either* term.
- *NOT* excludes search terms so that the retrieval set will not contain any of the terms that follow the operator NOT. For example, *St John's wort NOT adolescent* will retrieve results containing the term *St John's wort* without the term *adolescent*. Searchers should apply the NOT operator with caution, since it often excludes relevant results with only a passing mention of the term *NOTed* out.

For more efficient searching using Boolean operators, parentheses (brackets) can be used to nest search terms within other search terms. By nesting terms, searchers can specify the order in which the database interprets the search. It is generally recommended that synonyms (that is, terms *ORed* together) should be nested; for example,

(St John's wort OR hypericum) AND (depression OR depressive disorder).

Advanced Versus Basic Search Modes
Several resources offer the searcher an option of using a *basic* search interface with limited and rudimentary options for conducting and refining a search or a more *advanced* mode that will provide more

sophisticated search features and allow searchers to employ many of the techniques discussed in this section. The advanced search mode is the only choice for earnest researchers.

Utilize Filters and Limits

To aid in retrieval relevancy and precision, databases may offer options to filter and/or limit searches by certain parameters. Several databases have devised valuable and effective filters for researchers and clinicians specifically for finding the evidence to answer clinical questions. One example is MEDLINE's *Clinical Queries*, which offers essential built-in evidence-based medicine search filters to retrieve systematic reviews (and meta-analyses, evidence-based guidelines, etc.) and individual studies at the highest tier of the evidence hierarchy (e.g., randomized controlled trials for therapy scenarios). Other examples include the *evidence-based practice* special interest limit or the *systematic review* publication type limit within CINAHL. These filters can be particularly helpful in finding the best evidence on a topic.

Literature databases also offer several ways to limit the retrieval set. Common limits include the following:

- Date—Allows searchers to restrict the publication dates of the articles retrieved. Keep in mind that newer literature is not always better.
- Language—Articles from many countries and languages are included in databases, so it may be helpful to limit the results of a search to a specific language.
- Publication type—Journal articles are not created equal. Case reports, cohort studies, controlled trials, editorials, systematic reviews, comments, practice guidelines, audiovisuals, book chapters, dissertations, and so forth are found in the journal literature.
- Age—Some databases offer the ability to retrieve articles involving specific age groups. For example, by selecting the *infant* limit in CINAHL or MEDLINE, only articles concerning infancy will be retrieved.
- Full text—Several literature databases include a small selection of free full-text (entire) articles. Use of the full-text limit will restrict the results to only items that include, or provide links to, the full text. Selecting this option will often greatly reduce the retrieval set and give no guarantee in the quality of items retrieved. In addition, many health organizations, centers, academic institutions, etc. have the ability to embed a much larger set of full-text content into a database that would not be picked up by the generic full-text option. If the purpose of a literature search is to produce a comprehensive set of relevant articles, this limit should not be applied. However, if the purpose is simply to get a quick grasp of a clinical topic, this option might prove useful because whole articles could be obtained.

Phase III—Beyond the Literature Databases: Mining the Internet

Target Health Websites for Guidelines, Reviews, and Reports

There are plenty of health-related websites that provide quality information for both researchers and clinicians. It is often necessary to venture beyond the literature databases to find guidelines, reports, consensus statements, and other documents not published in the commercial literature. Table 2.3 presents a selective list of valuable sites for EBP.

Some websites look and act much like commercial literature databases and provide access to information created by others (called meta-sites). TRIP Database, for example, is a sophisticated tool, which searches dozens of evidence-based resources (in addition to the millions of articles in MEDLINE). SUMSearch 2 also searches the Internet for evidence-based medical information by scanning literature databases and high-impact medical journals, and employs a unique method of searching and filtering for the best results.

Whereas large meta-sites include citations from a wide variety of documents, others are designated as repositories for specific publication types. Practice guidelines are valuable components in the delivery of evidence-based health care practice. Therefore, clinicians and researchers should have some familiarly with sites specifically focusing on guidelines, such as National Guidelines Clearinghouse (NGC).

Government agencies and professional associations that have developed clinical guidelines may include them on their websites. For example, the National Kidney Foundation website offers a collection of its Kidney Disease Outcomes Quality Initiative (KDOQI) guidelines and the American Heart Association offers statements, guidelines, and clinical updates.

Websites of health agencies and associations organized around specific diseases or conditions also frequently post valuable reviews, reports, and studies that may or may not be included in the pages of journals. For example, the website for the Agency for Healthcare Research and Quality delivers agency-funded evidence-based research reports on clinical topics, health care services, and research methodologies. The National Cancer Institute and the National Kidney Foundation websites offer summaries of recently released results from clinical trials.

Search the Whole Internet

There is never one perfect location to find information on a health topic. Some people quickly turn to the ease of the Internet as a starting place, which can be quite useful if you know where to look or how to search for pertinent and reliable information. There are benefits to exploring a topic on the Internet as a complement to a formal search within relevant literature databases; websites are

TABLE 2.3 Select Examples of Websites

WEBSITE	NOTES
ACP Clinical Recommendations http://www.acponline.org/clinical_information/guidelines	ACP Clinical Recommendations cover many areas of internal medicine, including screening for cancer or other major diseases, diagnosis, treatment, and medical technology. Included are clinical practice guidelines, clinical guidance statements, and best practice advice.
Agency for Healthcare Research and Quality **Evidence-Based Practice Centers** http://www.ahrq.gov/clinic/epcix.htm	A collection of high-quality reports, reviews, and technology assessments based on rigorous, comprehensive syntheses and analyses of the scientific literature on topics relevant to clinical, social science/behavioral, economic, and other health care organization and delivery issues.
Agency for Healthcare Research and Quality **U.S. Preventive Services Task Force** http://www.ahrq.gov/clinic/uspstfix.htm	The U.S. Preventive Services Task Force is an independent panel of experts in primary care and prevention that systematically reviews the evidence of effectiveness and develops recommendations for clinical preventive services.
American Heart Association **Scientific Statements and Guidelines** http://my.americanheart.org/professional/index.jsp	A collection of AHA's scientific statements and practice guidelines that are published in *Circulation; Stroke; Arteriosclerosis, Thrombosis, and Vascular Biology; Hypertension; Circulation Research*, or other journals.
Bandolier http://www.medicine.ox.ac.uk/bandolier	A quirky independent online electronic journal and database written by Oxford University scientists. Each month PubMed and the Cochrane Library are searched for systematic reviews and meta-analyses, the reviews that look interesting are read and discussed in bullet points in Bandolier, first in the paper version and, after 6 months, on the website.
CMA Infobase http://www.cma.ca/cpgs	Guidelines produced or endorsed in Canada by a national, provincial/territorial, or regional medical, or health organization, professional society, government agency, or expert panel.
The Community Guide http://www.thecommunityguide.org	Developed by the nonfederal Task Force on Community Preventive Services, whose members are appointed by the director of the Centers for Disease Control and Prevention (CDC), the Community Guide summarizes what is known about the effectiveness, economic efficiency, and feasibility of interventions to promote community health and prevent disease.

Infectious Diseases Society of America Practice Guidelines
http://www.idsociety.org/Guidelines_Patient_Care

Includes standards, practice guidelines, and statements developed and/or endorsed by the Infectious Disease Society of America (IDSA).

Institute for Clinical Systems Improvement
http://www.icsi.org/guidelines_and_more

Institute for Clinical Systems Improvement (ICSI) is collaboration by medical groups, hospitals, and health plans that provide health care services to people who live and work in the Midwest. Included on the website are guidelines, order sets, protocols, guideline impact studies, patient education resources, and technology assessment reports.

The Joanna Briggs Institute
http://www.joannabriggs.edu.au

The Joanna Briggs Institute (JBI) is an initiative of Royal Adelaide Hospital and the University of Adelaide. The Institute provides "a collaborative approach to the evaluation of evidence derived from a diverse range of sources, including experience, expertise and all forms of rigorous research and the translation, transfer and utilization of the 'best available' evidence into health care practice." Many resources are available only to member institutions, although selected systematic reviews and best practice information sheets are available to nonmembers.

National Cancer Institute Clinical Trials
http://www.cancer.gov/clinicaltrials

Allows users to search and browse recent clinical-trial results by type of cancer or topic or search NCI's list of thousands of clinical trials now accepting participants. Also included are educational materials about clinical trials, a list of noteworthy clinical trials, and more information for research teams interested in conducting clinical trials.

National Guidelines Clearinghouse
http://www.guidelines.gov

Developed by the Department of Health and Human Services, the National Guidelines Clearinghouse (NGC) collects best practice guidelines produced by medical facilities, agencies, and organizations around the world. The site is searchable by disease, and there is a guideline comparison tool that allows different guidelines for the same disease to be compared.

National Kidney Foundation
http://www.kidney.org/professionals/kdoqi

The National Kidney Foundation website includes several clinical practice guidelines published under NKF's KDOQI brand. All guidelines follow the rigorous KDOQI process, are developed by independent volunteer work groups, and funded by more than a dozen companies within the kidney-disease field.

(continued)

TABLE 2.3 Select Examples of Websites (*continued*)

WEBSITE	NOTES
Nursing Best Practice Guidelines http://rnao.ca/bpg	Best practice guidelines for client care developed for Ontario nurses. Includes almost 50 published guidelines as well as a toolkit and educator's resource to support implementation.
Royal College of Nursing Clinical Guidelines http://www.rcn.org.uk/development/practice /clinicalguidelines	Several practice guidelines from the Royal College of Nursing (RCN) in the UK.
SUMSearch 2 http://sumsearch.org	A free meta-search engine for evidence-based medical information, scanning databases (MEDLINE, DARE, and NGC) as well as various high-impact medical journals. To automate searching, SUMSearch 2 combines meta- and contingency searching. Meta-searching is designed to scan multiple databases and sites simultaneously, and returns one single retrieval document to the user. If a high number of results are obtained, more restrictive searches (called contingency searches) are conducted by activating additional filters. Conversely, if the result is small, more databases are added to the search.
TRIP http://tripdatabase.com	A free meta-search engine that aims to provide quick access to a collection of evidence-based and other high-quality medical information resources via a single interface. TRIP identifies and searches numerous high-quality Internet resources that allow access to their content such as MEDLINE, Cochrane, National Guidelines Clearinghouse, ACP Journal Club, and top peer-reviewed journals. These resources are then categorized by type: Evidence-based synopses, clinical questions, systematic reviews, guidelines, core primary research, e-textbooks, and calculators.
VHL (Virginia Henderson Library) Repository http://www.nursinglibrary.org/vhl	The VHL Repository is an online digital service that collects, preserves, and disseminates digital materials in both abstract and full-text format. Submissions may be made by individual nurses, nursing students, and nursing organizations and may include preprints, working papers, theses, dissertations, conference papers, presentations, faculty-created learning objects, data sets, and so on.

often very current. The capability for "publishers," whether health care institutions, corporate entities, government agencies, or even individuals, to quickly and inexpensively publish permits immediate information transfer to the Internet user. This also allows groups to distribute potentially important relevant information that may go unpublished through commercial channels. This type of literature is often referred to as *grey literature*. Examples include scientific and technical reports, guidelines, care plans, patent documents, conference papers, internal reports, government documents, newsletters, factsheets, and theses.

The information available via the Internet is neither trustworthy nor well organized. There are numerous popular search engines that scour the Internet to retrieve materials that match keywords entered in the search box. These search engines use specific algorithms to sort retrieved results. In many cases, retrieval order depends on a mixture of keyword matches, currency, and other factors (not necessarily quality of content). To eliminate some of the vagaries of Internet searching, there are techniques to improve the quality and reliability of the retrieval set. The first is to try a selective search engine. A good example of a selective multidisciplinary search engine is Google Scholar (http://scholar.google.com), which restricts an Internet search to "scholarly" publications such as journal articles, technical reports, preprints, theses, books, and vetted web pages from academic publishers, professional societies, preprint repositories, universities, and other scholarly organizations. Another good technique is to seek and employ search tools or an *advanced search* option, which may offer numerous choices for making searches more precise and results relevant. Google, for instance, offers search tools that will restrict your results by date, reading level, and so forth.

Do keep in mind, however, that much of the Internet is not peer-reviewed or vetted in any way, so the searcher carries the burden of evaluating the quality and accuracy of the information presented. Strategies to assess website quality are presented in Exhibit 2.3.

Be Aware of Emerging Resources

Searching for, perusing, and validating either the review or the primary literature takes skill and precious time. New practical resources to support evidence-based decisions are becoming readily available to health care practitioners. Clinical summary databases (CSDs) are designed to act as quick, single-stop, point-of-care tools that quickly connect users to evidence-based information on treatment and diagnostic options for common conditions. The best CSDs summarize and synthesize current high-quality research for answers to specific clinical questions, often adding practice implications specifically supported by a rationale and pertinent, current evidence. The centerpiece of these products includes

Exhibit 2.3
Strategies to Determine Website Quality

1. Identify the website sponsor and author. Ascertain the credentials of the author.
2. Identify the date when the page was produced or revised.
3. View the HTML (hypertext markup language) or page source of web pages to look for author identification and/or publication date.
4. If you are not already knowledgeable about the topic, ask an expert to review the information.
5. Find reviews of Internet resources by reviewers in reputable print and online sources, or use selective subject directory/electronic library collections you trust to identify resources.
6. Peruse related trustworthy websites to see whether there is a link to the site you are questioning.
7. E-mail the author or responsible organization/sponsor and ask about credentials.

Source: Kovacs and Carlson (2000)

a database of hundreds of entries on the treatment and prevention of medical conditions, which are developed from synthesized information obtained by searching quality evidence-based medicine resources and health-related literature databases. Creation of these entries is generally overseen by recognized experts and clinical specialists. Most CSDs tend to be updated monthly although some are updated quarterly and/or will insert news items and urgent updates as needed. Although there is great variation in searchability, most interfaces offer browsable tables of contents and rudimentary search boxes; some include means to target or narrow search results. Examples of CSDs are listed in Table 2.4.

Most researchers and practitioners commonly scan a fairly narrow set of journals to find articles of interest. To broaden their radar, readers should consider using specialty resources that survey large sets of journals in selected disciplines. These *surveillance tools* summarize important articles that warrant the attention of their readership. In general, editors associated with these resources scan the health literature (often hundreds of journals) and highlight published topic reviews and individual studies from prominent journals. With few exceptions, reviews or studies that appear in these sources are sound and have met established quality criteria. Much like the CSDs, these resources boil down lengthy systematic reviews and detailed studies to a consumable package of value-added information. Selected examples of sources that provide this service are listed in Table 2.5.

TABLE 2.4   Clinical Summary Database Examples

- Mosby's Nursing Consult (evidence-based nursing section)
  http://www.nursingconsult.com/nursing/index
- UpToDate
  http://uptodate.com
- Clinical Evidence (*BMJ*)
  http://clinicalevidence.bmj.com/x/index.html
- ACP PIER
  http://pier.acponline.org/index.html
- DynaMed
  https://dynamed.ebscohost.com

TABLE 2.5   Surveillance Tool Examples

- Evidence-based nursing
  http://ebn.bmj.com
- ACP Journal Club
  http://www.acpjc.org
- EvidenceUpdates
  http://plus.mcmaster.ca/EvidenceUpdates
- Essential Evidence Plus: Daily POEMs (patient-oriented evidence that matters)
  http://www.essentialevidenceplus.com/content/poems

Phase IV—Pulling It All Together

The search for evidence does not end with successful retrieval from a database or website. The relevant information needs to be retained and organized for further analysis and full-text copies of articles, reports, and guidelines, and similar documents need to be obtained and stored. In addition, any search queries used should be retained and available for future searches on the topic.

Save Your Search Query

Experienced searchers are well aware of the benefits of saving database search queries at the conclusion of a search. One good motivation to do so is to prevent that sting of frustration when a literature search gets interrupted or misplaced and the entire search progression needs to be retraced. Another reason is simply to be in a position to quickly rerun a search at designated intervals to keep abreast of the literature on the particular topic. As a valuable convenience, databases now allow users to create individual accounts that will retain user information, search queries, and search results. MyNCBI (MEDLINE) and My EBSCOhost (CINAHL) are examples of user-created personal accounts within databases.

Invest in a Citation Manager

Databases allow searchers to output their retrieval sets in a variety of displays and a range of output formats. The most common display options are citation only, citation with abstract, or full record, which includes descriptors, accession numbers, and other useful data. Databases also offer different output options such as a text file and a Microsoft Word file, preserved in an e-mail, or sent to a printer. Websites, on the other hand, give virtually no output choice other than the browser-supported PRINT and SAVE AS options.

The most efficient researcher, however, will enlist the help of commercial software called a *citation manager* to transfer, store, and manage the bibliographic references/citations retrieved from databases or websites. Commonly used citation managers in the health sciences include the following:

- EndNote—http://www.endnote.com
- Reference Manager—http://www.refman.com
- Zotero—http://www.zotero.org
- Mendeley—http://www.mendeley.com

These products consist of a database in which full bibliographic citations (abstracts and subject headings) can be entered or imported, as well as a system for generating selective lists or articles in the different formats required by publishers. Citation managers can be integrated with word processors so that a list of citations in the appropriate format (e.g., MLA [Modern Language Association], APA [American Psychological Association], etc.) is produced automatically as an article is written. There are many citation managers available on the market and the best of them allow the following:

- Direct export from online databases such as MEDLINE, CINAHL, PsycINFO, ERIC into the citation manager
- Folders and subfolder organization of citations
- Output to formatted bibliographies in all major styles (MLA, APA, etc.)
- Automatic integration with word processor formats (e.g., Microsoft Word, RTF (rich text format), and HTML)
- Attachments, such as image files, Adobe PDFs, and Microsoft Word docs, to be embedded into a record within the database for opening at a later time

Find the Full Article (Full Text)

One of the barriers to conducting a successful literature search is simply obtaining the entire (full-text) articles of the retrieved results. Access to full-text articles has improved dramatically with the growth of electronic publishing; yet, this usually remains a multistep process. The majority of databases and websites tend to provide only citations and abstracts to items of interest, but entire articles are not always immediately available online. Certain databases are making an effort to assist the user by allowing publishers and academic institutions to insert links within item records to lead users to the full article. Keep in mind that commercial and academic publishers rarely give anything away for free and often charge fees, some exorbitant, to grant access to articles. A searcher may want to first contact a library associated with a local clinic, hospital, or school, or even turn to the public library. Libraries often have established access to journal collections or offer interlibrary loan services. If none are available in your area, an inexpensive alternative is the National Library of Medicine's Loansome Doc service for ordering documents through MEDLINE (PubMed).

Keep Up With the Topic

Keeping abreast of the published information on any given topic is no longer difficult. Several databases now offer *alert* or *current aware-ness* services that allow users to automatically receive new results (via e-mail) from saved search queries at prescribed intervals. Search queries can involve topics of interest, or can pertain to specific authors or a set of relevant journals.

Really simple syndication (RSS) is an emerging technology that many predict will revolutionize the way researchers and practitioners retrieve information from favorite sources. RSS is more or less an electronic table of contents service where one can quickly scan the contents (called feeds) of any number of the latest journals, headlines from favorite news sources, news from relevant organizations, entries from blogs and websites, and even updates from literature searches, at one personalized location (called a feed reader) with no nagging e-mail clutter. The most popular free feed reader is Google Reader (http://www.google.com/reader). Getting started with RSS is relatively easy, and it is likely to become an indispensable tool for keeping a researcher or clinician current and for saving time.

SUMMARY

In summary, literature reviews are not mysterious manifestations of scholarly pursuits. Nor should they be merely academic exercises. They are, and are increasingly required to be, vital components of quality health care. Literature reviews are the sum of many definable parts and the application of systematic procedures illustrated in this chapter in four phases: (1) presearch preparations and planning; (2) mining major literature databases for evidence-based information; (3) mining additional resources across the Internet; and (4) using new technologies to organize, store, and update found information. This systematic process builds a researcher's toolkit and can be adapted to meet the demands of EBP.

Above all, remember that one size does not fit all research situations. Allow for slippage, expect some detours, and reach out for help before spinning those research wheels needlessly. Timely consultations with subject experts, faculty, and medical librarians can decrease frustration. The process of conducting a literature review will, with time, actually become an interesting and rewarding journey of discovery.

SUGGESTED ACTIVITIES

1. You are planning a research study to determine adherence to diet by diabetic patients. Perform a literature search to locate articles published in the past 3 to 5 years that describe how diabetics conform to their prescribed diets. Use at least two appropriate databases (e.g., CINAHL and MEDLINE [PubMed]) to find pertinent articles. Compare and contrast articles you retrieve for levels of evidence, strength of evidence presented, and their usefulness for defined needs.
2. Locate practice guidelines on the treatment of foot ulcers in diabetics. Use at least two appropriate resources (e.g., NGC and MEDLINE [PubMed]). How do the search results compare?

REFERENCES

Bastian, H., Glasziou, P., & Chalmers, I. (2010). Seventy-five trials and eleven systematic reviews a day: How will we ever keep up? *PLoS Medicine, 7*(9), e1000326.

Brancato, V. C. (2006). An innovative clinical practicum to teach evidence-based practice. *Nurse Educator, 31*(5), 195–199.

Dee, C., & Stanley, E. E. (2005). Information-seeking behavior of nursing students and clinical nurses: Implications for health sciences librarians. *Journal of the Medical Library Association, 93*(2), 213–222.

Downs, F. S. (1969). Some critical issues in nursing research. *Nursing Forum, 8*(4), 393–404.

Klein, G. A. (2003). *Intuition at work: Why developing your gut instincts will make you better at what you do* (1st ed.). New York, NY: Currency/ Doubleday.

Kovacs, D. K., & Carlson, A. L. (2000). *How to find medical information on the internet: A print and online tutorial for the healthcare professional and consumer.* Berkeley, CA: Library Solutions Press.

Lyman, P., & Varian, H. R. (2003). *How much information? 2003.* Berkeley, CA: University of California. Retrieved February 21, 2008 from http://www.sims .berkeley.edu/how-much-info-2003

Mellon, C. A. (1984). Process not product in course-integrated instruction: A generic model of library research. *College & Research Libraries, 45*(6), 471.

Melnyk, B. M., Fineout-Overholt, E., Fischbeck Feinstein, N., Li, H., Small, L., Wilcox, L., & Kraus, R. (2004). Nurses' perceived knowledge, beliefs, skills, and needs regarding evidence-based practice: Implications for accelerating the paradigm shift. *Worldviews on Evidence-Based Nursing, 1*(3), 185.

Melnyk, B. M., Fineout-Overholt, E., Stillwell, S. B., & Williamson, K. M. (2009). Evidence-based practice: Step by step. Igniting a spirit of inquiry: An essential foundation for evidence-based practice. *American Journal of Nursing, 109*(11), 49–52.

Mulrow, C. D. (1994). Rationale for systematic reviews. *British Medical Journal (Clinical Research Ed.), 309*(6954), 597–599.

Polit, D. F., & Beck, C. T. (2008). *Nursing research: Generating and assessing evidence for nursing practice* (8th ed.). Philadelphia, PA: Wolters Kluwer Health/Lippincott Williams & Wilkins.

Pravikoff, D. S., Tanner, A. B., & Pierce, S. T. (2005). Readiness of U.S. nurses for evidence-based practice. *American Journal of Nursing, 105*(9), 40–51 (Quiz 52).

Skiba, D. J. (2005). Preparing for evidence-based practice: Revisiting information literacy. *Nursing Education Perspectives, 26*(5), 310–311.

Tanner, A., Pierce, S., & Pravikoff, D. (2004). Readiness for evidence-based practice: Information literacy needs of nurses in the United States. *Medinfo, 11*(Pt 2), 936–940.

Research and the Mandate for Evidence-Based Practice, Quality, and Patient Safety

Kathleen R. Stevens

The development of science for nursing and health care is a response to needs for knowledge to address the health of the public. The applied science of nursing has the ultimate aim of discovering effective interventions to resolve actual and potential health problems and to provide knowledge about effectiveness of interventions in producing desired health-related outcomes. Although nursing research has been well institutionalized since 1984, with the establishment of the National Institute for Nursing Research (NINR; originally, National Center for Nursing Research), only in the recent past has health care's research interests swung dramatically to examine how to move research findings into practice. Not only is there public demand for moving new knowledge into practice, but also there is demand for doing this in ways that increase quality and safety of care and increase the likelihood of realizing the intended health outcomes. In the past 10 years, research to build the science of quality and safety has grown.

This chapter presents events and findings that have influence on this new scientific interest in health care quality and safety. Included are descriptions of the underlying reasons for the new emphasis on quality improvement and safety, frameworks for conceptualizing and studying improvement and safety, methods used for such investigations, and new resources and future trends in improvement and safety research.

In addition, this chapter explores how evidence-based practice (EBP), quality, and safety in health care are reflected in nursing theory, research, and science in meeting the mandate for quality and safety. To provide a broad context, our discussion first presents an overview of the relationship among research, EBP, quality, and safety, providing a framework through which to view these facets of health care. Sections of the chapter are devoted specifically to quality and to safety, highlighting the dominant thinking and research advances in each area. The chapter concludes with a look to the future of quality and safety, examining recent advances and suggesting directions in theory, research, and science.

OVERVIEW: RESEARCH, EBP, QUALITY, AND SAFETY

Quality and safety are top priorities in contemporary health care. The responsibility and accountability for ensuring effective and safe care are inescapable for all health professionals and are a social obligation to every health care agency. Delivering the right care at the right time in the right setting is the goal of efforts to advance safety and quality. This challenge requires that well-prepared nurses play key roles in moving research into action to overhaul today's health care system.

For nurses to effectively guide the movement for quality and safety, skills are required that reflect improvement science and principles of high-reliability industries.

The morbidity and mortality toll of both ineffective care and unsafe care requires that all health professionals take a serious look at what must be done to address lapses in quality and to avoid the cost of hundreds of thousands of lives. To meet this challenge, it is vital to ensure that health care is error free, that all existing best (research-based) practices are used, and that everyone implements the highest quality and most reliable processes for every patient. The narrow notion of safety as the absence of medication errors or falls has been broadened. This is the challenge of quality and patient safety in health care. The foundation of success is translation of research results into clinical care; the infrastructure of success is conducting research to elucidate change interventions that improve clinical care processes at the individual clinician, organization, system, environment, and policy levels. Thus, research is the key to determining clinical effectiveness of care and translation is the key to redesigning health care systems that are safe and effective.

SEVERE PROBLEMS IN HEALTH CARE QUALITY

Research has built a large body of science about "what works" in health care, yet actual care lags behind what has been reported to be effective (Institute of Medicine [IOM], 2001). The end result is health care that is ineffective in producing intended patient health outcomes and care that is unsafe. These circumstances are prevalent in nursing and across all health professions, even though massive numbers of research reports provide "best evidence" for care. Health care processes and outcomes could be greatly improved if research results were put into practice.

QUALITY AND EBP

The quality of health care is based on the degree to which decisions about patient care are guided by "conscientious, explicit, and judicious use of current best evidence" (IOM, 2008, p. 3). The definition of health care quality emphasizes this point.

Definition
Quality of Health Care

Degree to which health services for individuals and populations increase the likelihood of desired health outcomes and are consistent with current professional knowledge. (IOM, 1990)

This definition makes clear that evidence is a core element in producing intended health outcomes. Unless patient care is based on the most current and best evidence, it falls short of quality.

The aim of EBP is to standardize health care practices to science and best evidence and to reduce illogical variation in care, which leads to unpredictable health outcomes. Development of EBP is fueled by public and professional demand for accountability in safety and quality improvement in health care. It is imperative that health care is based on current professional knowledge in order to produce the quality necessary for intended patient outcomes.

Leaders in the field have defined EBP as the "integration of best research evidence with clinical expertise and patient values" (Sackett, Straus, Richardson, Rosenberg, & Haynes, 2000, p. ii). Therefore, EBP melds research evidence with clinical expertise and encourages individualization of care through incorporation of patient preferences and the circumstances of the setting.

Just as evidence and quality are linked, so are safety and quality. The ties among safety, errors, quality, and caring are explained as concentric circles or subsets of a common flaw (Woolf, 2004). The innermost concentric circle is safety, followed by errors, then quality, and, finally, caring as the outermost circle. The model suggests that safety is a subcategory of health care errors. Such errors include mistakes in health promotion and chronic disease management that cost lives but do not affect safety—these are errors of omission. Following this model, errors are a subset of quality lapses, which result from both errors and systemic problems. Systemic problems that reduce quality in health care may stem from lack of access, inequity, and flawed system designs. Finally, this model suggests that lapses in quality are a subset of deficient caring; such deficiencies can be seen in lack of access, inequity, and faulty system designs (Woolf, 2004). In nursing research, such a model can serve to frame investigations of health care safety and quality.

Health care quality and safety have emerged as a principal concern relatively recently. In 1990, interprofessional opinion leaders began an intensive initiative to improve the quality of health care (IOM, 1990). These leaders proclaimed that there is a chasm between what we *know* (through research) to be best health care and what we *do*. In a series of influential reports, these national advisers called for one of our nation's most far-reaching health reforms, called the IOM Quality Initiative. A series of reports known as the *Quality Chasm Series* dissected health care problems and recommended fundamental and sweeping changes in health care (IOM, 2001). The directions set by the *Quality Chasm Series* continue to have marked impact on every aspect of health care. Each of the trendsetting IOM reports (2001, 2003a, 2003b, 2008, 2011) identifies EBP as *crucial* in closing the quality chasm. This movement is likely to continue beyond the next decade. Because of their enduring impact on the transformation of health care, we offer the following summary of some of the IOM *Chasm* reports.

In 2000, the IOM reviewed studies and trends and concluded that 48,000 to 98,000 Americans die annually in hospitals due to medical errors caused by defective systems rather than caregivers themselves. *To Err Is Human* (IOM, 2000) offered impressive documentation regarding the severity and pervasive nature of the nation's overall quality problem. In fact, using statistical approaches, the report documented that more people die from medical mistakes each year than from highway accidents, breast cancer, or AIDS. In addition to deaths, it was noted that medical errors cause permanent disabilities and unnecessary suffering. This report raised the issue of patient safety to high priority for every health care provider, scientist, agency leader, and policymaker.

The next report in this series further unfolded the story of quality in American health care. In *Crossing the Quality Chasm: A New Health System for the 21st Century* (IOM, 2001), health care leaders reviewed research that highlighted other widespread defects in our health care system. Defects included overuse, misuse, and underuse of health care services and described a wide gulf between ideal care (as supported by research) and the reality of the care that many Americans experience. The *Quality Chasm* report presented research evidence documenting a lack of quality in health care, cost concerns, poor use of information technology, absence of progress in restructuring the health care system, and underutilization of resources. Throughout these analyses of health care safety and quality, a deep-rooted problem was highlighted: although health science and technology were advancing at a rapid pace, the health care delivery system was failing to deliver high-quality health care services (IOM, 2001). The reports emphasized that a major part of the problem is that research results are not translated into practice and that practice lags behind research-generated knowledge.

The profession of nursing is central to many of the interprofessional and discipline-specific changes that must be accomplished to provide safe and effective care. The Interdisciplinary Nursing Quality Research Initiative (INQRI) supported by the Robert Wood Johnson Foundation (RWJF) funded studies to discover how nurses contribute to and can improve the quality of patient care (RWJF, 2008).

After a series of public input meetings, the IOM issued the 2011 report, *The Future of Nursing: Leading Change, Advancing Health.* The report identified the 3 million nurses in the profession as the largest segment of the nation's health care workforce. Of the eight recommendations was the urging for nurses to lead and manage collaborative efforts within an interdisciplinary team to redesign and improve practice and health care systems (IOM, 2011).

Because the purpose of research ultimately is to uncover causal relationships, the primary goal is to determine which interventions are most effective in assisting patients and clients to resolve actual and potential health problems. In other words, research shows us "what works" best to produce the intended health outcome for a given health problem. Knowledge discovered through research is then translated into practice guidelines and ultimately affects health policy through commonly accepted health care practices.

NURSING, RESEARCH UTILIZATION, AND EBP

In health professions, research is conducted to build a case for specific practices and interventions. Because the very reason for conducting research is to illuminate effective (best) practices, then it follows that research must be translated into clinical decision making at the point of care. Although this goal is clear, nurses have struggled to achieve research utilization since the 1970s.

Nursing has struggled with ways to move research results into practice; however, early attempts were not fully successful. Barriers to knowledge translation became a crucial topic of investigation in nursing in the early 1990s. A number of research utilization models were developed to explain the barriers and challenges in applying research results in practice. One program of study established a dissemination model (Funk, Tornquist, & Champagne, 1989) and developed a scale with which to quantify nurses' perception of barriers to applying research in practice (Funk, Champagne, Wiese, & Tornquist, 1990). Still widely used today, the BARRIERS scale is framed in the old paradigm of research utilization, in which results of a single study were examined for direct application, and clinical nurses were expected to read, critique, and translate primary research reports into point-of-care practice, and to devote time to these activities.

This early work in research utilization resulted in a clearer focus on clinical investigations. Nurse scientists who conducted research, largely in academic settings, were criticized for their shortcomings in making research results clinically meaningful. Such criticism included claims that research did not address pressing clinical problems, results were not expressed in terms understood by clinicians, and clinicians were not in positions to apply the results in care. In tandem, nurse scientists gathered momentum to establish what is today the National Institute for Nursing Research, dedicated to funding clinical research.

Initial research utilization models were developed prior to the emergence of EBP. The Stetler Model (Stetler, 1994) mapped a step-by-step approach that could be used by individual clinicians to critique research, restate findings, and consider the findings in their own decision making. The model focuses on a bottom-up approach to change in clinical practice. The Iowa Model outlined a process to guide implementation of research results into clinical practice in the context of provider, patient, and infrastructure (Titler et al., 2001). The Iowa Model gives heavy emphasis to nurse managers as key instruments of change. Both models have moved from their original roots in research utilization to reflect a broader approach used in EBP. These early efforts underscored the importance of moving research into direct patient care.

SHIFT FROM RESEARCH UTILIZATION TO EBP

Frequently, research results are either inadequately translated into clinical practice recommendations or applied inconsistently in the delivery of health care. Additionally, poor health care system design contributes to the chasm; health care design inadequacies include a lack of interprofessional teams to provide comprehensive and coordinated care and a complex system that is a maze to patients and that fails to provide patients the services from which they would likely benefit (IOM, 2001).

As growth in the EBP movement grew, it became apparent that the hurdles to translating research to practice required complex answers not yet discovered. The EBP movement has provided new scientific means with which to overcome these hurdles.

Until recently, much importance in the use of research was placed on what it was we *did not know,* and this became the basis for the clinician's action: designing and conducting research studies. In the EBP approach to the use of research, the knowledge itself has become the basis for action: improving care processes and outcomes with knowledge about clinical effectiveness. In EBP, the importance is placed on what we *do know* and on increasing the clinical utility and usefulness of the knowledge. It became clear that knowledge transformation must occur as research results are translated into practice (Stevens, 2004).

As the health care quality paradigm shifted to EBP, additional hurdles in transforming research results into common practice became apparent. Evidence-based practice approaches, derived from clinical epidemiology, provided new insights and changed the paradigm for thinking about translating research. With the paradigm shift, hurdles became apparent. Two primary hurdles include (a) the large volume and complexity of health research literature and (b) the low clinical utility of the form of knowledge that is available to the clinician (Stevens, 2004). The EBP movement offers techniques to overcome these two hurdles, including the transformation of knowledge reflected in the ACE Star Model: evidence summary, translation into clinical guidelines, integration into practice, and evaluation of outcomes and impact (Stevens, 2004).

Evidence Summary

To overcome the hurdle posed by the large volume of research, a new approach was developed in the mid-1990s. Evidence summaries became a key to bridging knowledge to practice. The most rigorous scientific method for synthesizing all research into a single summary is called a *systematic review* (SR). An SR is defined as a scientific investigation that focuses on a specific question and uses explicitly, preplanned scientific methods to identify, select, assess, and summarize similar but separate studies.

These EBP approaches produce a concise and comprehensible statement about the state of the science regarding clinical effectiveness. The new research method, SR, is the keystone to understanding whether a clinical intervention works (IOM, 2008). Indeed, it is now known that an evidence summary is requisite to "getting the evidence [about intervention effectiveness] straight" (Glasziou & Haynes, 2005). The sobering flip side of this logic is that *not* conducting an evidence summary or conducting a nonsystematic review (*not* getting the evidence straight) leads to a misinformed clinical decision. Nursing care must be driven by research evidence—not knowing the state of the science about clinical effectiveness results in ineffective, unnecessary, or harmful care. From EBP, we now realize that basing care on results of a single primary research study can lead to the selection of a wrong intervention. With this new realization, we have moved away from using single research studies to change practice to a much more rigorous knowledge form—the evidence summary.

SRs serve two important knowledge functions in health care. First, an SR provides evidence about the clinical effectiveness of a particular intervention in relation to specified outcomes. Second, an SR provides a view of gaps in the scientific field and points to further research needed to fill these voids. A prime advantage of an evidence summary, such as an SR, is that all research results on a given topic are transformed into a single, harmonious statement (Mulrow, 1994). In this way, the state of the science on a given topic is placed at the fingertips of the clinician in terms of what is known and what remains to be discovered. With regard to providing evidence-based direction for clinical care, an SR offers other advantages (Mulrow, 1994) as outlined in Exhibit 3.1.

Exhibit 3.1
Advantages of a Systematic Review

1. Reduces information into a manageable form
2. Increases power in cause and effect
3. Assesses consistencies across studies
4. Integrates information for decisions
5. Establishes generalizability—participants, settings, treatment variations, and study designs
6. Reduces bias and improves true reflection of reality
7. Reduces time between research and implementation
8. Offers basis for continuous update as new knowledge is discovered
9. Points to further research to address gaps

Source: Mulrow (1994)

Guidelines

The next stage of knowledge transformation is in the form of the evidence-based clinical practice guidelines (CPGs). To overcome low point-of-care use of research, evidence-based CPGs are used to translate the evidence summary into recommendations for clinical practice. Clinical practice guidelines are defined as "systematically defined statements that are designed to help clinicians and patients make decisions about appropriate health care for specific clinical circumstances" (IOM, 1990, p. 38). The utility of CPGs is enhanced by inclusion of specification and rating of supporting evidence. Evidence-based CPGs have the potential to reduce illogical variations in practice by encouraging use of clinically effective practices (IOM, 2008).

Integration

Once the evidence is straight-through summaries and guidelines, it becomes necessary to introduce the EBP into ongoing care. The challenges of changing the provider's practices are many and complex. New approaches to studying organizational change, complex adaptive systems, and culture shifts are adding to our understanding of the challenge of integration. Research will fill the gap in what we know about "getting the straight evidence used" (Glasziou & Haynes, 2005) in practice.

Evaluation

Once integrated, the practice change is evaluated for its impact on the care process, the patient health outcome, or both. The quality of the care process is equal to the degree to which the care reflects best (evidence-based) practice. A number of important quality indicator research initiatives are discussed in the section on the future of quality.

MANDATE

In view of the size and pervasiveness of the problem of quality in America's health care system, leaders issued an urgent call for fundamental change to close the "quality gap." This call and accompanying actions were detailed in the *Quality Chasm* report (IOM, 2001). Sweeping systemic changes were recommended. A blueprint for change outlined immediate action to improve all aspects of care over the next decade.

The plan offered strategies to implement change and specified six aims to improve quality while redesigning the health care delivery system so that patients will experience safer, more reliable, more responsive, more integrated, and more available care. These six aims include making sure that health care is safe, effective, patient-centered, timely, efficient, and equitable (IOM, 2001). In the changes in health care, these six principles have been identified as the following.

Health care must be redesigned to be

Safe
Timely
Effective
Efficient
Equitable
Patient centered

The "STEEEP" redesign principles are now woven throughout quality and safety initiatives at many levels of our health care institutions. For example, the Institute for Healthcare Improvement (IHI) identifies the

STEEEP principles as foundational to their corporate philosophy (IHI, 2008), and the new Health Care Innovations Exchange of the Agency for Healthcare Research and Quality (AHRQ) identifies the STEEEP principles in its criteria for inclusion of improvement projects (AHRQ, 2008a).

In these reports, EBP was identified as foundational to quality of care and safety. Recommendations included creating an environment that supports EBP (IOM, 2001), emphasizing the need for EBP to reduce unwarranted variations in care where knowledge for improvement was available (IOM, 2003a), and establishing EBP as a basic competence in all health professions (IOM, 2003b). The most recent report sets a blueprint for the nation to assess clinical effectiveness and provide credible information about what really works in health care (IOM, 2008). The recommendations are to set priorities and manage SRs of clinical effectiveness and to generate credible CPGs.

Health care facilities are reacting to the new quality and safety health care agenda with unprecedented speed. Few other movements in health care have gained such widespread and rapid momentum. Nurses have risen to the occasion to join and lead evidence-based quality efforts through improvement efforts, development of explanatory models and science of EBP, educational program revision, and development of oversight and regulatory programs.

SHIFTS IN NURSING RESEARCH COMPETENCIES

Because of these forces and shifts in emphasis, the relationship between research and clinical care has changed. In the past, primary research was conducted to test the effectiveness of interventions; now, researchers investigate ways to render health care systems and processes effective and safe. In addition, clinicians are expected to integrate research into practice—to transform knowledge into clinical practice. Clients demand that health care be based on best scientific evidence in combination with client preferences and the clinician's expertise (the definition of EBP).

This new paradigm of EBP requires a shift in thinking about research competencies that are needed in clinical care. Prior to the new knowledge forms offered by EBP, education programs prepared nurses to "conduct" investigations that would discover new knowledge. Although an important function, conducting research is insufficient to achieve evidence-based quality improvement. Increasingly, advance practice nurses assume roles that emphasize evidence-based quality improvement—competencies not widely included in basic and professional development education. These competencies include both knowledge and the skill to translate research into practice (Stevens, 2009). Systematic identification of these new competencies makes clear the distinction between conducting research and translating research into practice. National consensus on 83 EBP competencies (Stevens, 2009) has galvanized changes in nursing education programs as EBP is integrated through undergraduate, graduate, and professional development education. Additional work is under way in identifying learning outcomes for quality and safety education (Cronenwett et al., 2007), which also will contribute to this growing effort toward a workforce that is prepared to translate research into practice. Given that, a recent survey indicated that nurses still face significant barriers in employing EBP (Melnyk, Fineout-Overholt, Gallagher-Ford, & Kaplan, 2012); it is imperative to continue efforts to embed these competencies into the core of our profession.

CHANGES IN NURSING RESEARCH

The focus of nursing research has recently expanded to include the study of health care quality and patient safety. In the past, nursing research produced knowledge about individual clients through primary research studies, largely based on research designs used to investigate individual client treatment and experiences (such as experimental psychology and anthropology). These research reports were found to be difficult to translate into practice.

Today's health care redesign and evidence-based quality initiatives call on nurse scientists and clinicians also to embrace what is known about best (effective) practices and system change to support quality health care. New research methods and models, such as SRs and complex adaptive systems (CASs), are being added to prior methods and models, such as true experiment and King's theory of mutual goal setting. New competencies to translate research into practice are being added to prior investigative competencies to conduct primary research studies. Nurse researchers are realigning previous research approaches and adopting new research designs as part of translational science teams that produce knowledge about effective health care and systems.

New fields of study have set about to study improvement strategies and to understand factors that facilitate or hinder implementation. The aim of improvement science is to determine which improvement strategies work as we strive to ensure safe and effective care, and it primarily focused on the health care delivery system and microsystem (Berwick, 2008; ISRN, 2013).

Implementation science is important to improvement in that it assess ways to link evidence into practice; it adds to our understanding of the effectiveness of strategies to "adopt and integrate evidence-based health interventions and change practice patterns within specific settings" (NIH, 2013). Together, improvement and implementation science add to an increased emphasis on the *system* aspects of the care we deliver.

Patient Safety

Safety research is rapidly emerging as the nation's top priority in health care research. Although the epidemiology of errors receives much attention, investigating the prevalence of adverse events is hindered by the prevalent culture of blame. This culture squelches adequate reporting of adverse events and prevents health care providers from making adverse events visible for further analysis and correction of causes of unsafe care.

Enhancing patient safety in health care includes three complementary actions: (1) preventing adverse events, (2) making adverse events visible, and (3) mitigating the effects of adverse events when they occur (World Health Organization [WHO], 2005). These three actions have stimulated development of theories to guide safety and the testing of those theories to produce safety science.

Safety science in health care is relatively new. *To Err Is Human* (IOM, 2000) raised awareness of the hazards associated with health care, identifying errors as the eighth leading cause of death in the United States. Safety science was well established in other industries, such as the airlines and the gas industries. Such high-risk industries are inherently dangerous and have developed safety management systems that nurture a culture of safety, thereby reducing errors and risks for errors. Safety practices established in these high-risk industries are now being adapted and tested in health care.

As in any new field of science, key concepts must be defined, theories generated to guide investigations, and new methods employed to study the topic. Likewise, theories and models with which to frame the investigation must be developed and tested.

An *adverse event* is defined as an untoward and usually unanticipated outcome that occurs in association with health care. *Patient safety* has been defined by AHRQ as the freedom from accidental injuries during the course of medical care and encompasses actions taken to avoid, prevent, or correct adverse outcomes that may result from the delivery of health care.

Reason (2000) advanced one of the most widely used theories on human error, one that has been used extensively in high-risk industries and cited in IOM reports. In Reason's model, human error is recognized as being inevitable. Reason identified two ways to view human error: the person approach and the system approach. The person approach has been the longstanding tradition in health care, which focuses on individual providers, blaming providers for forgetfulness, inattention, or moral weakness. The system approach holds as its basic premise that humans are fallible and errors are to be expected. The theory suggests that, to avert or mitigate errors, interventions must focus on conditions under which individuals work and must build defenses against error (Reason, 2000).

It is the management of errors and risks that becomes everyone's priority in a safety organization. Organizations that have fewer accidents than normal as a result of a change in organizational culture are high-reliability organizations.

Safety Cultures

A culture of safety has emerged as a crucial element in providing safe patient care. A culture shares norms, values, and practices associated with a nation, organization, or profession. The model of cultural maturity (Westrum, 2004) explains stages in the evolution of a safety culture. These stages progress from a pathological stage where safety is a problem of the worker; the business is the main driver and the goal is to avoid being caught by regulators. Reactive cultures take action only after an error occurs. In a calculative culture, safety is driven by management, which collects much data and imposes safety on the worker. In a proactive culture, workforce involvement begins to move away from the top-down approach, focusing instead on improving performance where the unexpected is a challenge. The final evolutionary stage of an organizational culture is the generative stage, where everyone participates in safety because all workers understand that safety is an inherent part of the business.

Safety Models in Nursing

There are four safety models that are seen as an integral part of the culture of safety. These models are Reason's Swiss Cheese Model of System Accidents; Helmreich's Threat and Error Management (TEM) Model for Medicine, which was developed from aviation's Crew Resource Management (CRM); Marx's Just Culture; and CASs.

The Swiss Cheese Model of System Accidents describes high-technology systems that have many defensive layers; when holes in these defenses momentarily line up, the opportunity for accidents occurs. The hole in any one defensive layer does not normally cause a bad outcome. There are two reasons that holes occur in the defensive layers: active failures and latent conditions. An active failure is an unsafe act committed by people who are in direct contact with the system. Latent conditions arise from decisions made by designers, builders, procedure writers, and management. Latent conditions may lie dormant in a system for years until they combine with active failures and local triggers create an accident opportunity (Reason, 2000). Human-error research in nursing has been valuable in examining barriers to safety in a neonatal intensive care unit (Jirapaet, Jirapaet, & Sopajaree, 2006).

Threat and error management (TEM) was developed to analyze adverse events, define training needs for medical personnel, and define organizational strategies to recognize and manage threat and error

(Helmreich, 2000). Threats are factors that can increase the likelihood of an error being committed. In this model, threats are either latent or overt and serve as settings or overarching variables that increase the potential for error to occur. Latent threats are aspects of the hospital or medical organization that are not always easily identifiable but that predispose it to the commission of errors or the emergence of overt threats; examples are failure to maintain equipment and high nurse–patient staffing ratios. Overt threats include environmental factors such as poor lighting and excessive noise, individual factors such as fatigue, team- and staff-related factors such as poor communication, and patient-related factors such as low acuity level. For example, Pape (2003) significantly reduced nursing distractions during medication administration by having staff use protocols from high-risk industries (Pape, 2003).

Marx's Just Culture describes four behavioral concepts (evils) that are necessary to the comprehension of the interrelationship between discipline and patient safety: human error, negligent conduct, knowing violation of rules, and reckless conduct (Marx, 2001). Human errors are the mistakes, slips, and lapses that occur in our everyday behaviors. *Negligence* is a legal term used when a person has been harmed by a failure to provide reasonable and safe care in a manner consistent with that of other prudent health care workers. Intentional rule violations occur when an individual knowingly works around policy and procedures while performing a task or skill. Reckless conduct is the conscious disregard of obvious and significant risk; it differs from negligence in that negligence involves a failure to recognize the risk. The purpose of a Just Culture is to promote nonpunitive reporting of errors, either anonymously or confidentially, without eliminating individual or organizational responsibility.

The most prominent theory in complexity science is the CAS theory. CASs are collections of different agents, individuals, or groups that interact with other groups and with their environment in a way that allows them to learn and act in ways that are not always predictable. These systems are dynamic and evolve over time. CASs encompass individual, interdisciplinary, and system facets of quality and safety. Characteristics of CASs are their ability to self-organize, the emergence of new patterns from nonlinear interactions, and their co-evolution as the agent and the environment mutually transform in response to the interactions (Stroebel et al., 2005). The complexity of the health care system has been a challenge to those trying to adapt safety models of other high-risk industries. Usually, in other high-risk industries, the individuals involved in the fatal error die themselves, unlike in health care, where the health care worker is not directly harmed by the actions or the error. A CAS helps researchers understand the complexity of the work of the clinician (Ebright, Patterson, Chalko, & Render, 2003; Ebright, Urden, Patterson, & Chalko, 2004).

Risk Management Models

Incident reports are the primary method for data collection on errors. Other high-risk industries have criticized health care for not having a standardized method of investigation, documentation, and dissemination of information on medication errors. Studies have been conducted on failures within the incident reporting system. The current incident reporting system is voluntary. The present rate of medical errors underestimates the full scope of the problem because of the incomplete reporting in the medical field. Studies have shown that nurses use the incident report system more frequently than physicians and other health care workers, which results in nurses appearing to commit a disproportionate number of medication errors.

Root cause analysis (RCA) is a retrospective approach to error analysis that has been widely used in high-risk industries. The Joint Commission mandated the use of the multidisciplinary RCA in 1997 to investigate sentinel events in hospitals. RCAs are uncontrolled case studies (qualitative approach) that predominantly use Reason's taxonomy of error to uncover the latent errors that underlie a sentinel event. The majority of RCAs reported were on serious adverse events that resulted in patient death. Limitations of the RCA are the hindsight bias of the investigators and the voluntary nature of reporting. The Joint Commission suggests that hospitals underreport incidents because they fear being put on probationary status and because of the legal implications of the disclosure of a sentinel event. Nursing researchers have used RCA to change current nursing practice in the transport of sick newborns in an effort to improve patient outcomes (Mordue, 2005).

Most errors that affect patient safety occur at the microsystem level within a hospital macrosystem. For example, as part of an effort to increase error reporting and to capture Reason's active failures, *near miss* or *close call* (errors that do not reach the patient) incident reporting has improved with the Good Catch Pilot Program at M. D. Anderson Cancer Center (AHRQ, 2008a). Three strategies were employed to improve reporting of close-call errors. First, the terminology for a potential error was changed to *good catch*. Second, an end-of-shift safety report was implemented that gave nurses an opportunity to identify and discuss patient safety concerns that had come up during the shift. Third, awards and other patient safety incentives were sponsored by executive leadership to recognize the efforts of individual nurses to improve patient safety. For example, in one hospital, scores based on the anonymous reporting by individual nurses on the various units were kept at the unit level. Buy-in by the upper level of nursing management was instrumental in promoting open discussions about patient safety and the distribution of "Good Catch" pins to unit team members. At 9 weeks, more than 800 potential errors were reported, and at 6 months that number had increased to 2,744, which represents an increase of 1,468% in the reporting of potential errors. Changes that occurred as a result of the Good Catch program were highlighted in a weekly nursing newsletter as a source of feedback to employees (Mick, Wood, & Massey, 2007).

The IHI failure modes and effects analysis (FMEA) tool has been adapted from high-risk industries outside health care. Its purpose is to assess risks of failures and harm within a system and to identify the most important areas for improvement. This process is conducted with a multidisciplinary team approach that identifies any and all possible failure modes and causes; assigns risk priority numbers to these failures; and then plans, implements, and evaluates interventions to reduce potential failures. The FMEA tool is available online (http://www.ihi.org/IHI/Topics/PatientSafety/SafetyGeneral/Tools/Failure+Modes+and+Effects+Analysis+%28FMEA%29+Tool+%28IHI+Tool%29.htm) through IHI, which also offers online monitoring and tracking of the FMEA tool (http://www.ihi.org/ihi/workspace/tools/fmea).

Instruments, Tools, and Resources for Measuring Patient Safety

There are various approaches to quantifying variables important in patient safety research. Through methodological research designs, scientists have developed and estimated psychometric qualities (reliability and validity) of a number of such instruments. The following describes several important instruments used in quality and safety research, including Hospital Survey on Patient Safety Culture (AHRQ, 2004). Some of the surveys have been adapted from other high-risk industries, as was the Safety Attitudes Questionnaire (SAQ). The SAQ was developed in partnership with AHRQ. The Practice Environment Scale of the Nursing Work Index (PES-NWI) was developed specifically to address issues relevant to nursing in Magnet hospitals (Lake, 2002).

A valuable instrument for assessing the system context for safety is the Hospital Survey on Patient Safety Culture (AHRQ, 2004). This widely used survey gathers data about staff opinions regarding patient safety issues, medical error, and event reporting. It provides hospitals with basic knowledge necessary to assess safety culture and to help them evaluate how well they have established a culture of safety in their institution. In addition, benchmarking based on data voluntarily provided by other, similar hospitals can be accomplished (AHRQ, 2008b). The highly reliable 42-item questionnaire measures 12 domains: openness of communication, feedback and communication of errors, frequency of events, handoffs and transitions, management support, nonpunitive response to error, organizational learning, overall perceptions of patient safety, staffing, manager expectations, actions that promote patient safety, teamwork across units, and teamwork within units.

The SAQ was adapted from the Flight Management Attitudes Questionnaire (FMAQ), which has been used in aviation worldwide. Six attitudinal domains that have been identified as necessary components of a safety culture are measured in the SAQ: teamwork climate, job satisfaction, perceptions of management, safety climate, working conditions, and stress recognition (Sexton et al., 2006).

The PES-NWI was developed to measure five subscale domains of the hospital nursing practice environment. Two of the subscales measure the hospitalwide environment: Nurse Participation Hospital Affairs and Nursing Foundations for Quality of Care. The other three subscales are more unit specific: Nurse Manager Ability, Leadership, and Support; Staffing and Resource Adequacy; and Collegial Nurse–Physician Relations. The PES-NWI is a component of the National Quality Forum list (NQF, 2007).

From a microsystem level, the performance of the care team is critical in safeguarding patient safety. Communication failures have been shown to be the leading cause of sentinel events, including preventable patient deaths, accounting for up to 80% of adverse events (AHRQ, 2008c). The evidence-based program, Team Strategies and Tools to Enhance Performance and Patient Safety (TeamSTEPPS®), is rooted in more than 20 years of evidence from human factor research and is a powerful solution to improving patient safety through team performance (AHRQ, 2008c).

THE FUTURE OF QUALITY IMPROVEMENT AND SAFETY RESEARCH

Research in health care quality improvement and safety is evolving at an unprecedented speed. As health care is redesigned, providers, administrators, and policymakers look to scientists to develop and evaluate sound approaches. In response, scientists are developing and evolving new research designs, theories, and measurement approaches. Top priorities for health care organizations include providing high-quality and safe patient care. The quality and patient safety movement is accelerating in health care organizations, and progress is evident (Buerhaus, 2007).

Key national quality reports have been a major impetus for health care improvements in quality and safety. The Institute of Medicine (IOM) report *Crossing the Quality Chasm: A New Health System for the 21st Century* (IOM, 2001) identified the need for fundamental change in the U.S. health care system. The redesign of the health care system involves providing health care that is safe, timely, effective, efficient, equitable, and patient centered. In addition, the IOM's *Health Professions Education: A Bridge to Quality* (2003b) was another key report that identified five core competencies needed by health care professions to provide quality care in the 21st century. The essential five core competencies identified were (1) providing patient-centered care, (2) working in multidisciplinary teams, (3) using EBP, (4) applying quality improvement, and (5) using informatics.

National agencies such as the AHRQ, The Joint Commission, and the IHI have been instrumental in setting initiatives designed to advance quality and safety in the health care arena. The AHRQ's 14 Evidence-Based Practice Centers (EPCs) and the AHRQ's Translating Research Into Practice (TRIP) initiatives are important resources that assist in translating evidence-based research into clinical practice promoting quality and patient safety in health care. In addition, the AHRQ Health Care Innovations Exchange project is an exciting new program created to support health care professionals in sharing and adopting innovations that improve the quality of health care. The AHRQ Health Care Innovations Exchange website provides resources and guidance to assist health care organizations in stimulating innovations and promoting quality and safety (AHRQ, 2008a). Summary snapshots of innovations provide vital information such as the description of the innovation, the results, the evidence rating, factors regarding the planning and development process, resources used and skills needed, and adoption considerations related to getting started with the innovation and, more important, sustaining the innovation (AHRQ, 2008a).

The IHI's 100,000 Lives and 5 Million Lives campaigns are outstanding examples of how national initiatives can improve quality and safety and incorporate evidence-based knowledge into clinical practice. The 100,000 Lives campaign focused on six interventions to reduce morbidity and mortality. The six interventions were (1) deployment of rapid response teams, (2) improvement of care of patients with acute myocardial infarction by delivering reliable evidence-based care, (3) prevention of adverse drug events through medication reconciliation, (4) prevention of central line infections, (5) prevention of surgical site infections, and (6) prevention of ventilator-associated pneumonia. This initiative involved the participation of 3,100 hospitals and saved an estimated 122,000 lives in 18 months (IHI, 2008).

IHI expanded the quality and safety focus with the 5 Million Lives campaign to address the issue of protecting patients from 5 million incidents of medical harm between December 2006 and December 2008. The 5 Million Lives campaign continues with the six interventions in the 100,000 Lives campaign, in addition to six new interventions targeted on harm: (1) preventing harm from high-alert medications (i.e., anticoagulants, sedatives, narcotics, and insulin); (2) reducing surgical complications; (3) preventing pressure ulcers; (4) reducing methicillin-resistant *Staphylococcus aureus* (MRSA) infection; (5) delivering reliable, evidence-based care for congestive heart failure; and (6) defining the roles of hospital boards of directors in promoting and sustaining a culture of safety. Frequent new initiatives introduced by IHI are adding greatly to the nation's quality movement.

The Joint Commission is another national agency that focuses on improving quality and safety of health care. The Joint Commission's annual National Patient Safety Goals are reviewed by health care organizations to ensure that their clinical practices are addressing these quality and safety areas. In addition, The Joint Commission's Patient Safety Practices is an online resource providing more than 800 links that health care professionals can use to address patient safety issues (The Joint Commission, 2008). These goals have stimulated many innovative interventions, the impact of which is evaluated using research approaches.

QUALITY INDICATORS, MEASURES, AND REPORTING

Performance measures are necessary to determine the impact of ongoing quality improvement efforts. Such efforts require that specific quality indicators be identified and measurement approaches validated through research. In the recent past, a number of health care entities have responded to the need for such indicators by developing consensus on indicators that should be tracked and by launching annual quality reports from national surveys. These efforts are reflected in the work of the AHRQ and the National Quality Forum (NQF). Other groups have undertaken efforts to create nursing-sensitive quality indicators reflected in the following sources: National Database of Nursing Quality Indicators (NDNQI), Veterans Affairs Nursing Sensitive Outcomes Database, Military Nursing Outcomes Database, and California Nursing Outcomes Coalition Database.

These groups note that many barriers to the widespread adoption of consensus standards exist and that overcoming them will require significant resources. Despite progress in quality improvement, challenges remain. These include inadequately developed measures, lack of standardization of performance measures and quality indicators, the need to refine measures, misalignment of measures of outcomes and baseline measures, and the burdens of data collection.

AHRQ NATIONAL HEALTHCARE QUALITY REPORTS

Since 2003, AHRQ has reported on progress and opportunities for improving health care quality. One of the key functions of the AHRQ *National Healthcare Quality Report* (NHQR) is to track the nation's progress in providing safe health care. For 8 years, the reports have presented a snapshot of the safety of health care provided to the American people. NHQR surveys the health care system through quality indicators, such as the percentage of heart attack patients who receive recommended care when they reach the hospital or the percentage of children who receive recommended vaccinations. In all, 218 measures are used, categorized across four dimensions of quality—effectiveness, patient safety, timeliness, and patient centeredness (AHRQ, 2012).

As a result of such research efforts in improvement science, a clearer picture of health care safety is beginning to emerge. The 2011 report assessed the state of health care quality using core report measures that represent the most important and scientifically credible measures of quality for the nation (AHRQ, 2012). The report shows that, 5 years after the first NHQR and 7 years after the IOM's landmark publication *To Err Is Human* (2000), it is still difficult to document progress, although more information on patient safety is now available. The report reflects slow progress in improvements in quality and safety. Between 2000 and 2011, patient safety improved at an annual rate of only 2.3% a year. The report identifies four themes:

- Health care quality and access are suboptimal, especially for minority and low-income groups.
- Quality is improving; access and disparities are not improving.
- Urgent attention is warranted to ensure continued improvements in quality and progress on reducing disparities with respect to certain services, geographic areas, and populations, including:
  - Diabetes care and adverse events
  - Disparities in cancer screening and access to care
  - States in the South
- Progress is uneven with respect to national priorities identified in the National Quality Strategy and the Disparities Action Plan.

Variation in quality of care is decreasing, but not for all measures, and although the safety of health care has improved since 2000, more needs to be done (AHRQ, 2012).

QUALITY INDICATORS: THE NATIONAL QUALITY FORUM

The NQF is a nonprofit organization with diverse stakeholder membership from the public and private health sectors, including consumers, health care professionals, providers, health plans, public and private purchasers, researchers, and quality improvement organizations. Established in 1999, the NQF seeks to implement a national strategy for health care quality measurement and reporting. The NQF mission includes improving health care by "setting national goals for performance improvement, endorsing national consensus standards for measuring and publicly reporting on performance, and promoting the attainment of national goals through education and outreach programs" (NQF, 2013).

Since the formation of the NQF, health care quality has become a major public policy issue. The diverse NQF stakeholders agreed on standards by which the health care industry would be measured, and data on these measures are publicly reported. Together with the other forces in effect, the NQF has fostered public reporting of performance. Such reporting, once a rare event, is becoming the norm. NQF-endorsed voluntary consensus standards are widely viewed as the "gold standard" for the measurement of health care quality.

SELECTED NURSING PERFORMANCE QUALITY INDICATORS

Because of the sheer number of nurses and the frequency of contact with patients, nurses have a major impact on patient safety and health care outcomes (NQF, 2007a). Research points to the influence of nursing on patient outcomes (e.g., IOM, 2004); however, only recently have advances in building a platform for public reporting reflecting nursing-sensitive performance measures been made.

National Quality Forum 15

The NQF endorsed a set of 15 consensus-based nursing-sensitive standards. These uniform metrics will increase understanding of nurses' influence on inpatient hospital care and advance internal quality improvement. The measures are recommended to evaluate the impact that nurses in acute care settings have on patient safety, health care quality, and professional work environment (NQF, 2007a).

Definition
Nursing-Sensitive Performance Measures

Nursing-sensitive performance measures are processes and outcomes—and structural proxies for these processes and outcomes (e.g., skill mix, nurse staffing hours)—that are affected, provided, and/or influenced by nursing personnel—but for which nursing is not exclusively responsible. Nursing-sensitive measures must be quantifiably influenced by nursing personnel, but the relationship is not necessarily causal. (NQF, 2007a)

The "NQF-15" includes measures from three perspectives: patient-centered outcome measures, nursing-centered intervention measures, and system-centered measures. The NQF-15 is expected to grow as nursing research continues to advance other measurement and reporting initiatives (NQF, 2007a).

NQF undertook a 15-month study to better understand the adoption of NQF-15 and to identify the successes, challenges, and technical barriers experienced by those implementing the measure. In 2006 and 2007, interviews were conducted with critical leaders, hospital representatives, quality organization leaders, and representatives of implementation initiatives. Interview data were augmented with a web-based survey. Content and descriptive analyses led to recommendations to accelerate adoption of the NQF-15. The 10 recommendations focus on aligning the NQF-15 with priorities, advancing science, improving regulatory and reporting requirements, fostering adoption of the standard through education, holding nurses accountable for public reporting, and creating a business case for nursing quality measurement (NQF, 2007b). The NQF-15 measures were drawn largely from existing nursing performance measurement databases, including NDNQI, and from several other initiatives.

National Database of Nursing Quality Indicators

Another major quality and safety measurement effort is reflected in the NDNQI. The American Nurses Association developed the NDNQI in 1998. The NDNQI is designed to assist health care organizations in patient safety and quality improvement initiatives by supplying research-based national comparative data on nursing care and its impact on patient outcomes. The NDNQI reflects nursing-sensitive indicators related to the structure, process, and outcomes of nursing care. Structure of nursing care is reflected by the supply, skill level, and education and certification of nursing staff. Process indicators reflect nursing care aspects such as assessment, intervention, and RN job satisfaction. Outcome indicators reflect patient outcomes that are nursing sensitive; these improve with both greater quantity and greater quality of nursing care (e.g., pressure ulcers, falls, and IV infiltrations) (NDNQI, 2008).

KEY INITIATIVES IN FUTURE QUALITY AND SAFETY

A number of initiatives are proving to be the key in the forefront of quality and safety. These include additional IOM reports, the Magnet Recognition Program®, and the INQRI, each of which is described here.

The IOM report *Keeping Patients Safe: Transforming the Work Environment of Nurses* (2004) identified mandates for quality and safety. The report emphasized a call for change for health care organizations, federal government, state boards of nursing, educational institutions, professional organizations, labor organizations, and professional nurses and urged them to take an active role in improving quality and safety in health care. This report identified essential patient safeguards in the work environment of nurses, calling for (1) governing boards that focus on safety, (2) leadership and evidence-based management structures and processes, (3) effective nursing leadership, (4) adequate staffing, (5) organizational support for ongoing learning and decision support, (6) mechanisms promoting multidisciplinary collaboration, (7) work designs promoting safety, and (8) organizational culture that enhances patient safety. Additional research addressing patient safety is necessary in the following areas: information on nurse's work, including on how nurses divide their time among various activities; information on nursing-related errors; safer nursing work processes and workspace design; standardized measurements of patient acuity; and safe nursing staff levels on various nursing units (IOM, 2004).

Magnet Recognition Program

The Magnet Recognition Program developed by the American Nurses Credentialing Center has been a driving factor urging nursing to develop a research agenda focused on evidence-based practice, quality, and safety. The Magnet Recognition Program was developed to recognize health care organizations that provide nursing excellence and to provide a channel for spreading successful nursing practices. Providing high-quality and safe patient care and integrating evidence-based knowledge into clinical practice are important components in achieving the esteemed Magnet Recognition certification (ANCC, 2008). The program has had a significant impact on quality and safety in nursing and in increasing the amount of attention paid to employing evidence-based practice and conducting research.

Interdisciplinary Nursing Quality Research Initiative

Robert Wood Johnson Foundation is a leading funder of research on nursing quality care. The primary goal of the INQRI was to "generate, disseminate and translate research to understand how nurses contribute to and can improve the quality of patient care" (RWJF, 2008). The program of research began to fill the gap in what is known about nurses' effect on quality and on keeping patients safer and healthier. Forty interdisciplinary research teams examined nurses' practices, processes, and work environments to determine the impact that nurses have on the quality of patient care. The ultimate goal is to support research to reduce health care errors and improve patient care. These studies comprised the first large-scale effort to identify the ways in which nurses can improve the quality of patient care and the contributions that nurses make to keep patients safer (INQRI, 2013). Lessons learned from this program have paved the way for future work in nursing quality research.

SUMMARY

Patient safety and the national effort to ensure that health care systems provide quality and safe care will continue to be top priorities for health care professionals. Nurses are essential in creating and sustaining a culture of safety, translating evidence-based research into clinical practice in health care, and creating the science of safety and quality to improve the quality of health care and maximize positive health outcomes.

SUGGESTED ACTIVITIES

1. Explore the AHRQ Health Care Innovations Exchange. Search and locate the profile of an innovation of interest. Review the section "Did It Work," and analyze the approach to evaluating the impact of the innovation. How was the resulting evidence rated? What does the rating mean?
2. Search a bibliographic database such as CINAHL. Locate a research study using "complex adaptive systems" or chaos theory as a framework. List the primary variables in the investigation. Relate the results to quality and/or safety in health care.

ACKNOWLEDGMENTS

The author is grateful for the contributions of Katherine McDuffie and Paula C. Clutter to the original chapter.

REFERENCES

Agency for Healthcare Research and Quality (AHRQ). (2004, November 10). *New AHRQ survey helps hospitals measure and improve patient safety culture* [Press Release]. Retrieved from http://archive.ahrq.gov/news/press/pr2004/hospcult2pr.htm

AHRQ. (2008a). *AHRQ health care innovations exchange.* Retrieved June 2008, from http://www.innovations.ahrq.gov

AHRQ. (2008b). *Patient safety culture surveys.* Retrieved April 26, 2009, from http://www.ahrq.gov/professionals/quality-patient-safety/patientsafety culture/hospital

AHRQ. (2008c). *TeamSTEPPS national implementation project.* Available from http://teamstepps.ahrq.gov/ (Accessed March 7, 2013).

AHRQ. (2012). *2011 National healthcare quality report.* Available from http://www.ahrq.gov/research/findings/nhqrdr/nhqr11/index.html (Accessed March 1, 2013).

American Nurses Credentialing Center (ANCC). (2008). *Magnet recognition program.* Retrieved June 2, 2008, from http://www.nursecredentialing.org/Magnet.aspx

Berwick, D. M. (2008). The science of improvement. *Journal of the American Medical Association, 299*(10), 1182–1184.

Buerhaus, P. (2007). Is hospital patient care becoming safer? A conversation with Lucian Leape. *Health Affairs, 26*(6), w687–w696.

Cronenwett, L., Sherwood, G., Barnsteiner, J., Disch, J., Johnson, J., Mitchell, P., … Warren, J. (2007). Quality and safety education for nurses. *Nursing Outlook, 55*(3), 122–131.

Ebright, P. R., Patterson, E. S., Chalko, B. A., & Render, M. L. (2003). Understanding the complexity of registered nurse work in acute care settings. *Journal of Nursing Administration, 33*(12), 630–638.

Ebright, P. R., Urden, L., Patterson, E., & Chalko, B. (2004). Themes surrounding novice nurse near-miss and adverse-event situations. *Journal of Nursing Administration, 34*(1), 531–538.

Funk, S. G., Champagne, M. T., Wiese, R. A., & Tornquist, E. M. (1990). BARRIERS: The barriers research utilization scale. *Applied Nursing Research, 4*(1), 39–45.

Funk, S. G., Tornquist, E. M., & Champagne, M. T. (1989). Application and evaluation of the dissemination model. *Western Journal of Nursing Research, 11*(4), 486–491.

Glasziou, P., & Haynes, B. (2005). The paths from research to improved health outcomes. *ACP Journal Club, 142*(2)(Suppl.), A-8–A-10.

Helmreich, R. L. (2000). On error management: Lessons from aviation. *British Medical Journal, 320*(7237), 781–785.

Improvement Science Research Network (ISRN). (2013). *What is improvement science?* Retrieved from http://www.isrn.net/about/improvement_science.asp (Accessed March 7, 2013).

Institute for Healthcare Improvement (IHI). (2008). *About us.* Retrieved April 2, 2008, from http://www.ihi.org/ihi/about

Institute of Medicine (IOM). (1990). *Clinical practice guidelines: Directions for a new program.* In M. J. Field & K. N. Lohr (Eds.). Washington, DC: National Academies Press.

IOM. (2000). *To err is human: Building a safer health system.* In L. T. Kohn, J. M. Corrigan, & M. S. Donaldson (Eds.). Washington, DC: National Academies Press.

IOM. (2001). *Crossing the quality chasm: A new health system for the 21st century.* Washington, DC: National Academies Press.

IOM. (2003a). *Priority areas for national action: Transforming health care quality.* Washington DC: National Academies Press.

IOM. (2003b). *Health professions education: A bridge to quality.* In A. Greiner & E. Knebel (Eds.). Washington, DC: National Academies Press.

IOM. (2004). *Keeping patients safe: Transforming the work environment of nurses.* In A. Page (Ed.). Washington, DC: National Academies Press. Retrieved from http://www.iom.edu/?id=19376

IOM. (2008). *Knowing what works: A Roadmap for the nation.* In J. Eden, B. Wheatley, B. L. McNeil, & H. Sox (Eds.). Washington, DC: National Academies Press.

IOM. (2011). *The future of nursing: Leading change, advancing health* (prepared by Robert Wood Johnson Foundation Committee Initiative on the Future of Nursing). Washington, DC: National Academies Press.

Interdisciplinary Nursing Quality Research Initiative (INQRI). (2013). *Program overview.* Available from http://www.inqri.org/ (Retrieved March 1, 2013).

Jirapaet, V., Jirapaet, K., & Sopajaree, C. (2006). The nurses' experience of barriers to safe practice in the neonatal intensive care unit in Thailand. *JOGNN: Journal of Obstetric, Gynecologic, & Neonatal Nursing, 35*(6), 746.

Joint Commission. (2008). *National patient safety goals.* Retrieved June 7, 2008, from http://www.jointcommission.org/patientsafety/nationalpatient safetygoals/

Lake, E. T. (2002, June). Development of the practice environment of the Nursing Work Index. *Research in Nursing & Health, 25*(3), 176–188.

Marx, D. (Ed.). (2001). *Patient safety and the "Just Culture": A primer for health care executives.* New York, NY: Trustees of Columbia University.

Melnyk, B. M., Fineout-Overholt, E., Gallagher-Ford, L., & Kaplan, L. (2012). The state of evidence-based practice in US nurses: Critical implications for nurse leaders and educators. *Journal of Nursing Administration, 42*(9), 410–417.

Mick, J. M., Wood, G. L., & Massey, R. L. (2007). The Good Catch pilot program. *Journal of Nursing Administration, 37*(11), 499–503.

Mordue, B. C. (2005). A case report of the transport of an infant with a tension pneumo-pericardium. *Advances in Neonatal Care, 5*(4), 190–200.

Mulrow, C. D. (1994). Systematic reviews: Rationale for systematic reviews. *British Medical Journal, 30*(6954), 597–599.

National Dataset of Nursing Quality Indicators (NDNQI). (2008). Retrieved March 20, 2013, from www.nursingquality.org

National Institutes of Health (NIH). (2013). *Dissemination and implementation research in health.* PAR 10-038. Available from http://grants.nih.gov/grants/guide/pa-files/PAR-10-038.html (Accessed February 12, 2013).

National Quality Forum (NQF). (2007a). *Nursing voluntary consensus standards for nursing-sensitive care: An initial performance measure set.* Washington DC: National Quality Forum. Retrieved March 14, 2013, from http://www.qualityforum.org/Project_Details.aspx?id=1139

NQF. (2007b). *Tracking NQF-endorsed consensus standards for nursing sensitive care: A 15-month study.* Washington DC: National Quality Forum. Retrieved March 7, 2013, from http://www.qualityforum.org

NQF. (2008). *National Quality Forum endorses National Consensus Standards promoting accountability and public reporting.* Retrieved March 7, 2013, from http://www.qualityforum.org/news/releases/080508-endorsed-measures.asp

NQF. (2013). *Mission and vision.* Retrieved March 7, 2013, from http://www.qualityforum.org/About_NQF/Mission_and_Vision.aspx

Pape, T. M. (2003). Applying airline safety practices to medication administration. *Med-surg Nursing, 12*(2), 77–94.

Reason, J. (2000). Human error: Models and management. *British Medical Journal, 320*, 768–770.

RWJF Interprofessional Nursing Quality Research Initiative. Available at http://www.inqri.org/about-inqri/program-overview. Accessed June 20, 2013.

Sackett, D. L., Straus, S. E., Richardson, W. S., Rosenberg, W., & Haynes, R. B. (2000). *Evidence-based medicine: How to practice and teach EBM* (2nd ed.). Edinburgh: Churchill Livingstone.

Sexton, J. B., Helmreich, R. L., Neilands, T. B., Rowan, K., Vella, K., Boyden, J., Roberts, P. R., & Thomas, E. J. (2006). The safety attitudes questionnaire: Psychometric properties, benchmarking data, and emerging research. *BMC Health Services Research, 3,* 6.

Stetler, C. B. (1994). Refinement of the Stetler/Marrram model for application of research findings to practice. *Nursing Outlook, 42*(1), 15–25.

Stevens, K. R. (2004, October). *ACE star model of knowledge transformation: Utility in practice and education.* Proceedings of the NIH State of the Science Conference.

Stevens, K. R. (2009). *Essential competencies for evidence-based practice in nursing* (2nd ed.). San Antonio, TX: Academic Center for Evidence-Based Practice (ACE), University of Texas Health Science Center.

Stroebel, C. K., McDaniel, R. R., Crabtree, B. F., Miller, W. L., Nutting, P. A., & Stange, K. C. (2005). How complexity science can inform a reflective process for improvement in primary care practices. *Journal on Quality and Patient Safety, 31*(8), 438–446.

Titler, M. G., Kleiber, C., Steelman, V. J., Rakel, B. A., Budreau, G., Everett, L. Q., ... Goode, C. J. (2001). The Iowa model of evidence-based practice to promote quality care. *Critical Care Nursing Clinics of North America, 13,* 497–509.

Westrum, R. (2004). A typology of organizational cultures. *Quality and Safety in Health Care, 13*(2), ii22–ii27.

Woolf, S. H. (2004). Patient safety is not enough: Targeting quality improvements to optimize the health of the population. *Annals of Internal Medicine, 140,* 33–36.

World Health Organization (WHO). (2005). *WHO draft guidelines for adverse event reporting and learning systems.* Geneva, Switzerland : WHO Document Production Services.

4

Establishing and Sustaining an Evidence-Based Practice Environment

Elizabeth A. Carlson and Beth A. Staffileno

There are numerous reasons to establish an evidence-based practice (EBP) program for nursing staff. First, patients have complex care needs coupled with shortened lengths of stay and an increase in new therapies. Nurses must deliver care that is based on evidence of its effectiveness, safety, and currency. An EBP program is a proven way to move nursing care toward these desired outcomes (Barrett, 2011; Geotz, 2011; Wurmser, 2009). In addition, use of EBP methods empowers the nurses to address questions and problems they encounter in a systematic manner. Not only does it improve patient care, but allows for dissemination both internally and to the broader nursing community.

Second, many organizations understand the positive influence that results from seeking accreditation. Ensuring that the processes and structure are in place to move toward positive outcomes allows an organization to establish, confirm, and codify goals and behaviors that result in exemplary practice. One such designation is the Magnet Recognition Program® awarded by American Nurses Credentialing Center (ANCC). Magnet-Recognized organizations have "strong leadership, empowered professionals and exemplary practice" as their "essential building blocks." EBP not only contributes to exemplary practice but empowers nurses to provide strong leadership (http://www.nursecredentialing.org /MagnetModel.aspx). The use of EBP and the supports and structures needed to improve practice and contribute to the profession results in an organization that values these contributions and those who make them.

Third, the American Nurses Association (ANA) Standard 9: Evidence-Based Practice and Research (2010) states that evidence-based practice is a core competency for professional nurses. The ANA (2010, p. 51) states that "evidence-based nursing knowledge, including research findings, guide practice" and that evidence needs to be incorporated when initiating changes in practice.

Fourth, in 2001, the report, *Crossing the Quality Chasm: A New Health System for the 21st Century,* presented the need to improve the health care delivery system by providing safe, effective, patient-centered, timely, efficient, and equitable care. One of the components of this needed redesign of health care was the use of "evidence-based decision making" (p. 8). Coupled with the 2001 report is the Institute of Medicine's (IOM) report of 2011, *The Future of Nursing,* which stated that nursing is the key to improving health care. Three of the four key messages pertain to EBP. The first, that nurses should practice to the full extent of their education and training, which includes the knowledge and skills needed to practice evidence-based care. Second, that nurses should attain higher levels of education and training, addresses not only the world of academe but also the need for organizations to continually educate their staff. The third message, that nurses should be full partners in redesigning health care, again supports the need for nurses to be fluent in evidence-based approaches to problems.

As a result, changes have occurred in both nursing education and nursing clinical practice. In academia, two key changes in educational preparation at the entry into practice level are evolving. At the baccalaureate level, the expectation of preparation for EBP is apparent as indicated by AACN's Essential III: Scholarship for Evidence-Based Practice. "Baccalaureate education provides a basic understanding of how evidence is developed, including the research process, clinical judgment, interprofessional perspectives, and patient preference as applied to practice" (http://www.aacn .nche.edu/education-resources/BaccEssentials08.pdf). Thus, nursing programs have incorporated EBP into their curriculum as they focus on educating the student to use national standards based on evidence (Newhouse, 2006).

In addition, a new certification, clinical nurse leader (CNL), has at its core the knowledge and ability to oversee the care coordination for a group of patients and provide direct patient care. As stated by AACN, "this master's degree–prepared clinician puts evidence-based practice into action to ensure that patients benefit from the latest innovations in care delivery" (http://www.aacn.nche.edu/cnl/CNLFactSheet.pdf). As more nursing programs offer this curriculum, organizations will have CNLs as staff members.

These key changes in the education of new graduates just entering practice affect where they look for their first job as a nurse. Newhouse (2006) states the importance of new nurses working in an environment "that is evidence enhanced" (p. 441) for the benefit this type of environment offers to their professional development. This results in new graduates having the expectation that the organizations at which they seek employment will incorporate an EBP approach to the delivery of care and would support their practice and leadership through an EBP approach.

As a consequence of this organizational expectation, new graduates will expect the staff with whom they work to be conversant with and use EBP in their patient-care approaches. With the emphasis on EBP for recent graduates and their expectations of the EBP approach being used in organizations, it is critical that all members of the nursing staff who have not had the opportunity to learn the EBP approach during their educational programs, obtain the necessary knowledge and skills. As the emphasis on teamwork and interprofessional approaches to care increases, it is important that a common approach to patient care delivery is used. It is therefore incumbent upon the nurse leader to set the EBP vision for the organization.

INFRASTRUCTURE

Setting the Vision

Evidence-based practice will not be successful unless it is clear that this is a priority of the organization and, most critically, the chief nursing officer (CNO). The CNO must be the EBP champion for the organization. As with any program that is implemented, for EBP to be successful, it must be part of the nursing vision for the organization. A strong and ongoing EBP program takes time to establish and integrate into the culture of how nursing functions. Without strong and visible support from leadership, use of EBP and incorporation of the principles into the thought process of the nursing staff will not occur. The concept of continual inquiry and seeking to provide care that has been shown to result in improved patient outcomes must be interwoven into the structure and language of the organization for EBP to be successful. In addition, as indicated, the ANA (2010) states that EBP is a core competency for professional nurses. Therefore, the use of EBP is not optional. The CNO must actively lead the organization to using an evidence-based approach to patient care.

An EBP program requires additional support from executive leadership throughout the organization. Merely including EBP as a goal is not sufficient for success. EBP needs to be a high priority in the nursing strategic plan and embedded into the organization's strategic plan. Hauck, Winsett, and Kuric (2013) assessed the impact of leadership facilitation strategies on the establishment of EBP in an organization. One of their findings was that transformational leadership was required to drive organizational change. Leadership provides vision, resources, and facilitation. A transformational leader establishes the vision, sells the vision, provides the way forward, and leads others toward that vision (Marshall, 2011). For example, the CNO must develop the case for the institutional acceptance, endorsement, and funding of an EBP program.

Prior to presenting the need for and benefits of EBP for inclusion in the organizational strategic plan, the CNO must get others on board with the vision. The creation of support requires a multipronged approach and work at both the organizational executive level and the care delivers' level is necessary. Not only does the organizational executive leadership's support need to be cultivated but nursing leadership and influential staff nurses need to be on board as well. Information and literature demonstrating the benefits of EBP must be discussed and provided to these key individuals. Multiple and disparate methods of communicating the benefits of EBP are required such as newsletters, town hall meetings, discussions with nursing staff, informational boards either electronic or paper, as well as cultivating the support and encouragement of any grassroots interest.

Having organizational executive support alone will not guarantee success, nor will strong nursing support alone result in success. Without the support of those who determine the strategic goals and what programs are funded, those who must enable the staff members to participate, and support from the caregivers who will be the ones implementing EBP, success is not ensured. All three legs to the stool need to be in place: (1) the CNO needs to establish the expectation, (2) the organizational executive leadership needs to support the use of resources for EBP, and (3) the staff needs to see this as integral to how they practice nursing and not as a discrete action divorced from their professional practice. The CNO needs to present a logical and comprehensive assessment of the risk-to-benefit ratio resulting from care based on evidence. The benefits to the organization and thus to the key decision makers must be presented and discussed. Concerns voiced during these discussions need to be considered and addressed. Organizational concerns may include the cost of the program, including needed personnel, support services, time away from patient care while learning, and any potential risks. Nursing leadership concerns may parallel these concerns and include issues of costs to the unit budgets, coverage for caregivers when in educational sessions, impact on staffing, seasoned staff responses, and the addition of "one more thing" to the nurses' workload. Influential nursing staff may voice concerns about obsolescence of their skills; impact on workload; expectations of accomplishment without support to be successful; and the impact on the evaluation, reward, and compensation systems. The CNO needs to be prepared to listen and address these concerns and offer mitigating solutions.

Subsequent to creating support for EBP and the costs and requirements involved, the CNO needs to have EBP included as an organizational goal within the strategic plan. Funds are allocated based on organizational priorities and unless EBP is an organizational priority, funding may fall on nursing alone to provide or be nonexistent. Because EBP will not only improve nursing care but also patient outcomes, organizational support is the ideal. An EBP culture provides an opportunity for interdisciplinary dialogue and information exchange thus leading to collaborative patient care. Organizational benefits include higher quality patient care, which contributes to greater patient and family satisfaction as well as decreased length of hospital stay (Melnyk & Fineout-Overholt, 2005). Many CNOs recognize the need for an EBP facilitator, but face resistance in acquiring the financial resources needed to support such services. Given the quality and financial benefits to the entire organization, the organization needs to support an EBP program and position. It is not appropriate for a program that benefits the organization to be assumed to be the financial responsibility of nursing alone.

Loss of payments for hospital-acquired conditions (HACs) and proposed incentive pay for better outcomes should be a driving force to incorporate the EBP facilitator's role in health care settings as part of operational costs (Staffileno, Wideman, & Carlson, in press). Because the positive results of EBP have been shown to have impact, reducing the cost of falls (Oberman, Pawluk, Staffileno, & McCullum-Smith, 2011), use of indwelling catheters and urinary tract infections (Conklin, 2004), and hospital-acquired pressure ulcers (McInerney, 2008), which benefit the entire organization, a case can be made that the cost of implementing and maintaining EBP is an organizational one.

Necessary Resources

Establishing and implementing an EBP environment requires essential resources, such as personnel, time, money, and space (Cullen & Adams, 2012; Schulman 2008; Staffileno & Carlson, 2010). However, during times of cost containment, allocating these resources can be challenging and thereby may require creative and intentional planning (Beck & Staffileno, 2012). The benefits of EBP include: nursing care driven by evidence improves patient care and clinical outcomes, nursing satisfaction increases as nurses become more empowered and engage in clinical inquiry to drive excellence and quality care, and the organization experiences improvement in reimbursement as patients experience fewer complications resulting in reduced resource utilization (Geotz, 2011; Maljanian et al., 2002; Melnyk & Fineout-Overholt, 2005; Staffileno et al., in press). Despite the well-documented benefits of EBP, nurses continue to experience difficulty incorporating EBP into daily practice because of insufficient time, lack of administrative support and mentoring, resistance in changing practice, and lack of education on the EBP process (Barrett, 2011; Melnyk & Fineout-Overholt, 2012; Staffileno & McKinney, 2011).

Raising Awareness

Raising awareness and developing excitement about EBP often require a change in culture to move from tradition-based care to evidence-based care that is embraced by nurses at all levels of preparation. Several strategies can be implemented for building a foundation and stimulating enthusiasm for incorporating the EBP process. For instance, facilitating staff participation in EBP-related activities can be introduced through interactive sessions such as doing a version of the Great Cookie Experiment or conducting a mock trial. The original Great Cookie Experiment introduced concepts of the research process to nursing students by comparing two chocolate chip cookies (Hudson-Barr, Weeks, & Watters, 2002; Thiel, 1987). Student nurses gained insight into methodology, data collection, data analysis, and dissemination of research findings. Modifications of the Great Cookie Experiment have been done using other comparisons (such as hand sanitizer, lotions, breakfast bars, music, etc.) (Bennett, Raupers, Hicks, & Schoener, 2009; Hagle & Millenbruch, 2011; Morrison-Beedy & Cote-Arsenault, 2000; Sternberger, 2002) and with incorporating newer technology (Staffileno, Brown, & Kleinpell, 2012). Nurses can become engaged in the experiment using "real time" sequencing of events using online-survey software (i.e., SurveyMonkey) and data-management tools (i.e., Excel), or by using audience response systems that allow for greater interaction, immediate feedback, and anonymous participation (Cain & Robinson, 2008; Caldwell, 2007; Dangel & Wang, 2008; DeBourgh, 2008; Staffileno et al., 2012; Zurmehly & Leadingham, 2008).

Another interactive approach used to raise awareness about EBP is a mock trial. Mock trials have been used by other disciplines as an educational platform (Biddinger, 1999; Phillips et al., 2006; Staffileno & McKinney, 2010; Warden, Brockhopp, Alfred, & Holbrook, 1994; Werth, 2002) and more recently in nursing as a venue to highlight concepts of how to incorporate EBP into clinical practice. For example, a mock trial can engage nurses to use available evidence when making clinical practice decisions. A topic that is relevant to nurses housewide, such as moral distress or safe patient handling can be selected as a "case" to argue. To develop the pros and cons of the case, nurses gain experience reviewing literature, critiquing the evidence, and presenting an argument for or against the issue at hand. Thereby, nurses gain critical-thinking skills using a problem-solving, systematic method for addressing clinical practice issues.

Education

Building an EBP infrastructure begins with staff education, which requires adequate personnel. Education promotes awareness and enables nurses to become professionally literate and develop necessary skills to critically appraise evidence prior to implementing findings into their practice. A doctoral-prepared or advanced practice nurse can serve as an EBP facilitator, whether employed by the organization or brought in as a consultant, and often has a dual appointment within a clinical and academic setting (Currey, Considine, & Khaw, 2011; Jamerson & Vermeersch, 2012; Staffileno & Carlson, 2010; Staffileno & McKinney, 2011). The EBP facilitator enables others to initiate, conduct, and integrate EBP projects into clinical practice. The EBP facilitator serves as an educator, mentor, and change agent within the organization by: (1) assessing the needs of nursing related to EBP, (2) raising awareness and developing excitement about EBP, (3) presenting EBP-related information and education in a way that is understandable and meaningful to direct-care nurses, (4) building confidence and empowering nurses to engage in EBP-related activities, (5) assisting nurses with interpreting unit-specific data trends and facilitating EBP initiatives, (6) networking within the community and facilitating interdisciplinary collaboration, (7) facilitating the development of EBP proposals and project implementation, and (8) facilitating policy changes with intended plans for dissemination. Table 4.1 outlines an action plan that an EBP facilitator may use when establishing a foundation for an EBP environment.

Depending on the needs of the organization, the EBP facilitator may assist with developing a formal EBP program that can be presented in one of two ways: (1) an EBP-condensed curriculum, or (2) an EBP fellowship training (Albert, 2008; Barret, 2011; Ingersoll, Witzel, Berry, & Qualls, 2010; Staffileno & Carlson, 2010; Staffileno & McKinney, 2011). The EBP-condensed curriculum provides EBP education using a systematic approach and well-defined objectives (Table 4.2). The condensed curriculum can be offered using face-to-face classroom, online module, or podcast instruction. The curriculum can be designed with weekly content to include: review of EBP concepts, how to find and evaluate available evidence, how to manage and interpret data, and how to apply evidence to practice changes. The EBP Training Fellowship offers a slightly different approach in that the program provides education and practical experiences. The EBP Fellowship provides an infrastructure for nurses, educators, and researchers to collaborate in promoting an evidence-based environment to improve the delivery of patient care. It offers nurses additional support and training that is needed for them to identify a clinical problem, develop a project proposal, and integrate an evidence-based practice change at the point of care. The scope of the EBP fellowship may vary depending on the organization, but can span 6 to 18 months. The key focus is to provide direct-care nurses with dedicated release time for education and facilitated time to implement an EBP change. Consistently, lack of time has been cited as a major barrier preventing nurses from implementing EBP in their daily practice (Fink, Thompson, & Bonnes, 2005; Hutchinson, 2006;

TABLE 4.1 EBP Action Plan

ACTIVITY	STRATEGY
1. EBP needs assessment	▪ Assess organizational readiness ▪ Conduct a survey to assess staff knowledge and current state of EBP within the organization* ▪ Conduct focus groups
2. Raising EBP awareness	▪ Gather an EBP team/committee and develop a campaign to market EBP culture ▪ Create a logo to be displayed throughout the hospital and used as a screen saver on computer terminals ▪ EBP team/committee review EBP models ▪ Display posters/flyers/billboard
3. Information and education	▪ Executive meetings ▪ Unit meetings ▪ Brown-bag sessions ▪ "How to" sessions (literature search, evaluating the evidence, critiquing research) ▪ E-mails/newsletters/announcements ▪ Journal clubs (e-journal clubs) ▪ Roving carts moving from unit to unit ▪ Offer continuing-education credit as educational programs
4. Building confidence	▪ Set goals that are realistic and attainable ▪ Create EBP decisional algorithm showing step-by-step process ▪ Train the trainer and identify champions ▪ Highlight accomplishments
5. Evaluating unit-specific data	▪ Review key metrics with unit manages and staff ▪ Identify monthly and quarterly triggers
6. Networking	▪ Develop relations with local colleges and/or universities ▪ Develop relations with health department, senior citizen groups, etc.
7. Implementing EBP	▪ Develop a template and EBP protocol ▪ Start with one EBP project to showcase the process and then build on it ▪ Facilitate EBP practice change and evaluate
8. Disseminating	▪ Assist with presenting EBP projects internally (establish an annual EBP day) and externally (local, regional, and national meetings) ▪ Assist with presenting educational programs

EBP, evidence-based practice.

*There are a few EBP assessment scales that can be used; Barriers: the barriers to research utilization scale (Funk, Champagne, Wiese, & Tornquist, 1991); Evidence-Based Practice Beliefs Scale (Melnyk & Fineout-Overholt, 2003); and Evidence-Based Practice Implementation Scale (Melnyk, 2003).

TABLE 4.2   Structured EBP Programs

	CONDENSED EBP CURRICULUM	EBP FELLOWSHIP TRAINING
Format	Face to face or online	Face to face
Length	~8 weeks	~12–18 months
Content	▪ EBP concepts ▪ Searching for evidence ▪ Evaluating evidence ▪ Managing/interpreting data ▪ Applying evidence at the point of care	▪ EBP concepts and practical experiences ▪ Identifying clinical questions ▪ Forming a team ▪ Proposal development ▪ Project implementation ▪ Dissemination and clinical practice changes
Continuing education	Awarded	Awarded
Outcome	▪ Ability to seek and critically evaluate evidence ▪ Incorporate EBP into delivery of patient care	▪ Conduct an EBP project ▪ Incorporate EBP project change to practice ▪ Serve as EBP role model

EBP, evidence-based practice.

Karkos & Peters, 2006; Majid et al., 2011; Melnyk et al., 2012; Pravikoff, Tanner, & Pierce, 2005). Therefore providing dedicated time for EBP training and implementation sends a clear message supporting the importance of an EBP environment. Dedicated release time can range from 4 to 16 hours per month and may vary with respect to organizational setting. Interestingly, emerging evidence shows successful patient and financial outcomes with dedicated Training Fellowship programs (Hinds, Gattuso, & Morrell, 2000; Staffileno & McKinney, 2011; Staffileno et al., in press; Turkel, Ferket, Reidinger, & Beatty, 2008; Turkel, Reidinger, Ferket, & Reno, 2005). Continuing-education certificates can be awarded as part of either of these EBP programs, which serves as incentive for nurses and demonstrates a professional development commitment on behalf of the organization.

Organizational Support

The success of an EBP environment requires organizationwide support involving personnel from various departments, such as executive leaders, nurse managers, Information Services (IS), Operational Development, and Professional Development. Identifying key personnel is necessary for developing and implementing an EBP environment (Table 4.3). For example, the CNO is needed to support the EBP vision and align strategic goals with the organization's mission. The CNO and other senior executives are needed to garner support and financing for

TABLE 4.3 Personnel Resources and Roles

Chief nursing officer	▪ Assess organizational need or gap analysis ▪ Identify core EBP team ▪ Set EBP vision to align with strategic plan ▪ Establish EBP council/committee ▪ Identify funding sources
Senior executives	▪ Support EBP infrastructure as part of the organization's mission ▪ Endorse EBP culture
Nurse managers	▪ Provide active endorsement and accountability ▪ Provide opportunities to learn about EBP and pose clinical questions ▪ Identify EBP champions ▪ Budget time and resources for creative EBP environment
Medical librarian	▪ Educate users on search methods ▪ Serve as resource ▪ Establish links to EBP websites, national guidelines, and specialty organizations ▪ Assist with searches
Information services	▪ Assist with implementing interactive educational sessions ▪ Coordinate with medical librarian to establish EBP links and resources on unit work stations for 24-hour access ▪ Update electronic health record with practice changes
Operational development	▪ Implement new technologies to support EBP projects ▪ Establish link to policy and procedures and mechanism for updating ▪ Provide data management and statistical support ▪ Establish a link to IRB education and processes
Professional development	▪ Offer EBP education and human subject training ▪ Include EBP exemplars as part of performance appraisal and clinical ladder ▪ Incorporate annual EBP competencies and skill appraisal ▪ Incorporate evidence-based standards into policy and procedures ▪ Review current practices and establish an audit and feedback system ▪ Develop database to track and share housewide EBP projects, including ongoing and completed ▪ Develop database posting conferences and call for abstracts

EBP, evidence-based practice; IRB, Institutional Review Board.

an EBP environment. Although initially creating an EBP infrastructure may require upfront expenditures for the organization, fostering an EBP environment increases patient safety and ultimately minimizes cost. The resultant EBP model of care helps improve the financial status of the organization by enhancing patient safety, improving patient outcomes and care efficiencies, and reducing the cost of care (Geotz, Janney, & Ramsey, 2011). Other key personnel resources needed include: (1) nurse managers to implement the EBP culture, support staff for EBP education, release time, and practice changes; (2) medical librarian to assist with literature searches and using research databases, and identifying web-based resources; (3) IS to assist with interactive sessions and technological distribution of EBP-blasts, blogs, e-logos, and update reminders; (4) Operational Development to assist with data management, statistical applications, updates in practice in electronic health record, and coordination with the Investigation Review Board process; and (5) Professional Development to integrate EBP skills and competencies, patient-care changes related to EBP project outcomes, documentation, and policy changes.

Time, money, and space are additional resources necessary for successfully establishing an EBP environment. As noted previously, lack of time is a common and major barrier for nurses adopting EBP principles (Melnyk, 2012). Time is a commodity needed in all aspects of establishing an EBP environment. For example, time is needed by executive leaders to start the EBP transformation and identifying key stakeholders. Time is needed for mentoring, and nurses need time allocated for EBP training, integration, and evaluation. Nurse managers need to dedicate release time for nurses to attend educational sessions and for nurses to effectively implement EBP projects. There is a trickle-down time effect involving personnel whether it is the medical librarian providing instruction on doing a literature review, Professional Development staff providing EBP competency skills, or Operational Development staff assisting with data monitoring.

Money is another commodity necessary for establishing an EBP infrastructure and aligns hand in hand with personnel and time. However, many organizations are faced with limited resources, which pose challenges, especially for those nursing leaders interested in implementing EBP but who must do so while staying budget neutral. Frequently the Division of Nursing underwrites the cost for initiating the EBP initiative; there is evidence showing a return on investment for the organization through adopting results/changes from nurse-driven evidence-based projects (Geotz et al., 2011; Ingersoll et al., 2010; Staffileno, Wideman, & Carlson, 2013; Wurmser, 2009). As evidence for the financial benefits of an EBP environment increases, the CNO will have greater leverage to demonstrate why this is an organizationwide cost. Additionally, the CNO may consider alternative financial resources through both internal and external funding, such as identifying with foundation, philanthropic, community, or professionally related sponsorships. An ongoing process of EBP enables nurses' rapid adoption of scientific knowledge for the purpose of improving patient care. Moreover, using EBP standards in the delivery of care improves quality, increases health care value, and reduces costs (Geotz et al., 2011; Ingersoll et al., 2010; Wurmser, 2009).

Providing adequate space, both physical and virtual, is a necessary resource for an EBP environment. Classrooms and conference centers are needed to conduct education, seminars, and presentations, provide one-on-one consultation, and support other EBP initiatives. Access to a medical library via hardcopy or electronic resources should be available within the organization and/or at the unit level. Nurses should have a designated area to store EBP-related supplies, toolkits, and equipment that may be associated with an EBP project.

Interweaving EBP Into the Organization's Structure and Culture for Sustainability

Implementing EBP into the organization is a beginning step of fully embedding the process into the environment. Sustaining EBP requires not only continuation of initial personnel and resources, as noted in Table 4.3, but additional efforts and approaches are needed (Table 4.4).

The key to sustainability and integration into the organization's culture is the demonstration of clinical and financial successes resulting from EBP. Therefore, evaluation of the outcomes must be a primary component of any EBP project. Improvement in nurse-sensitive indicators, report card indicators, and cost savings is a way to demonstrate

TABLE 4.4   Elements for EBP Sustainability

EBP outcomes	▓ Maintain a database of EBP projects ▓ Track EBP outcomes and trend results ▓ Showcase projects and distribute clinical outcomes ▓ Public recognition
Reward and compensation	▓ Annual competencies and performance evaluation ▓ Merit improvements ▓ Individual and unit acknowledgments
Policy and procedures	▓ Update policy and procedures and track all EBP revisions
Interprofessional engagement	▓ Include health care members from various domains (physicians, pharmacists, physical and respiratory therapists, etc.)
Continuation of support and resources	▓ Regularly evaluate EBP implementation strategies and resources (as noted in Table 4.3) ▓ Maintain momentum

EBP, evidence-based practice.

success. Nursing-initiated projects incorporating research and/or EBP processes can produce favorable outcomes for the organization (such as interventions to minimize the occurrence of pressure ulcers, which lead to decreased length of stay for patients or safe patient handling to reduce falls).

Leadership includes incorporating EBP into the reward or compensation system. If use of EBP is not one of the aspects on which staff are evaluated, it will be seen by the staff as an add-on versus an integral aspect of how they practice nursing. In leading organizations (Murphy, Hinch, Llewellyn, Dillon, & Carlson, 2011), use of EBP in the care of the patient is an expectation for promotion via a clinical ladder system. Behaviors are incorporated into the pertinent aspects of professional practice that are expected by the organization from its nursing staff. This links the rewards to the expectations and to the professional competencies. Documentation of how the nurse used an evidence-based-structured approach to problem solving and care given is required. Having EBP as one of the criteria on which a nurse is evaluated clearly sends the message that the organization values this approach and rewards employees who incorporate this behavior into their work.

Another leadership approach to incorporating, and thus sustaining, the use of EBP in the organization's way of doing business is to insist that both new and revised policies and procedures use EBP approaches as the underlying and determinant rationale. Because policy and procedures are the basis for how the care is delivered, or what the organizational standard is, having the policies and procedures based on evidence not only reinforces to the nursing staff that this is the expected approach to care and problem solving, but it also strengthens the policy and procedure. Because many policy and procedure committees are interprofessional, taking this approach also offers the benefit of demonstrating to all staff the benefits of EBP, thus increasing the likelihood that the organization will continue to use this approach and support it.

SUMMARY

Leadership, starting with the CNO, is essential for implementing and sustaining an EBP environment. Not only must the CNO provide leadership within nursing's domain, but engagement of the entire executive team is warranted as the accrued benefits of an EBP environment impacts the organization overall. Numerous resources and processes are required to implement and sustain a strong EBP infrastructure, and the deployment of these resources is an organizational responsibility. Continued efforts to: (1) minimize barriers that impede clinical inquiry, (2) implement strategies to enhance nurses' EBP knowledge and skills, (3) implement evidence-based project changes, and (4) acknowledge and reward EBP successes will generate enthusiasm and maintain momentum for a sturdy EBP environment.

REFERENCES

Albert, N. M., & Siedlecki, S. L. (2008). Developing and implementing a nursing research team in a clinical setting. *Journal of Nursing Administration, 38*(2),90-96.

American Nurses Association (ANA). (2010). *Nursing scope and standards of practice* (2nd ed.). Silver Spring, MD: Nursesbooks.org

Barrett, R. (2011). Strategies for promoting the scientific integrity of nursing research in clinical settings. *Journal for Nurses in Staff Development, 26*(5), 200–205.

Beck, M., & Staffileno, B. A. (2012). Implementing evidence-based practice during an economic downturn. *Journal of Nursing Administration, 42*(7/8), 350–352.

Bennett, S., Raupers, D., Hicks, M., & Schoener, L. (2009). One hospital's 'peanutty' path to magnet designation. *American Nurse Today, 4*(8), 59–60.

Biddinger, L. (1999). A mock trial at nursing grand rounds. *Journal for Nurses in Staff Development, 15*(3), 111–115.

Cain, J., & Robinson, E. (2008). A primer on audience response systems: Current applications and future considerations. *American Journal of Pharmaceutical Education, 72*(4), 1–6.

Caldwell, J. E. (2007). Clickers in the large classroom: Current research and best-practice tips. *CBE-Life Science Education, 6,* 9–20.

Conklin, S. A. (2004). Collaborative practice model reduces indwelling urinary catheter use and risk for nosocomial urinary tract infections. *Worldviews on Evidence-Based Nursing, 1*(4), 232–242.

Cullen, L., & Adams, S. L. (2012). Planning for implementation of evidence-based practice. *Journal of Nursing Administration, 42*(4), 222–230.

Currey, J., Considine, J., & Khaw, D. (2011). Clinical nurse research consultant: A clinical and academic role to advance practice and the discipline of nursing. *Journal of Advanced Nursing, 67*(10), 2275–2283.

Dangel, H. L., & Wang, C. X. (2008). Student response systems in higher education: Moving beyond linear teaching and surface learning. *Journal of Educational Technology Development and Exchange, 1*(1), 93–104.

DeBourgh, G. A. (2008). Use of classroom 'clickers' to promote acquisition of advanced reasoning skills. *Nursing Education Practice, 8,* 76–87.

Fink, R., Thompson, C. J., & Bonnes, D. (2005). Overcoming barriers and promoting the use of research in practice. *Journal of Nursing Administration, 35*(3), 121–129.

Funk, S. G., Champagne, M. T., Wiese, R. A., & Tornquist, E. M. (1991). Barriers: The barriers to research utilization scale. *Applied Nursing Research, 4*(1), 39–45.

Geotz, K., Janney, M., & Ramsey. (2011). When nursing takes ownership of financial outcomes: Achieving exceptional financial performance through leadership, strategy and education. *Nursing Economics, 29*(4), 173–182.

Hagle, M. E., & Millenbruch, J. L. (2011). Retooling the great American cookie experiment for nursing grand grounds. *Clinical Nurse Specialist, 25*(5), 220–223. doi: 10.1097/NUR.0b013e3182299606

Hauck, S., Winsett R. P. & Kuric J. (2013). Leadership facilitation strategies to establish evidence-based practice in an acute hospital. *Journal of Advanced Nursing.* Mar;69(3):664-74. doi: 10.1111/j.1365-2648.2012.06053.x. Epub June 15, 2012.

Hinds, P. S., Gattuso, J., & Morrell, A. (2000). Creating a hospital-based nursing research fellowship program for staff nurses. *Journal of Nursing Administration, 30*(6), 317–24.

Hudson-Barr, D., Kenney Weeks, S., & Watters, C. (2002). Introducing the staff nurse to nursing research through the great American cookie experiment. *Journal of Nursing Administration, 32*(9), 440–443.

Hutchinson, A. M., & Johnston, L. (2006). Beyond the BARRIERS scale. Commonly reported barriers to research use. *Journal of Nursing Administration, 36*(4), 189–199.

Ingersoll, G. L., Witzel, P. A., Berry, C., & Qualls, B. (2010). Meeting Magnet research and evidence-based practice expectations through hospital-based research centers. *Nursing Economics, 8*(4), 226–235.

Jamerson, P. A., & Vermeersch, P. (2012). The role of the nurse research facilitator in building research capacity in the clinical setting. *Journal of Nursing Administration, 42*(1), 21–27.

Karkos, B., & Peters, K. (2006). A Magnet community hospital. Fewer barriers to nursing research utilization. *Journal of Nursing Administration, 36*(7/8), 377–382.

Maijanian, R., Caramanica, L., Taylor, S. K., MacRae, J. B., & Beland, D. K. (2002). Evidence-based nursing practice, Part 2: Building skills through research roundtables. *Journal of Nursing Administration, 32*(2), 85–90.

Majid, S., Foo, S., Luyt, B., Zhang, X., Theng, Y. L., Chang, Y. K., & Mokhtar, I. A. (2011). Adopting evidence-based practice in clinical decision making: nurses' perceptions, knowledge, and barrier. *Journal of the Medical Library Association, 99*(3), 229–236.

Marshall, M. (2011). *Transformational leadership in nursing: From expert clinician to influential leader.* New York, NY: Springer Publishing Company.

McInerney, J. (2008). Reducing hospital-acquired pressure ulcer prevalence through a focused prevention program. *Advances in Skin & Wound Care, 21*(2), 75–78.

Melnyk, B. M., & Fineout-Overholt, E. (2003). *Evidence-based practice implementation scale.* Gilbert, AZ: ARCC LLC Publications.

Melnyk, B. M., & Fineout-Overholt, E. (2005). *Evidence-based practice in nursing and healthcare.* Philadelphia, PA: Lippincott Williams & Wilkins.

Melnyk, B. M., & Fineout-Overholt, E., Gallagher-Ford, L., & Kaplan, L. (2012). The state of evidence-based practice in U.S. nurses. Critical implications for nurse leaders and educators. *Journal of Nursing Administration, 42*(9), 410–417.

Morrison-Beedy, D., & Cote-Arsenault, D. (2000). The cookie experiment revisited: Broadened dimensions for teaching nursing research. *Nurse Educator, 25*(6), 294–296.

Murphy, M., Hinch, B., Llewellyn, J., Dillon. P. J., & Carlson, E. (2011). Promoting professional nursing practice: Linking a professional practice model to performance expectations. *NCNA, 46*(1), 67–79.

Newhouse, R. (2006). Examining the support for evidence-based nursing practice. *Journal of Nursing Administration, 36*(7/8), 337–340.

Oberman, K., Pawluk, H. S., Staffileno, B. A., & McCullum-Smith, D. (2011). Safe fall prevention program: How well did we do? 2011 National Teaching Institute Research Abstracts. *American Journal of Critical Care, 20*, e48–e66.

Phillips, J. M., Heitschmidt, M., Joyce, M. B., Staneva, I., Zamansky, P., Francisco, M. A., . . . Kranzer, S. F. (2006). Where's the evidence? An innovative approach to teaching staff about evidence-based practice. *Journal for Nurses in Staff Development, 22*(6), 296–301.

Pravikoff, D. S., Tanner, A. B., & Pierce, S. T. (2005). Readiness of U.S. nurses for evidence-based practice. *American Journal of Nursing, 105*(9), 40–51.

Schulman, C. S. (2008). Strategies for starting a successful evidence-based practice program. *AACN Advanced Critical Care, 19*(3), 301–311.

Staffileno B. A. & Mckinney C. (2010) Utilizing a mock trial todemonstrate evidence-based nursing practice – a staff development process. *Journal for Nurses in Staff Development, 26*(2), 73–76.

Staffileno, B. A., Brown, F. M., & Kleinpell, R. (2012). Promoting nursing research: It's just a click away. *Journal for Nurses in Staff Development, 28*(3), 143–145

Staffileno, B. A., & Carlson, E. (2010). Providing direct care nurses research and evidence-based practice information, an essential component of nursing leadership. *Journal of Nursing Management, 18,* 84–89. http://www.mdlinx.com/nurselinx/news-article.cfm/2942001

Staffileno, B. A., & McKinney, C. (2011). Getting 'research rich' at a community hospital. *Nursing Management, 42*(6), 10–14.

Staffileno, B. A., Wideman, M., & Carlson, E. (2013). The financial and clinical benefits of a hospital-based PhD nurse researcher. *Nursing Economics, 31*(4), 194–197.

Sternberger, C. (2002). Research strategies. The great music experiment: Taking the cookie experiment to the Web. *Nurse Educator, 27*(3), 106–108.

Thiel, C. A. (1987). The cookie experiment: A creative teaching strategy. *Nurse Educator, 12*(3), 8–10.

Turkel, M. C., Ferket, K., Reidinger, G., & Beatty, D. E. (2008). Building a nursing research fellowship in a community hospital. *Nursing Economics, 26*(1), 26–34.

Turkel, M. C., Reidinger, G., Ferket, K., & Reno, K. (2005). An essential component of the magnet journey. Fostering an environment for evidence-based practice and nursing research. *Nursing Administration Quarterly, 29*(3), 254–262.

Warden, S., Brockhopp, D. Y., Alfred, M., & Holbrook, P. (1994). The effect of a mock trial on nursing students' ability to make clinically sound legal judgments. *Nurse Educator, 19*(3), 18–22.

Werth, J., Harvey, J., McNamara, R., Svoboda, A., Gulbrandson, R., Hendren, J., . . . Leybold, C. (2002). Using controversial mock trials in "psychology and law" courses: Suggestions from participants. *Teaching Psychology, 29*(1), 20–24.

Wurmser, T. (2009, February). The financial case for EBP. *Nursing Management,* pp. 12–14.

Zurmehly, J., & Leadingham, C. (2008). Exploring student response systems in nursing education. *CIN: Computers, Informatics, Nursing, 26*(5), 265–270.

PART II

Building Blocks for Evidence

5

Appraising a Single Research Article

Mary Schira

Whether one is reading a research article for translation of findings into evidence-based practice or as a building block for a proposed study, the process begins with a single research article. Advanced practice nurses frequently read the data-based literature to answer questions related to diagnosis, therapeutic interventions, and prognosis of individual patients (Facchiano & Snyder, 2012). One of the barriers, noted by individuals to translating research findings (and therefore providing evidence-based care) into practice is a lack of confidence in their ability to read and interpret research findings. The critical-thinking skills nurses use in practice every day provide a foundation for developing the skill of reading and evaluating research.

Reading and evaluating data-based literature is a critical skill in translating research into clinical practice. Previous chapters have addressed how to locate the research literature and ensure that once the literature is located, it can be retrieved; chapters that follow provide additional details regarding elements of a research study and the article in which the results are published. The purpose of this chapter is to review the sections of a single research article and to provide an organized approach to reading and interpreting the strength and relevance of the information presented in the data-based article.

The critical appraisal of a data-based article determines the strengths, weaknesses, and usefulness of the findings. The goal of the appraisal is to evaluate the quality and clinical relevance of the evidence for use in practice (Facchiano & Snyder, 2012) or for additional research. As a result, understanding the components of a data-based article and important questions to consider while reading each section is needed.

Research articles are written with a similar organization. Components of a research article include the abstract, background, and significance of the study, methods, data analysis, findings and results, discussion, and implications for practice. The logic of the researcher's thinking should be clear enough so that the reader has few questions about how and why the study was conducted. By the end of the article, the reader should be able to determine how the research results fit into current knowledge and how (or whether) the findings translate to the practice environment for implementation or further testing and validation. As the reader progresses through the report, each section builds on the previous information. Table 5.1 provides a summary of key elements to consider as the reader appraises a research article and may be helpful as a guide or checklist in reading the literature.

Appraisal guides and tools are also available online to assist in critically appraising the data-based literature. Two such online resources are Critically Appraised Tool (CAT)maker and BestBETs. CATmaker is a software tool available through the Center for Evidence-Based Medicine (http://www.cebm.net). CATmaker guides the reader through determining the key information in the study and assessing the validity and usefulness of the research. The guides are formatted in appraisal sheets with questions that relate to types of studies (e.g., questions related to appraising diagnostic study-related research differ from those appraising therapy-related research). At the end of the guided process, a summary is created that the reader may store, retrieve, share, and continue to update as additional research on the same topic is appraised.

BestBETs (http://bestbets.org/links/BET-CA-worksheets.php) uses a slightly different approach from CATmaker but also provides appraisal tools targeted at the type of study. Like CATmaker, questions are provided so that the reader focuses on and evaluates key aspects of the study. Readers have an option to submit their appraisal of a study to the CA database and can review appraisals that have been submitted in a specific topic area. Both BestBETs and CATmaker have numerous other resources to assist in reading and translating the data-based literature into practice and are strong resources for further reading and guidance in the research-appraisal process.

THE ABSTRACT

The first part of a research article is the abstract. The abstract is a brief, targeted summary of the full article that follows. The targeted summary provides the reader initial information about the study to evaluate whether the study is of interest or applies to the reader's practice setting or population (DiCecco, 2007). Most readers use the abstract as a screen to determine whether or not to read the entire research article.

Table 5.1 Evaluating a Single Research Article—Questions to Consider

Problem Statement/Purpose

What was studied? What variables were measured (independent and dependent)?

Does the purpose (or research question) clearly address the problem?

Literature Review

Is the literature current? Relevant?

Is the research literature summarized and evaluated?

Are gaps in the literature noted?

How likely is it that the current study will close the gaps in current knowledge?

Design

What is the overall design of the study? Quantitative or qualitative?

Is the design a good match with the problem statement or purpose of the study?

Method

Ethics—How was the protection of human subjects ensured?

Sample—How was the sample identified? Do the subjects have characteristics that can answer the research question?

Instruments—What instruments were used? Were they reliable? Valid?

Study Procedure

Was the procedure realistic?

If an independent variable was manipulated, was it done consistently?

How were instruments/tools administered? In what environment? Was the environment consistent?

Over how much time were data collected?

Data Analysis

How were data analyzed?

Were statistical tests used appropriately?

If the research is a qualitative study, how were themes and meaning elicited?

Findings/Results

What were the outcomes of the study?

Were all aspects of the problem statement/purpose addressed?

How do the findings fit with previous research? Support or not support?

Discussion

What conclusions did the researcher draw from the findings?

Do the findings make sense, relate to the problem?

How do the findings compare with other research findings in the literature?

Can the results be generalized to other populations? Settings?

What limitations are noted? How will limitations affect generalizability of the findings?

Implications

Are implications for practice and research noted?

Do the implications flow directly from the findings?

BACKGROUND AND SIGNIFICANCE

The beginning of a research report provides an overview of and a context for the research. The aim of the first few paragraphs is to provide the reader with an understanding of the background of the study, why the study was conducted, and why the study was important (significance). The reader should be able to identify gaps in current knowledge, and how the study proposed to fill the gaps should specifically be addressed. Near the end of the section (or set apart), the purpose or problem statement of the study is also presented. Both or only one may be included in a published report, as they are closely related. The purpose or problem statement should be clearly stated and provide the variables (independent and dependent) studied. The author may also include research questions, hypotheses tested in the study, or both. In any case, the reader will know the population (who) and the phenomenon (what) that were studied. The reader can use the information to assess the rest of the report.

LITERATURE REVIEW

In some cases, the background section includes a review of the literature. In other articles, the literature review is set apart as a separate section in the article. The review of the literature should be appraised for both content and relevance. The literature presented should be relevant to the study, relate to the variables that were studied, and be current. The literature review often includes both theoretical and data-based sources. The previous research studies included in the discussion should at the minimum address the purpose, sample, design, and findings and a brief critique of the study's strengths and weaknesses (Burns & Grove, 2011). Another approach in reporting the research literature is to present a synthesis of numerous studies and an overall evaluation of the body of knowledge. Whichever approach is used, the reader should have an understanding of the current knowledge and how the study plans to address gaps in knowledge or expand current knowledge to a different population or practice setting. The existing research literature included in the review may be directly or indirectly related to the purpose of the study. Indirectly related studies should be linked for relevance.

The reader should specifically check the dates of the literature cited in the article's literature review and reference list and judge whether or not it is (at least reasonably) current. Although some studies are considered classics, much of the cited literature should be recent and reflect up-to-date thinking and understanding of the study's focus. This is especially important in practice areas undergoing rapid change (e.g., genetics and genomics) and in areas that are time sensitive (e.g., attitudes and opinions). The reader's personal knowledge and level of expertise in the content area are valuable in determining the currency and strength of the literature review included in the research report.

METHOD

A large section of the research report is the method section, which describes how the study was conducted. The method section includes design, sample, instruments, and specific procedures for data collection (Russell, 2005). The method section is a critical part of a research article and deserves careful attention. While reading the method section, the reader should be alert for any problems in the way the study protocol was implemented, such as sample bias, inconsistencies in data collection among subjects, loss of subjects, and weaknesses of the instruments or tools used to collect the data. The strength of the method section helps the reader determine the overall usefulness and generalizability of the results that will follow.

Design

The study design is identified early in the method section if it has not already been implied in the purpose or problem statement. The author should identify whether the study used a quantitative, qualitative, or *mixed-method* design. Quantitative studies use designs that result in numerical data that can be used in statistical (mathematical) analysis and assess the size of relationships among variables (DiCecco, 2007). Variables of interest in quantitative designs may be measured using physiologic instruments (e.g., blood pressure and weight), questionnaires with fixed responses (e.g., scale of 1 to 5), or variables that can be assigned a number (e.g., gender). Quantitative research designs may be further identified as experimental, quasi-experimental, or nonexperimental, depending on how subjects were chosen, whether and how study variables were manipulated, and how the data to measure the variables were collected.

Qualitative studies also identify a specific study approach but do not result in numbers for statistical analysis. The most common qualitative designs are ethnographic, phenomenological, historical, and grounded theory approaches. Just as in quantitative designs, there are specific and distinguishing elements among the qualitative designs. The goal of studies that use qualitative designs is to explore or explain the phenomenon of interest from the perspective of individuals experiencing the phenomenon. As a result, qualitative designs yield descriptions that can then be analyzed for themes, common elements, and shared meaning among subjects (Vishorevsky & Beanlands, 2004). The end result of a qualitative design may be new knowledge or the beginning of a theory, whereas the end result of a quantitative study is often acceptance or rejection of current knowledge or theory.

In some instances, the study design may include both qualitative and quantitative elements, resulting in a mixed-method design. In such a design, the reader should evaluate whether the design was appropriately used and followed in gathering the specific data. The specific qualitative and quantitative design aspects must be compatible. For example, sample size in a mixed-method study may be a challenge. Quantitative and qualitative design approaches can differ greatly, with quantitative designs often seeking large sample sizes and random selection or assignment to treatment groups whereas some qualitative designs have small samples obtained from a narrowly recruited group of individuals.

The design of the study should be sufficiently detailed so that the reader can determine how the study was actually conducted. The timeline and sequence of the study procedures should be clear and concise so that the study can be replicated. Regardless of the overall research design, the key question for the reader to consider is how well the design used is likely to fulfill the purpose of the study and answer the research question.

Sample

The number of subjects who participated in the study (sample size) should be clearly stated and described in the article. Additional information in the article should describe how the sample size was determined. In a quantitative study, sample size is determined by completing a power analysis, a mathematical determination based on the researcher's desired level of statistical significance, estimates of variability, and effect size. In a pilot study, this detail is not included because a primary purpose of a pilot study is to obtain beginning information to justify and guide larger studies (Oliver & Mahon, 2006). In many qualitative studies, the researcher describes how it was determined that the (often small) sample size was sufficient to answer the research question.

The article should also provide details regarding specific inclusion and exclusion criteria for participants accepted as subjects. Careful attention to potential subjects excluded from the study will assist in determining whether findings may be translated to clinical practice. The reader should be especially alert for any apparent bias in selecting the sample and exclusions that can limit generalizability of the findings beyond the study's individual sample and/or setting. A description of potential subjects who were approached for inclusion but refused to participate should also be included to determine how closely the study population represents the population of interest as a whole.

The demographic characteristics of study participants (e.g., age and gender) are usually presented and help the reader evaluate to what degree the study sample is congruent with the reader's population of interest. Sample characteristics are also important in determining whether or not the study findings might be applicable for translation into practice. The more closely the sample matches the reader's population, the more likely the reader is to implement the findings into practice if all other criteria are met (no contradictory study results and other studies with similar results). In addition, the number of subjects and a brief description of subjects who did not complete the study or study procedures should be included so that the reader can make a judgment whether individuals who completed the study were different from those who did not complete the study, which is a potential source of bias called *attrition*.

In quantitative studies, random selection of subjects and random assignment of subjects to treatment groups are ideal but often difficult to accomplish because of the constraints that accompany research on human subjects in a clinical environment. As a result, a convenience sampling method that does not contain apparent selection bias is often appropriate and is strengthened when the design incorporates random assignment to treatment groups. The reader needs to make a judgment regarding bias in the sample and the appropriateness of the sampling plan in answering the problem.

Research Instruments and Data Collection Tools

Each research tool or instrument used in the study should be described in detail. The instruments should measure the variables of interest. If an existing tool or instrument was used (e.g., Depression Scale), the number of items and a brief description of what the tool measures should be described. Measures of reliability, the consistency of the tool or instrument, and validity, whether the tool actually measures the phenomenon under study, are important considerations and should be reported in the article. The choice of the specific tool used should be explained in the context of the study variables, previous research that used the tool(s), and any subject characteristics considered in choosing the tool (e.g., reading level and short administration time in a population likely to experience fatigue with a long tool). An advantage of using research instruments that have already been used is that reliability and validity data may already be established (Oliver & Mahon, 2006). If the researcher had developed a tool for the study, a full description of the instrument and a discussion of how reliability and validity were established should be included. Whether an existing research instrument was used or a tool was created for the study, a lack of information regarding reliability and validity leads to questions regarding whether or how well the variables in the study were actually measured.

Ethics

The method section should also include a short description of how ethical considerations in conducting the study were addressed. Alternatively, the protection of human subjects may be addressed as the first part of the description of the study procedure. In either case, a statement regarding review of the study by an institutional review or research ethics board prior to the beginning of the study is generally included. In addition, procedures for obtaining subjects' consent to participate in the study and how consent was obtained should be detailed. If the subjects were minors or were incompetent to provide informed consent personally, the author should fully describe consent procedures, mention whether any difficulties were encountered, and if difficulties were encountered, how they were managed.

Study Procedures

The procedure section provides a detailed description of how the study was conducted, including exactly how and when data were collected and under what conditions. The information should be clearly presented so that the reader could replicate the study by following the description. The reader should see a logical flow in the data collection process and consider any extraneous variables in the setting that may affect the data.

DATA ANALYSIS

By the time the reader comes to the data analysis section of the research article, he or she will know a great deal about the study. The reader has formed beginning opinions about the strength and potential usefulness of the study and is looking forward to reading the findings and results. The data analysis section begins with a description of how the data obtained from the research instruments were summarized and analyzed. The intent of this section is to tell the reader how the data were analyzed and is a straightforward presentation of information. In a qualitative study, the data analysis approach is described, including how themes or patterns were elicited from the data. In a quantitative report, the data are analyzed using statistical methods and tests. There are numerous statistical procedures and tests available. The key issue in evaluating the statistical analysis is to determine that the method used is appropriate for the research question and how the data were measured (Burns & Grove, 2011; DiCecco, 2007). For the novice reader, the data analysis section may be the most intimidating part of the research article. This discomfort is often due to limited exposure to and understanding of the statistical tests used and uncertainty about whether the appropriate test has been applied to the data. Resources that will aid the reader as skills develop include a basic statistics book and colleagues with an understanding of data analysis techniques. As with any skill, the more the reader gains in understanding, the easier reading the analysis section becomes.

FINDINGS AND RESULTS

For many, the most enjoyable section of a research article to read is the findings of the study. Each previous section has been laying the foundation for this part of the article. The findings tell the reader what the researcher discovered as a result of the data that were collected and analyzed. As the findings of a study are presented, whether a qualitative or quantitative design was used, the reader learns whether the research question was answered and how completely the question or problem statement was addressed. All results and data that address the research question or problem statement are included in a discussion of the findings. If the study was analyzed using statistical methods, the statistical significance of the results is noted. In the results section, the data and outcomes of statistical analysis are presented but generally not explained or discussed. The intent of the findings section is to present the factual outcome of data analysis, rather than explain the meaning of the data. Although this section may seem dry or unimaginative, the advantage of this approach is to allow the reader to make beginning judgments regarding the study outcomes in the absence of the opinion or interpretation of meaning from others. In addition to a narrative summary of the results, most articles present findings in a table for easier review.

Qualitative study findings, depending on the specific qualitative design used in the study, are presented quite differently from quantitative results. In a qualitative study, direct quotes or summaries of participant responses are often included in the results section or may be presented in a combined Results/Discussion section. The author may group the findings according to themes or patterns that became apparent during the data analysis. As a result, many qualitative studies provide data using a narrative approach and describe results in terms of richness and depth of the data.

Some readers prefer to read the results section immediately after reading the problem or purpose of the study. This may be due to curiosity about the outcome or to a wish to decide whether or not to read the entire article. The dedicated reader will then go back to the beginning of the article and read it entirely. There is nothing inherently wrong with reading the results out of sequence as long as the reader recalls that, in order to use the findings in practice or to build additional research studies, the previous sections of the article are critical in evaluating the strength of the findings. In addition, this approach may encourage a reader to fully read only those articles that report significance or that reinforce current ways of thinking. Studies that do not demonstrate statistical significance are often as revealing as those that do and encourage us to challenge existing perceptions. Finally, because the results section presents but does not discuss the findings, the reader may overlook studies with clinical (but not statistical) significance.

DISCUSSION

In the discussion section of an article, the author presents the conclusions he or she drew from the findings, acknowledges any limitations of the study, and suggests how findings may be generalized to individuals or groups beyond the study sample. In the discussion, a description of how the results fit into the current body of knowledge in general and previous research in specific should be presented. The author should compare and contrast the study findings with those of the previous research that was cited in the review of the literature presented earlier in the article. A critical comparison by the author demonstrates to the reader that the researcher evaluated the findings with an open mind.

CONCLUSIONS

The author's conclusions provide the researcher's interpretation of the study findings. In contrast to the factual presentation of the study outcomes in the findings section, the conclusions present the meaning of the results from the author's perspective. The conclusions drawn by the researcher should flow from the scope of the study and directly relate to the purpose of the study; they should be confined to the variables that were studied. The reader should evaluate the author's perspective as well as his or her own to determine whether the findings answer questions in the reader's clinical experience and/or provide information that explains phenomenon previously unexplained.

LIMITATIONS

The author's identification of the study's limitations recognizes that, although no study is perfect, results can make a contribution and provide valuable information for future researchers (Facchiano & Snyder, 2012; Oliver & Mahon, 2006). At the same time, limitations cannot be used as an excuse for a poor design or flawed study procedures. Among the limitations often cited in research reports are problems with data collection (e.g., unexpected intervening variable that occurred during data collection), small sample size, problems with how the sample was obtained (e.g., convenience sample), and limitations inherent in the study's research design (e.g., nonrandom assignment of subjects to groups). In most cases, the reader has already identified limitations and is not surprised by those noted by the author. The limitations will affect the reader's confidence in translating the findings into clinical practice.

GENERALIZABILITY

The generalizability of study findings is an essential evaluation of a study's outcome. Studies are conducted with subjects who have specific characteristics and in settings with unique environments. In addition, manipulation of the independent variable and measurement of the dependent variable may be done in more than one way, and researchers may use comparable research instruments or tools or very different ones. As a result, the meaning of the findings and how the findings may be implemented with other populations and in other settings must be addressed in the article. An understanding of the limitations of the study also affects generalizability. A study with numerous or key limitations results in findings that have minimal or narrow generalizability beyond the population or setting in the study. This is especially likely when bias is present in the sample. Bias may be a design flaw or may be unintentional and discovered during data analysis.

IMPLICATIONS

The final major aspect of a research article is its implications for practice and research. An important goal of research is to provide evidence to further explain phenomena, validate current thinking and practice, or change current practice and approaches. Depending on the purpose of the study, the strength of the study's design, and the statistical and clinical significance of findings, it is important for the author to suggest to the reader how the findings may actually be used. Implications may be noted for direct patient care practice, education, or the delivery of health care services. The implications should have direct links to the findings, be realistic, and be suggested within the limitations of the study as previously noted by the author. Again, the reader will critically evaluate the information presented and determine the extent to which the reader agrees or disagrees with the author's perspective.

Implications for future research are similarly important. Authors commonly cite a need for replication of the study, recognizing that changes in clinical practice are rarely made on the basis of a single study. In addition, the author should make suggestions for further studies that might expand understanding of the phenomenon or problem studied. In the case of an article based on a pilot study, the author should make specific recommendations for a larger study that may incorporate additional variables, change the study design, or revise or change the research tools.

SUMMARY

Reading a single research article is the first step in progressing down the path of translating evidence into practice, planning a research study, or both. Like most skills in nursing, comfort and proficiency in reading research studies increase with diligent practice. The critical-thinking skills that nurses use in clinical practice are the building blocks for critically evaluating each section of a research article.

SUGGESTED ACTIVITIES

Read two research articles—one quantitative and one qualitative—in your area of expertise or interest. Compare and contrast the two studies in the following areas.

1. Evaluate the method sections of the articles and note the following:

   ▪ What specific type of design did the research use?
   ▪ Does the design "match" the purpose of the study? Will the design provide the information to achieve the purpose or answer the problem stated?
   ▪ How was the sample obtained? Based on the specific quantitative/qualitative design of the study, was the sampling plan appropriate?
   ▪ In the quantitative study, were the reliability and the validity of the research instrument(s) described? In the qualitative study, how did the researcher record and organize the data?
   ▪ Were data obtained in the same manner from all subjects?

2. Evaluate how the data were analyzed.

   ▪ In the quantitative study, were the statistical tests appropriate to the type of data collected?
   ▪ In the qualitative study, were the data analyzed in a way consistent with the type of qualitative design?

3. In both studies, are conclusions consistent with the data? Are limitations identified?
4. How could the study's findings be used, in practice, to plan further research?

REFERENCES

Burns, N., & Grove, S. (2011). *Understanding nursing research: Building an evidence based practice* (5th ed.). Philadelphia, PA: Elsevier.

DiCecco, K. (2007). Medical literature. Part II: A primer on understanding scientific design. *Journal of Legal Nurse Consulting, 18*(2), 3–11.

Facchiano, L., & Snyder, C. (2012). Evidence-based practice for the busy nurse practitioner. Part III: Critical appraisal process. *Journal of the American Academy of Nurse Practitioners, 24,* 704–715.

Oliver, D., & Mahon, S. (2006). Reading a research article. Part III: The data collection instrument. *Clinical Journal of Oncology Nursing, 10,* 423–426.

Russell, C. (2005). Evaluating quantitative research reports. *Nephrology Nursing Journal, 32,* 61–64.

Vishnevsky, T., & Beanlands, H. (2004). Qualitative research. *Nephrology Nursing Journal, 31,* 234–238.

6

Identifying a Focus of Study

Lea Ann Matura and Vivian Nowazek

There are numerous sources of ideas for identifying the focus of an inquiry. The literature review presents what is currently known about the topic of interest and the gaps in the literature. Once a thorough search and evaluation of the available evidence have been conducted, the focus of the study can be defined in the form of a purpose, objectives, and specific aims, along with well-developed research questions. This chapter delineates the components needed to define a research topic. Examples are included to illustrate the concepts and to facilitate practice in critically evaluating material from an evidence-based perspective.

SOURCES OF TOPICS AND PROBLEMS

When a researcher is identifying a topic of inquiry, several sources can provide guidance in determining the question or problem to investigate. Some areas previously identified as starting points include clinical practice, continuous quality improvement, the research literature, professional organizations, and conferences (Mateo & Kirchhoff, 1999). Likewise, there are multiple examples from varying clinical settings or domains of health care where ideas may be generated: clinical problems or questions, the literature, regulatory agencies, new diagnoses, media coverage, sentinel events, and legislative issues are only a few possibilities, but, these examples may stimulate thoughtful reflection on practice as we look forward to future studies. Once an idea is generated, a search of the literature is the next step in discovering what is already known and not known about the topic.

Clinical Problems or Questions

The clinical setting is an excellent place to generate research questions. For example, a nursing unit may have protocols that define "routine vital signs," or perhaps a health care provider's order reads "Vital signs every 4 hours." Where is the evidence to support how often vital signs should be recorded? Are there studies that have explored the relationship between how often or when vital signs are recorded and patient outcomes?

Another pervasive problem in health care is the prevention of pressure ulcers. Standard practices recommend turning patients every 2 hours, although there continues to be little support for this practice. A recent review purports that patients need to be turned frequently, every 2 hours (House, Giles, & Whitcomb, 2011). Few studies have focused solely on frequency of turning and pressure ulcer prevention and/or development. A recent study found that turning every 3 hours was effective in preventing pressure ulcers in the elderly compared to the usual care of turning every 6 hours (Moore, Cowman, & Conroy, 2011). This study only included Caucasians and patients 65 years or older, thereby limiting the generalizability of these findings. One study found that turning every 4 hours on a specialty mattress reduced the number of pressure ulcers (Defloor, Bacquer, & Grypdonck, 2005). A study compared lateral and supine positioning to positioning at a 30-degree and a 90-degree angle (Young, 2004). The investigators did not find any difference between the two groups. These studies demonstrate no support for the common practice of repositioning patients every 2 hours and suggest the need for more research.

Literature

Reading and critiquing the literature are other mechanisms for identifying gaps in what is known and not known in clinical practice. For example, researchers conducted a randomized controlled trial (RCT) to investigate whether telephone-only motivational interviewing increased physical activity among rural adults (Bennett, Young, Nail, Winters-Stone, & Hansen, 2008). They found that the intervention did not increase physical activity, but they suggested that more investigation was needed to determine whether winter weather negatively influenced the physical activity or whether a longer intervention period would have provided a positive result. Because a telephone intervention is a relatively inexpensive method to improve care, especially in rural areas, more investigation is needed, and this area offers an ideal opportunity for more nursing research.

Regulatory Agencies

Regulatory agencies such as The Joint Commission (TJC) (http://www.jointcommission.org) and the Centers for Medicare and Medicaid Services (CMS) (http://www.cms.hhs.gov) are rich sources for research ideas. The Joint Commission collaborated with the American Heart Association and the American College of Cardiology to develop performance measures, or core measure sets, for acute myocardial infarction (AMI). These measures specify evidence-based interventions necessary to provide patients with quality care. These measures include such interventions as smoking-cessation education. Nursing is in an excellent position to test interventions that assist patients in their smoking-cessation efforts.

Technology

Advances in technology, such as electronic health records (EHRs) and telemedicine, afford opportunities for nurses to use technology in caring for patients. One of the largest challenges in health care is implementing electronic medical records (EMR) for patients. Researchers described how primary care practices within the Practice Partner Research Network implemented EMRs in a national quality improvement project, Accelerating Translation of Research into Practice. They evaluated performance on 36 process and outcome indicators across eight domains common to primary practice, such as cardiovascular disease, diabetes, and cancer. They found that nursing plays an important role in facilitating quality improvement within primary care practices (Nemeth et al., 2007). More research is necessary to determine whether the use of EMRs improves health care delivery. Additionally, research to determine how to overcome barriers to adopt EMRs is needed. One study found that only 1.5% of hospitals have integrated EMRs (Jha et al., 2009). Research assessing processes and barriers could be a gap that researchers should identify and investigate.

Telehealth is another area that is expanding to provide improved health care, especially for chronic conditions such as heart failure. An RCT was conducted to determine whether telehomecare, a telephone-based data transfer, could affect outcomes such as hospitalization and mortality (Dansky, Vasey, & Bowles, 2008). They found that patients in the telehomecare group had lower rates of both hospitalization and emergency department visits at 1- and 2-month follow-up periods and fewer symptoms than the control group. A limitation to this study is that the power analysis suggests that a larger sample was needed; therefore, this study should be replicated with a larger sample size. There are many more patient populations with chronic illnesses that need to be studied to determine whether telemedicine can help deliver and improve health care. Replication could also be used to better specify the dose, frequency, and duration of the "intervention" necessary to positively affect patient care outcomes.

New Diagnoses

Discoveries in health care are persistent, including new diagnoses, especially because of research in genetics. As new syndromes are defined and new diseases and diagnoses are discovered, there will be an increasing need for research in these areas. Infectious diseases are continuing to emerge and evolve. For example, the World Health Organization (WHO) in October 2008 investigated an unknown disease in South Africa and Zambia (World Health Organization, 2008). An employee of a safari tour company in Zambia died from an unknown cause. The paramedic and the nurse caring for the patient also became ill and died. The reported signs and symptoms were fever, headache, diarrhea, myalgia, a rash, and liver dysfunction. To date, the infection does not seem to be a type of hemorrhagic fever. Nursing can play a key role in assisting in the care of, and infection control practices for, these patients, which are all sources for investigation.

An example of a new genetic syndrome is a microdeletion of 15q13.3, which causes mental retardation, epilepsy, and facial and digital dysmorphisms (Sharp et al., 2008). Although this disorder is thought to affect about 3 out of 1,000 individuals with mental retardation, there is a need for further investigation to determine the impact of this syndrome on patients and their caregivers. This again gives nursing an excellent opportunity to investigate the impact of this syndrome and possible interventions to improve patient care.

Similarly, researchers discovered a new genetic syndrome, which revealed a microduplication of chromosome 22q11.2 in patients previously diagnosed with DiGeorge/velo-cardio-facial (DG/VCFS) syndrome (Naqvi et al., 2011). The phenotypic features of this new syndrome are widely spaced eyes and superior placement of the eyebrows with increased distance from the eyebrow to upper eyelid crease, downslanting palpebral fissures, and a long narrow face. These features are different from the DG/VCFS syndrome, which led researchers to conclude that this is a new syndrome. The genotype was discovered in 2003 making this a new disorder that needs research. Nursing would be especially poised to conduct research to improve the care and lives of these patients and patients' families.

Media

The media represent another avenue for generating ideas for investigation. Media include television, radio, newspapers, and the Internet. The media report issues that are important to patients and providers.

For example, an online and television report in the summer of 2012 reported a new phlebovirus transmitted from ticks to humans (McMullan et al., 2012). This virus causes fever, fatigue, diarrhea, and loss of appetite. At this point, they are not certain whether this can be transmitted from human to human although no family members or caregivers have shown signs or symptoms of infection. This disease sparks a number of questions from an epidemiological point of view. It is unknown how widespread this infection may become or whether there are any long-term effects.

Sentinel Events

Unfortunately, untoward, or sentinel, events sometimes occur. TJC defines a sentinel event as "an unexpected occurrence involving death or serious physical or psychological injury, or the risk thereof. Serious injury specifically includes loss of limb or function" (Joint Commission, 2007). These events may be related to system problems, knowledge deficits, equipment malfunction, or a variety of other related problems. Some examples of sentinel event alerts issued in 2008 concerned the prevention of errors relating to commonly used anticoagulants, behaviors that undermine a culture of safety, the prevention of pediatric medication errors, and the prevention of accidents and injuries in the magnetic resonance imaging (MRI) suite. Nurses are well poised to study how these important occurrences happen and to develop effective interventions for prevention.

Several studies have described disruptive behavior or workplace bullying and how it potentially affects patient safety and nurse retention (Johnson & Rea, 2009; Vessey, DeMarco, Gaffney, & Budin, 2009). The next few steps, as outlined by the Joint Commission, can be skills-based training for management on relationship building, collaborative practice, and conflict resolution. Cultural assessment instruments can be used to determine whether attitudes are changing over time as a result of the training. Another potential study might focus on the development of a system for assessing staff perceptions of the seriousness of unprofessional behavior and the risk of harm to patients. All of these are areas that need further investigation to keep patients and the health care team safe and to improve the delivery of quality care.

Legislative Events

Other opportunities for nursing research are related to legislative and health policy issues. Nursing is an integral part of health policy discussions and should conduct research on legislative issues in order to promote and protect the public's health. The Affordable Care Act was passed in 2009. Nursing is well-positioned to examine outcomes related to the outcomes of the legislation. Is access to health care improved? Are patient-centered outcomes improved with health care reform? These are crucial questions that will need to be examined.

Similarly, nurse staffing ratios are a legislative issue that many states have been debating for decades. On January 1, 2008, California upgraded its staffing ratios to 1:3 on step-down units; 1:4 on telemetry units; and 1:4 in other specialty areas such as oncology. Other mandated ratios are 1:2 in critical care, 1:4 in pediatrics, and 1:4 in the emergency department (Coffman, 2002). Further research will be needed to determine whether these ratios improve patient care and patient safety. One problem with these ratios is that the term *nurse* is defined as a registered nurse (RN) or a licensed practical nurse (LPN). Previous research on nursing educational level and patient outcomes determined that having RNs, those with a bachelor's degree or higher, provide direct patient care improves care by decreasing mortality (Aiken, Clarke, Cheung, Sloane, & Silber, 2003). An initial study to determine how the ratios have affected outcomes concluded that there has not been a significant positive impact on nurse-sensitive quality indicators, such as pressure ulcers and patient falls (Bolton et al., 2007). In contrast, another study found that hospital nurse staffing ratios in California were associated with lower mortality and nursing units had better nurse retention in California and in other states where there are mandated nurse–patient staffing ratios (Aiken et al., 2010). Clearly, more research is needed on work environments and patient outcomes, including economic implications.

BACKGROUND

An exhaustive review of the literature is imperative to determine what is currently known about the subject or phenomenon. Well-written studies provide insight into the implications of the findings and suggestions for future research or directions for inquiry. A review of studies related to the topic helps to summarize the findings and thereby helps the reader to develop a sense of where the next inquiry should begin. The review also gives ideas on possible research designs, along with potential leads for experts or consultants for the study. The review should give a good suggestion of theories or conceptual models that have been applied or allude to possible conceptual frameworks for future studies.

The background section of the proposal for the study should give a concise overview of the body of science under investigation and how the studies contribute to knowledge development. The background should connect the literature and define the domains of the concepts under investigation. An explanation of how the literature search was conducted should also be provided. Common research databases include the Cumulative Index to Nursing and Allied Health Literature (CINAHL) and Medical Literature Analysis and Retrieval System Online (MEDLINE). CINAHL is primarily used by nurse scientists, but it is important not to limit oneself to only one research database as a tool for searches. MEDLINE is a search engine for biomedical research. It is important to use multiple search engines when exploring a topic. Limiting oneself to one database may mean that one does not find all available research on the topic. Research fields for nursing overlap with those of other disciplines, such as medicine, pharmacy, physical therapy, nutrition, and psychology.

When searching for relevant studies, one should employ a variety of methods, including searches by subject, keywords, and author. A subject search is a broad search in which one is looking for general information on a topic. This may be a good starting point when determining the breadth of a particular topic or phenomenon. Depending on the topic, a subject search may reveal literally thousands of papers. At this point, it can be helpful to narrow the topic area by using limits. These limits may include gender, race, human subjects, or other areas. Selecting a particular article may be helpful to determine Medical Subject Headings (MeSH) terms as created by the National Library of Medicine (NLM). MeSH terms are developed by NLM and consist of a preferred list of medical terms. These terms are helpful in finding other studies on the topic once a good study has been found to provide an exhaustive search on a particular topic. Chapter 2, on general searching, includes ways of maximizing the effectiveness of the literature search.

When reviewing the literature, one should review primary, not secondary, sources, that is, publications written by those who conducted the study, not publications that report on and summarize studies conducted by others. Reviewing primary sources allows the reviewer to determine the validity of the study rather than relying on another person's interpretation of the study. An exception to this recommendation is the systematic review, the purpose of which is to summarize all the research on a topic to determine the outcome across a number of studies, populations, and clinical settings.

SIGNIFICANCE

Determining the significance of a study is vital to deciding whether the topic is worthy of investigation. Is the topic timely? Will the topic add significant information to a body of knowledge? Does it provide new information, or does it help confirm previous results by replicating a previously done study? Is the study innovative? Does it describe a new phenomenon or a new way of studying a problem? The section on significance should point out the limited amount of information currently available or determine whether no information is currently published. On the other hand, the section on significance may indicate that there is conflicting evidence on the topic and that further investigation is needed to clarify what is known or unknown. The significance of a study may be related to testing a theory or furthering scientists' understanding of how the research will help a particular patient population. Following are examples of how the significance of a study may be articulated.

Researchers investigated the maternal background and intrapersonal predictors that were associated with timing of breastfeeding cessation (Tenfelde, Finnegan, Miller, & Hill, 2012).

Breastfeeding protects infants against many adverse health outcomes, including gastrointestinal infections, ear infections, diabetes, and obesity. Improved cognitive development has been shown in infants who were breastfed for longer periods of time. Therefore the study is significant by determining those factors that may be amenable to interventions to prolong breastfeeding.

In another example, investigators examined overall and specific symptoms in patients with multiple sclerosis (MS) and how the symptoms correlated with physical activity (Motl, Snook, & Schapiro, 2008). They presented an extensive review of previous literature investigating symptoms related to MS, followed by a discussion of why their study was significant. They determined that previous studies had evaluated the relationship between overall symptoms, rather than specific symptoms, and physical activity. Also, previous studies did not account for possible functional limitations related to patients' ability to perform physical activities. These limitations served as the foundation for determining the significance of their study.

PURPOSE, OBJECTIVE, AND AIMS

Once researchers have identified a topic of interest and conducted a thorough review of the literature, they can define the study further by developing its purpose, objectives, and specific aims. The purpose statement of a study is a statement of the essence of what the investigators are attempting to explore. The statement generally begins with, "The purpose of this study. . .". This statement will guide the development of the research project by denoting what the focus of the research is. Following is an example of a purpose statement: "The purpose of this study was to describe falls and injuries within assisted living communities and determine whether a function-focused care intervention increased the risk of falls and/or injuries" (Resnick, Galik, Gruber-Baldini, & Zimmerman, 2012). In one qualitative study, researchers wanted to determine the experience of nurses during the Persian Gulf combat. They stated the study's purpose as follows: "The purpose of the ongoing project is to gather accounts of nurses who have served their country during wartime, on the battle front or in supportive roles" (Rushton, Scott, & Callister, 2008).

The objectives of a study are very closely related to the purpose. Although some researchers may use the terms *purpose* and *objectives* interchangeably, they are distinct components in the research protocol. Objectives are components of the study that can be measured. Although the objectives should flow from the purpose statement and are closely related to it, they are distinctly different.

In this study, the objective of the study was stated as "The objective of this study is to examine the influence of diabetes self-care maintenance and management on number of hospitalizations and hospitalization days" (Song, Ratcliffe, Tkacs, & Riegel, 2012). The objectives help fulfill the purpose of the study: to describe the influence of self-care in people with diabetes on the hospital length of stay.

Similarly, the aim of a study and its purpose can be interchangeable. Although the purpose is the essence of what is being studied, the aim is more aligned with the goal of the study or what the researchers want to accomplish. Generally, the aim of the study is contained in a statement that begins like this: "The aim of this study. . .". In one qualitative study, researchers identified the need to investigate the relationships between parents and neonatal intensive care unit (NICU) nurses during the prolonged hospitalization of premature babies (Fegran, Fagermoen, & Helseth, 2008). The specific aim of the study was stated this way: "The aim of this study was to explore the development of relationships between parents and nurses in an NICU."

The decision whether to use a purpose statement or to present an aim may be based on the personal preference of the researcher, the audience that the researcher is presenting to, or the funding agency. For example, thesis or dissertation committees may require specific wording related to aims in a research proposal or protocol. When writing for publication in journals, one may encounter similar requirements. When one is writing a grant proposal, one may be required to provide a list of objectives for the research project. Whatever the requirements are, the researcher will need to state in some form the essence of the project and what the researcher wants to accomplish.

RESEARCH QUESTIONS

Once the topic of inquiry has been identified and the literature review conducted, the researcher can write the research questions. Research questions are interrogatives that bring out what is being studied specifically. Not all studies have specific research questions; some studies may have a hypothesis or hypotheses, which are discussed in the following section. The research questions contain the independent and dependent variable(s), which are also discussed in another section of this chapter. Another important factor related to research questions is the way the question is stated. The wording of the question in a quantitative study drives the statistical analysis.

Research questions are often restatements of the purpose. For example, researchers wanted to examine stress among pregnant Black women (Gennaro, Shults, & Garry, 2008). In their study, they identified three purposes: "(a) compare three commonly used measures of stress during pregnancy in Black women, (b) examine changes in stress in Black women over time to determine when stress is highest, and (c) provide exploratory information as to whether any of the stress measures help to predict Black women who might be more likely to deliver preterm infants than other Black women" (pp. 538–539). The three research questions were derived from the purpose statements: "(1) What is the relationship between three measures of stress in pregnant Black women: Corticotropin-releasing hormone (CRH) (a physiological measure), Prenatal Distress Questionnaire (PDQ), and Perceived Stress Scale (PSS)? (2) After 28 weeks, is stress highest in pregnant Black women? (3) Is there a difference in stress between Black women (a) in preterm labor who deliver preterm, (b) in preterm labor who deliver term, or (c) who experience normal term labor and deliveries?" (p. 539).

Qualitative studies also have research questions. Researchers used grounded theory methods to determine how women with potential cardiac symptoms made decisions about seeking treatment (Turris & Johnson, 2008). Their purpose statement was "to explore how women seeking treatment for the symptoms of potential cardiac illness interpreted their symptoms, made decisions about seeking treatment, and understood experiences of care in the emergency department." Their primary research question was derived from the purpose and was stated this way: "In the context of the symptoms of a potential cardiac event, what is the process by which women understand and make decisions about those symptoms?" In this qualitative study, there is a relationship between the purpose and the research question, although the research question is not an exact restatement of the purpose. Some researchers may decide to use hypotheses instead of research questions; these are discussed in the following section.

HYPOTHESES

A hypothesis is a prediction of outcomes between one or more variables (Mateo & Kirchhoff, 1999). Generally, in order to state a hypothesis, a researcher relies on previous literature or a theoretical framework to support the relationship between variables. Hypotheses can be directional, nondirectional, or null.

A directional hypothesis not only predicts the relationship between one or more variables but also states the direction of the relationship. Researchers conducted a pilot study to determine differences in temperature rhythms, rest and activity rhythms, melatonin rhythms, sleep percentages, and daytime sleepiness in older adults living in independent apartments and in nursing homes (Chaperon, Farr, & Lochiano, 2007). They had three research hypotheses. One of the hypotheses stated "Older age will be a predictor of increased negative effects of environmental cues" (p. 22). In this hypothesis, older age suggests a direction in the relationship between the variables; with increasing age, there is an increasing negative effect. Usually, theory or past findings enable the prediction.

In contrast, a nondirectional hypothesis does not predict the direction of the relationship. One of the hypotheses from the same researchers stated: "Apartment-dwelling residents will have different axillary body temperature rhythms, rest/activity rhythms, melatonin rhythms, sleep percentages, and daytime sleepiness than nursing home residents" (p. 22). The investigators stated that there would be a difference between apartment-dwelling residents and nursing home residents in relation to the defined outcome variables, but they did not state the direction of the association. Similarly, the other nondirectional hypothesis in this study stated: "Daytime or nighttime light exposure will be associated with differences in axillary body temperature rhythms, rest/activity rhythms, melatonin rhythms, sleep percentages, and daytime sleepiness" (Chaperon et al., 2007). The researchers stated that there would be an association but did not elaborate which direction the association would take.

A null hypothesis or statistical hypothesis is a statement that predicts that there is no relationship between variables (Mateo & Kirchhoff, 1999). The null hypothesis is not always explicitly written but can be derived from the hypotheses that are stated. The null hypothesis is what is accepted or rejected in relation to statistical procedures. In one study, researchers wanted to explore the effects of a 5-day tactile touch intervention on oxytocin levels in critical care patients (Henricson, Berglund, Määttä, Ekman, & Segesten, 2008). The directional hypotheses stated that tactile touch would increase oxytocin levels after the intervention and continue to increase the levels over a 6-day period. The null hypothesis would be stated this way: There is no difference in the levels of oxytocin in intensive care unit patients after a tactile touch intervention.

In another example, researchers investigated whether positioning of intubated infants affected the colonization of bacteria in the trachea, putting infants at risk for infections (Aly, Badawy, El-Kholy, Nabil, & Mohamed, 2008). They hypothesized that intubated infants positioned on their sides would be less likely to have bacterial colonization in their tracheas than those positioned supinely. This is an example of a directional hypothesis. The null hypothesis would be that there is no difference in the amount of tracheal bacterial colonization in those infants positioned on their sides and those positioned supinely.

VARIABLES

A research question is written in terms of the dependent variable (DV), also known as the observed outcome, and the independent variable(s) (IV), or the variable(s) hypothesized or thought to produce the dependent variable. Dependent variable values depend on the independent variable(s). Variables are operationally defined by what is measured, how the indicators are measured, and how the values are interpreted. In other words, an operational definition characterizes how the variable is measured.

Variables are classified according to the level or scale of measurement; the four scales are nominal, ordinal, interval, and ratio (NOIR). Knowing the level or scale of measurement provides the necessary information for readers to interpret the data from that variable. Certain statistical analyses are used only for data measured at certain measurement levels. The level of measurement of the IV, the question being asked, and the number of groups of the DV are key determinants for selecting the correct statistical test to analyze the research study data. In general, it is desirable to have a higher level of measurement (e.g., interval or ratio) than to use a lower one (e.g., nominal or ordinal). When in doubt as to the level of measurement, the rule of thumb is to treat the variable at the highest level of measurement that can be justified, that is, to use an interval rather than an ordinal scale and an ordinal scale rather than a nominal one. Statistics for higher levels of measurement are more powerful at detecting differences in the research data. Once the statistical test is determined, the sample size can be calculated.

SUMMARY

In summary, identifying a focus of study can be challenging. There are multiple sources for initially determining what to study, including, but not limited to, the literature and clinically derived questions. A thorough search of the literature will help determine what is already known on the subject and further define what the topic will be. Once the literature has been scrutinized, the purpose or aim of the study can be delineated. In conjunction with the purpose, research questions and or hypotheses are then formulated. The hypothesis describes a relationship between the independent and the dependent variable(s).

The independent and dependent variables determine the statistical test to be performed once the number of groups in the study and the level of measurement (nominal, ordinal, interval, or ratio) have been determined.

SUGGESTED ACTIVITIES

1. Suppose you were interested in determining how to manage dyspnea in patients with heart failure. Write down your strategy for determining what information is currently known and formulate a research question(s).
2. For the following research questions, write a directional, a nondirectional, and a null hypothesis:
   a. Does massage decrease anxiety in patients undergoing cardiac catheterization?
   b. Does mouth care in intubated adult patients decrease ventilator-associated pneumonia?
   c. Are maternal–infant bonding behaviors affected by the performance of initial newborn infant physical examination?

REFERENCES

Aiken, L., Clarke, S., Cheung, R., Sloane, D., & Silber, J. (2003). Educational levels of hospital nurses and surgical patient mortality. *Journal of the American Medical Association, 290*(12), 1617–1623. doi: 10.1001/jama .290.12.1617

Aiken, L. H., Sloane, D. M., Cimiotti, J. P., Clarke, S. P., Flynn, L., Seago, J. A., Spetz, J., & Smith, K. L. (2010). Implications of the California nurse staffing mandate for other states. *Health Services Research, 45*(4), 904–921. doi: 10.1111/j.1475-6773.2010.01114.x

Aly, H., Badawy, M., El-Kholy, A., Nabil, R., & Mohamed, A. (2008). Randomized, controlled trial on tracheal colonization of ventilated infants: Can gravity prevent ventilator-associated pneumonia? *Pediatrics, 122*(4), 770–774. doi: 10.1542/peds.2007-1826

Bennett, J., Young, H., Nail, L., Winters-Stone, K., & Hansen, G. (2008). *A telephone-only motivational intervention to increase physical activity in rural adults: A randomized controlled trial* (Vol. 57). Hagerstown, MD: Lippincott Williams & Wilkins.

Bolton, L. B., Aydin, C. E., Donaldson, N., Storer Brown, D., Sandhu, M., Fridman, M., & Aronow, H. U. (2007). Mandated nurse staffing ratios in California: A comparison of staffing and nursing-sensitive outcomes pre- and postregulation. *Policy, Politics, & Nursing Practice, 8*(4), 238–250. doi: 10.1177/1527154407312737

Chaperon, C., Farr, L., & Lochiano, E. (2007). Sleep disturbance of residents in a continuing care retirement community. *Journal of Gerontological Nursing, 10*(33), 21–28.

Coffman, J. M., Seago, J. A., & Spetz, J. (2002). Minimum nurse-to-patient ratios in acute care hospitals in California. *Heath Affairs, 21*(5), 53–64.

Dansky, K. H., Vasey, J., & Bowles, K. (2008). Impact of telehealth on clinical outcomes in patients with heart failure. *Clinical Nursing Research, 17*(3), 182–199. doi: 10.1177/1054773808320837

Defloor, T., Bacquer, D. D., & Grypdonck, M. H. F. (2005). The effect of various combinations of turning and pressure reducing devices on the incidence of pressure ulcers. *International Journal of Nursing Studies, 42*(1), 37–46. doi: 10.1016/j.ijnurstu.2004.05.013

Fegran, L., Fagermoen, M. S., & Helseth, S. (2008). Development of parent–nurse relationships in neonatal intensive care units—from closeness to detachment. *Journal of Advanced Nursing, 64*(4), 363–371. doi: 10.1111/j.1365 -2648.2008.04777.x

Gennaro, S., Shults, J., & Garry, D. J. (2008). Stress and preterm labor and birth in black women. *Journal of Obstetric, Gynecologic, & Neonatal Nursing, 37*(5), 538–545. doi: 10.1111/j.1552-6909.2008.00278.x

Henricson, M., Berglund, A.-L., Määttä, S., Ekman, R., & Segesten, K. (2008). The outcome of tactile touch on oxytocin in intensive care patients: A randomised controlled trial. *Journal of Clinical Nursing, 17*(19), 2624–2633. doi: 10.1111/j.1365-2702.2008.02324.x

House, S., Giles, T., & Whitcomb, J. (2011). Benchmarking to the international pressure ulcer prevalence survey. *Journal of Wound Ostomy & Continence Nursing, 38*(3), 254–259. doi: 10.1097/WON.0b013e318215fa48.

Jha, A. K., DesRoches, C. M., Campbell, E. G., Donelan, K., Rao, S. R., Ferris, T. G., Shields, A., Rosenbaum, S., & Blumenthal, D. (2009). Use of electronic health records in U.S. hospitals. *New England Journal of Medicine, 360*(16), 1628–1638. doi: 10.1056/NEJMsa0900592

Johnson, S. L., & Rea, R. E. (2009). Workplace bullying: Concerns for nurse leaders. *Journal of Nursing Administration, 39*(2), 84–90. doi: 10.1097/NNA .1090b1013e318195a318195fc

Mateo, M., & Kirchhoff, K. (1999). *Using and conducting nursing research in the clinical setting* (2nd ed.). St. Louis, MO: W.B. Saunders.

McMullan, L. K., Folk, S. M., Kelly, A. J., MacNeil, A., Goldsmith, C. S., Metcalfe, M. G., Batten, B. C., Albarino, C. G., Zaki, S. R., Rollin, P. E., Nicholson, W. L., & Nichol, S. T. (2012). A new phlebovirus associated with severe febrile illness in Missouri. *New England Journal of Medicine, 367*(9), 834–841. doi: 10.1056/NEJMoa1203378

Moore, Z., Cowman, S., & Conroy, R. M. (2011). A randomised controlled clinical trial of repositioning, using the 30° tilt, for the prevention of pressure ulcers. *Journal of Clinical Nursing, 20*(17–18), 2633–2644. doi: 10.1111/j.1365-2702.2011.03736.x

Motl, R. W., Snook, E. M., & Schapiro, R. T. (2008). Symptoms and physical activity behavior in individuals with multiple sclerosis. *Research in Nursing & Health, 31*(5), 466–475. doi: 10.1002/nur.20274

Naqvi, N., Davidson, S. J., Wong, D., Cullinan, P., Roughton, M., Doughty, V. L., Franklin, R. C., & Daubeney, P. E. (2011). Predicting 22q11.2 deletion syndrome: A novel method using the routine full blood count. *International Journal of Cardiology, 150*(1), 50–53. doi: 10.1016/j.ijcard .2010.02.027

Nemeth, L., Wessell, A., Jenkins, R., Nietert, P., Liszka, H. A., & Ornstein, S. (2007). Strategies to accelerate translation of research into primary care within practices using electronic medical records. *Journal of Nursing Care Quality, 22*(4), 343–349.

Resnick, B., Galik, E., Gruber-Baldini, A. L., & Zimmerman, S. (2012). Falls and fall-related injuries associated with function-focused care. *Clinical Nursing Research, 21*(1), 43–63. doi: 10.1177/1054773811420060

Rushton, P., Scott, J. E., & Callister, L. C. (2008). "It's what we're here for:" Nurses caring for military personnel during the Persian Gulf Wars. *Nursing Outlook, 56*(4), 179–186.e1 (quotation on p. 171).doi: 10.1016/j.outlook.2008.03.010

Sharp, A. J., Mefford, H. C., Li, K., Baker, C., Skinner, C., Stevenson, R. E., ... Eichler, E. E. (2008). A recurrent 15q13.3 microdeletion syndrome associated with mental retardation and seizures. *Nat Genet, 40*(3), 322–328. doi: 10.1038 /ng.93. Available from http://www.nature.com/ng/journal/v40/n3/suppinfo /ng.93_S1.html

Song, M., Ratcliffe, S. J., Tkacs, N. C., & Riegel, B. (2012). Self-care and health outcomes of diabetes mellitus. *Clinical Nursing Research, 21*(3), 309–326. doi: 10.1177/1054773811422604

Tenfelde, S. M., Finnegan, L., Miller, A. M., & Hill, P. D. (2012). Risk of breast-feeding cessation among low-income women, infants, and children: A discrete time survival analysis. *Nursing Research, 61*(2), 86–95. doi: 10.1097 /NNR.1090b1013e3182456b3182450a.

The Joint Commission. (2007). Sentinel Event. Sentinel Event Alert, Issue 40: Behaviors that undermine a culture of safety [Internet]. 2008 retrieved March 29, 2013 from http://www.jointcommission.org/sentinel_event_alert _issue_40_behaviors_that_undermine_a_culture_of_safety

Turris, S. A., & Johnson, J. L. (2008). Maintaining integrity: Women and treatment seeking for the symptoms of potential cardiac illness. *Qualitative Health Research, 18*(11), 1461–1476. doi: 10.1177/1049732308325824

Vessey, J. A., DeMarco, R. F., Gaffney, D. A., & Budin, W. C. (2009). Bullying of staff registered nurses in the workplace: A preliminary study for developing personal and organizational strategies for the transformation of hostile to healthy workplace environments. *Journal of Professional Nursing, 25*(5), 299–306. doi: 10.1016/j.profnurs.2009.01.022

World Health Organization. (2008). *Unknown disease in South Africa and Zambia*. Retrieved September 21, 2012, from http://www.who.int/csr/don /2008_10_10/en/index.html

Young, T. (2004). The 30-degree tilt position vs. the 90-degree lateral and supine positions in reducing the incidence of non-blanching erythema in a hospital inpatient population: A randomised controlled trial. *Journal of Tissue Viability, 14*(3), 80, 90, 92–96.

7

Conceptual and Theoretical Frameworks

Mary E. Johnson

Systematic reviews synthesize bodies of research findings to uncover the appropriate principles to be applied to practice (Coopey, Nix, & Clancy, 2006), but how does the advanced practice registered nurse (APRN) critically appraise a specific research study to determine whether the findings are appropriate for integration into practice? The APRN must have the skills necessary to scrutinize research findings to determine their usefulness in clinical practice, which is done by examining the findings for both validity and clinical applicability. An important consideration when making this determination is congruence between the research study and the theory or conceptual framework that guided the research design.

Research is vital to the expansion of nursing knowledge. Theories are an important link between research and knowledge development in that theories provide the researcher with a framework for designing the study, collecting data, and interpreting findings; the findings are then used to describe, explain, and predict nursing practice (McEwen & Wills, 2011). Without a theoretical framework, research studies lack coherence not only within the study, but also in relation to previous research about a given topic. Without a theoretical framework, research studies are often problem based and the findings may not be applicable to other settings (Verran, 1997). The APRN must be able to evaluate research reports to determine the applicability of the theory or conceptual model that was used to guide the study and the appropriateness for integration of new knowledge into practice. This chapter includes a discussion of the relationships among theory, practice, and research, the characteristics of theory, and criteria for evaluating a theory and its use in a published study.

THEORETICAL AND CONCEPTUAL FRAMEWORKS

Although there has been considerable debate about the definition of the different terms—theory, theoretical framework, and conceptual framework—the consensus among nursing authors is that conceptual frameworks are more abstract than theories. Conceptual frameworks link concepts in meaningful ways, but are usually not considered to be as fully developed as theoretical frameworks. This leads some to assert that the development of conceptual frameworks is a necessary step in the development of theories (Meleis, 2012). Other nurse theorists view conceptual frameworks, not as a step toward the development of theories, but as analogous to grand theories (McEwen & Wills, 2011). Still others use the three terms interchangeably (Meleis, 2012). In the end, Meleis proposes that the debate over the meaning of these terms is an academic issue of "semantics" (p. 128), which has led not only to confusion within the discipline, but also has delayed progress in the development of theories useful to research and practice. She suggests that the use of the term "theory" is sufficient.

A theory (or theoretical framework) is a "set of logically interrelated concepts, statements, propositions, and definitions" (McEwen & Wills, 2011, p. 26), which presents a systematic view of a phenomenon from which one may ask questions and specify relations among variables in order to explain and predict phenomena (McEwen & Wills, 2011; Peterson & Bredow, 2013). Theories help define and differentiate a discipline, explain events, structure and organize knowledge, and guide APRNs by identifying the goals and outcomes of practice, and contribute to a rational practice that questions and validates intuition and assumptions.

Over time, there has been considerable debate about whether nursing should only use theories developed by and for nursing or could also use theories that were developed in other disciplines. The rationale for the former is that theories help define the boundaries of a discipline. Thus, theories developed by and for nurses articulate the purpose of nursing and identify nursing interventions; research that uses theories developed within nursing contributes to the development of nursing knowledge. The widespread use of non-nursing theories in research and practice lends support to the assertion that the origin of the theory is less important than the theory's pragmatic utility. Those who find the use of theories developed in disciplines other than nursing (borrowed theories) acceptable assert that knowledge is not confined to a particular discipline, but rather is available to all. Moreover, in this day of interdisciplinary research and practice, knowledge and theories are shared within a team; theories provide a common language to frame research and practice. As an applied discipline, nurses use knowledge from the physical and social sciences. Likewise, theories developed within nursing may also contain concepts shared by other disciplines. In other words, the boundaries that separate disciplines may not be rigid and impenetrable. When theories from other disciplines are used in research or practice, they should be consistent with a nursing perspective and regardless of the term used or whether nursing or borrowed theories are employed, a theory must be meaningful and relevant (McEwen & Wills, 2011).

CLASSIFICATION OF THEORIES

There are two major ways of classifying theories. The first is by scope and the second is by purpose (McEwen & Wills, 2011). This section focuses on the two major ways of classifying theories.

Scope

Scope refers to the breadth of phenomena encompassed by the theory and is correlated with the degree of theoretical abstractness. In terms of scope, a theory may be classified as grand, middle range, or practice/situation specific. Grand theories focus on broad areas of a discipline. In nursing, the grand theories explain phenomena of central concern to nursing, such as the meta-paradigm concepts of person, health, nursing, and environment. Grand theories incorporate highly abstract concepts that often lack operational definitions. Therefore, the propositions are not considered to be accessible to testing (McEwen & Wills, 2011). However, there is evidence that grand theories are used as frameworks for nursing research (Im & Chang, 2012). Some examples include the Roy Adaptation Model (Bakan & Akyol, 2008), Watson's Theory of Human Care (Gillespie, Hounchell, Pettinichi, Mattei, & Rose, 2012), and Orem's Self-Care Theory (Peters & Templin, 2010).

Middle range theories are more focused and limited in scope than grand theories. Middle range theories encompass a limited number of concepts that tend to be more concrete than those found in grand theories. Thus, the concepts can usually be operationally defined. The theoretical properties are more specific and accessible to testing than those found in grand theories (McEwen & Wills, 2011). In the past 15 years, there has been a significant growth in the development of middle range theories (Peterson & Bredow, 2013). One reason may be their applicability to both research and practice. One theory that has been used extensively in research is Mishel's Uncertainty in Illness Theory (Mishel, 1990). Briefly, the theory proposes that when individuals experience increased uncertainty in the trajectory of their illness, they use a range of coping mechanisms, which then impact their adaptation to the illness.

Middle range theories may be developed in several ways. That is, they may be developed from grand theories (Lewandowski, 2004), reviews of the literature (Spratling & Weaver, 2012) and research (Sanford, Townsend-Rocchiccioli, Horigan, & Hall, 2011), or a combination of research and literature reviews (Siaki, Loescher, & Trego, 2013). For example, Barrett's theory of power was developed from Rogers's Science of Unitary Human Beings (Lewandowski, 2004). Major components of Barrett's middle range theory are the dimensions of awareness, choice, intentional action, and creating change. Humans are enhancing their own power when they are participating in change in their lives. In this study, Lewandowski sought to determine whether guided imagery reduces pain and increases a sense of power over the pain in people with chronic pain. Spratling and Weaver (2012) developed a theoretical framework of resilience in medically fragile adolescents from reviews of the risk and resilience literature in this population. Sanford et al. (2011) developed a theoretical model of decision making in heart failure from their grounded theory study of the ways caregivers of people with heart failure make decisions. Finally, Siaki et al. (2013) constructed a middle range theory of risk perception from their synthesis of the literature and qualitative and quantitative data from a study of Samoan Pacific Islanders who are at high risk for developing diabetes and cardiovascular disease.

Situation-specific or practice theories are the most focused and least complex theories. Situation-specific theories contain a limited number of concepts that are easily defined and explain a small aspect of reality. Situation-specific theories tend to be prescriptive (McEwen & Wills, 2011). Unlike grand or middle range theories that are generalizable across populations and situations, situation-specific theories are most applicable in specific contexts. Situation-specific theories are limited to specific populations or particular areas of interest and take sociopolitical, cultural, and historical contexts into consideration (Im, 2005). Situation-specific theories may be developed from middle range theories, research, and practice (Peterson & Bredow, 2013). An example of a situation-specific theory is the Asian Immigrant Menopausal Symptom (AIMS) theory (Im, 2010). This theory was developed using an integrative approach of literature synthesis and research and describes the process by which Asian women progress through menopause and the factors that influence how Asian women experience menopause and the symptoms they experience.

Purpose

Theories may be classified as descriptive, explanatory, predictive, or prescriptive. Descriptive theories describe or name concepts, properties, and dimensions, but do not explain how the concepts in the theory are related. Descriptive theories tend to be generated from descriptive research such as concept analyses, case studies, literature reviews, or grounded theory research (McEwen & Wills, 2011). Explanatory theories describe associations or relationships among concepts or propositions, explaining how and why these concepts are related. These studies are developed using correlational research (McEwen & Wills, 2011). Predictive theories describe the conditions under which particular outcomes will occur. These theories are generated and tested using research designs such as pretest, posttest design, and quasi-experimental and experimental designs (McEwen & Wills, 2011). Prescriptive theories describe interventions that will achieve a particular outcome (McEwen & Wills, 2011).

COMPONENTS OF THEORIES

Theoretical and conceptual frameworks are characterized by concepts that are organized in a coherent manner. Concepts are considered to be the building blocks of theories, and relational statements provide coherence within a theoretical framework. In other words, relational statements describe how concepts are related to each other. This section focuses on the components of theories.

Concepts

Concepts give meaning to an object, phenomenon, or idea by describing or naming them (Grove, Burns, & Gray, 2013). Concepts may be a single word, two words, or a phrase and are generally regarded as the building blocks of theories. Concepts may be classified as abstract or concrete, variable or nonvariable, and theoretically or operationally defined (McEwen & Wills, 2011). Concrete concepts are directly observable, whereas abstract concepts are inferred indirectly. Examples of concrete concepts include height or weight, which are directly measured. Highly abstract concepts such as pain, hope, or caring are more difficult to measure. The continuum from concrete to abstract is important to researchers because concepts that are more concrete are not only easier to measure, but are also less prone to measurement error than abstract concepts.

Variable concepts are those that exist on a continuum and are measured using an instrument that reflects the range of possibilities for the concept. For example, participants in a research study might be asked to rate pain on a scale from 1 to 10 or they might be given a validated self-report tool that indicates the degree to which the person feels hopeful or height or weight might be recorded. On the other hand, nonvariable concepts are discrete concepts for which there is not a range of possibilities; for example, one is either pregnant or not pregnant and one is either male or female. In research, important discrete variables are often recorded as demographic data.

When researchers use a theory to underpin a research study, they decide which concepts are useful for the study and how they are going to measure the concept. For example, in their study of patient satisfaction with postpartum teaching methods (Wagner, Bear, & Davidson, 2011), the researchers used a middle range theory, the Interaction Model of Client Health Behavior (IMCBH) as their theoretical framework. Although there are many concepts in the theory, the authors selected patient satisfaction as the main outcome concept. This concept was measured using a client satisfaction tool, which was determined to be both reliable and valid. This tool also contained measures of subconcepts that are central to the theory: affective support, health information, decisional control, professional competencies, and overall satisfaction with care.

Theoretical definitions of concepts indicate the meaning of a concept in the context of a theory. Theoretical definitions may be highly abstract, which entails the need for operational definitions, which indicate how the concept is defined and measured in the context of a particular research study. Operational definitions form the bridge between the theoretical and the empirical worlds. Because of the close relationship between theoretical and operational definitions, they need to be consistent. In other words, the link between theoretical definitions, operational definitions, and the measurement tools should be clear and congruent. For example, the Alhusen, Gross, Hayat, Woods, and Sharps (2012) study of the relationships among maternal–fetal attachment and health practices on neonatal outcomes in low-income urban women was grounded in two theoretical frameworks, Maternal Role Attainment (MRA) and an expansion of MRA, Becoming a Mother (BAM). Maternal–fetal attachment is a primary theoretical concept, which was defined as behaviors that indicate an affiliation between the woman and her unborn child. Maternal–fetal attachment was measured using the Maternal–Fetal Attachment Scale and although it was not directly stated, one can infer that maternal–fetal attachment was operationalized as the score on the Maternal–Fetal Attachment Scale.

Relational Statements

Relational statements describe the direction, shape, strength, symmetry, sequencing, probability of occurrence, necessity, and sufficiency of concepts within a theory (Grove et al., 2013). Understanding and articulating relational statements are important because these statements can form the basis for the hypotheses in research studies. Further testing will confirm the accuracy of these relational statements and will also determine the strength of the relationship and whether the nature of the relationships among concepts is positive or negative, linear or curvilinear, or symmetrical or asymmetrical. Positive relationships mean that as the strength or volume of one concept changes, the strength or volume of another concept will change in a similar direction. For example, if the number of calories one consumes increases, one's weight will also increase. Negative relationships indicate that as the strength or volume of one concept changes, the strength or volume of another concept will change in the opposite direction. For example, a significant drop in blood pressure is often accompanied by an increase in heart rate.

For example, in Mishel's Uncertainty Theory, which Jiang and He (2012) used as the framework for their study of the effects of an uncertainty management intervention on uncertainty, anxiety, depression, and quality of life in persons with chronic obstructive pulmonary disease (COPD), uncertainty increases when patients have a lack of information that is important to them. Also, when uncertainty increases because of exacerbations of symptoms, patients use behavioral strategies to manage the uncertainty. The authors proposed that their uncertainty intervention would decrease uncertainty experienced by those with COPD, which would consequently increase the participants' quality of life and decrease their depression and anxiety.

THEORY EVALUATION

Over time, multiple methods for describing and evaluating a theory have been proposed (Meleis, 2012; Peterson & Bredow, 2013). This section will focus on evaluating a theory for use in research (Peterson & Bredow, 2013) and evaluating theories for their use in published studies (Grove et al., 2013). Theory evaluation is an important step in evaluating the strength of a research study. Overall, when reading published research studies, the choice of theory should be clear and there should be a clear link among the theory, the hypotheses, the measures used, and the interpretation of the findings.

When selecting a theory for use in a research study, the theory should be reviewed in detail, scrutinizing it with the following questions. When reviewing a theory in a published research study, the theory should also be scrutinized for clarity and consistency, although the theory explanation in published studies will be less detailed than in the theorist's own works, which means all the following questions may not be addressed. If an APRN wants to use a theory for research or practice, one should return to the theorist's original works. Internal criticism refers to internal coherence of the theory's components; external criticism refers to the coherence between the theory and external factors such as the social context or nursing's meta-paradigm (Peterson & Bredow, 2013).

Internal Criticism

Questions the reviewer should ask regarding internal criticism pertain to the clarity, consistency, adequacy, logical development, and level of theory development (Peterson & Bredow, 2013).

- Clarity: Are the theory's main components clearly stated and easily understood?
- Consistency: Are definitions of the key concepts consistent? Is the use of terms, interpretations, principles, and methods consistent?
- Adequacy: Does the theory cover all that it purports to cover? Are there gaps? Does the theory require further development?
- Logical development: Has the theory been logically developed over time? Are statements and conclusions well supported or are assumptions and premises unsubstantiated?
- Level of theory development: What is the stage of development of the theory? Are the elements named? Has the theory been around for some time, and can it be used to explain or predict outcomes? How frequently have researchers applied the theory to different situations?

External Criticism

Questions the reviewer should ask regarding external criticism pertain to the theory's relation to the real world, significance, scope, and complexity (Peterson & Bredow, 2013).

- Reality convergence: Is the theory consistent with the reader's experience of the world of nursing? Do the assumptions ring true?
- Utility: Is the theory useful to the researcher in terms of explaining a phenomenon and generating hypotheses?
- Significance: To what extent does the theory address issues important to nurses?
- Discrimination: Does the theory generate hypotheses that are not adequately addressed by other theories?
- Scope: Is the focus of the theory narrow enough to produce relational statements that are testable? Is the theory applicable to practice?
- Complexity: How complex is the theory? Is the theory parsimonious, using as few concepts as possible to explain it? Can the theory be easily understood?

When evaluating the use of a theory in a published study, the following steps are recommended (Grove et al., 2013).

1. Describe the theory used in the study. This is easier if the theory is explicitly identified and summarized. If possible, diagram the major concepts and the relationships among the concepts. Are theoretical and operational definitions identified?
2. Appraise the logical structure of the theory. If the theory identified in the article is linked to a larger theory, are the definitions consistent with the theorist's definitions? Are the variables reflective of

the major theoretical concepts? Are the conceptual definitions supported by the literature? Are the relational statements logical?

3. Evaluate the relationship between the theory and the methodology. Are the conceptual and theoretical definitions consistent? Are the hypotheses, questions, or objectives consistent with the relational statements in the theory? Is the fit between the relational statements and research design appropriate?

4. Appraise the findings. Are the findings interpreted in relation to the theory? Are the findings for the hypotheses, questions, or objectives consistent with the relational statements?

THEORY/PRACTICE/RESEARCH

There is a cyclical relationship among theory, practice, and research in that theory can provide a framework for or be generated from research and a framework for or be generated from practice (McEwen & Wills, 2011; Meleis, 2012). Theory that is generated from practice may be validated through research and, based on the findings from research, modified for continued use in practice. Theory lends structure to practice by enabling the APRN to "see" what is happening in a particular way and directing the APRN toward focused interventions. Theories also enable clinicians to make sense of seemingly disparate pieces of clinical data.

For example, in the study previously cited, Jiang and He (2012) found that their uncertainty intervention significantly decreased the uncertainty, anxiety, and depression and increased the quality of life experienced by persons with COPD. Thus, an APRN who works primarily with this population might be interested in implementing this intervention. However, the APRN should also be aware of limitations of the study. For example, the sample included people who had moderate to severe COPD for less than 2 years. The population also consisted of outpatients in China. Thus one can see that further research is needed to determine whether the intervention is effective with a wider range of the population. In other words, this intervention seems very promising, but the APRN who will use the findings in practice needs to ask whether it would also be effective with people who have had COPD longer than 2 years or who live in the United States or Europe. The need for further research does not preclude the use of the intervention in practice, but further research would potentially increase one's confidence that the intervention would produce positive outcomes.

SUMMARY

A theoretical or conceptual framework is constituted by concepts (words or terms) that represent abstract ideas, which are linked in a manner that represents the relationship between the concepts. The scope and purpose of the theory may vary. Theories might be grand, middle range, or practice/situation specific. Theories are useful in describing, explaining, and predicting phenomena. Depending on the scope and purpose, the theory may provide only general guidelines for practice or may provide new knowledge suitable for specific guidelines (Fawcett & DeSanto-Madeya, 2012).

Theories comprise concepts and relational statements that indicate how the concepts are related to each other. When evaluating a theory for use in research or evaluating a theoretically grounded research study for use in practice, it is important to scrutinize whether the selected theory is congruent with the research design and whether the theory and the findings are useful and applicable to the APRN's particular practice setting.

SUGGESTED ACTIVITIES

1. Debate whether nurses should only use theories developed within nursing or whether it is acceptable to use theories developed in other disciplines and used in research conducted by nurses.
2. Select an article that focuses on a clinical intervention that has been implemented as part of a research study. Identify the theory that was used to guide the study. Use the guidelines presented in this chapter to determine the fit between the focus of the study and the selected theory.
3. Using the same article, describe how knowledge gained from the study might be used in APRN practice.
4. Select a theory and illustrate how it can be used to describe, explain, or predict a phenomenon.

REFERENCES

Alhusen, J. D., Gross, D., Hayat, M. J., Woods, A. B., & Sharps, P. W. (2012). The influence of maternal-fetal attachment and health practices on neonatal outcomes in low-income, urban women. *Research in Nursing and Health, 35,* 112–120.

Bakan, G., & Akyol, A. D. (2008). Theory-guided interventions for adaptation to heart failure. *Journal of Advanced Nursing, 61,* 596–608.

Coopey, M., Nix, M. P., & Clancy, C. M. (2006). Translating research into evidence-based nursing practice and evaluating effectiveness. *Journal of Nursing Care Quality, 21,* 195–202.

Fawcett, J., & DeSanto-Madeya, S. (2012). *Contemporary nursing knowledge* (3rd ed.). Philadelphia, PA: F.A. Davis.

Gillespie, G. L., Hounchell, M., Pettinichi, J., Mattei, J., & Rose, L. (2012). Caring in pediatric emergency nursing. *Research and Theory for Nursing Practice: An International Journal, 26,* 216–232.

Grove, S. K., Burns, N., & Gray, J. R. (2013). *The practice of nursing research. Appraisal, synthesis, and generation of evidence.* St. Louis, MO: Elsevier Saunders.

Im, E. (2005). Development of situation-specific theories. An integrative approach. *Advances in Nursing Science, 28,* 137–151.

Im, E. (2010). A situation-specific theory of Asian immigrant women's menopausal symptom experience in the United States. *Advances in Nursing Science, 33,* 143–157.

Im, E., & Chang, S. J. (2012). Current trends in nursing theories. *Journal of Nursing Scholarship, 44,* 156–164.

Jiang, X., & He, G. (2012). Effects of an uncertainty management intervention on uncertainty, anxiety, depression, and quality of life of chronic obstructive pulmonary disease outpatients. *Research in Nursing and Health, 35,* 409–418.

Lewandowski, W. A. (2004). Patterning of pain and power with guided imagery. *Nursing Science Quarterly, 17,* 233–241.

McEwen, M., & Wills, E. M. (2011). *Theoretical basis for nursing* (3rd ed.). Philadelphia: Wolters Kluwer Health/Lippincott Williams & Wilkins.

Meleis, A. I. (2012). *Theoretical nursing. Development & progress* (5th ed.). Philadelphia, PA: Wolters Kluwer Health/Lippincott Williams & Wilkins.

Mishel, M. H. (1990). Reconceptualization of the uncertainty in illness theory. *Image: Journal of Nursing Scholarship, 22,* 256–262.

Peters, R. M., & Templin, T. N. (2010). Theory of planned behavior, self-care motivation, and blood pressure self-care. *Research and Theory for Nursing Practice: An International Journal, 24,* 172–186.

Peterson S. J., & Bredow, T. S. (2013). *Middle range theories. Application to nursing research.* Philadelphia, PA: Wolters Kluwer Health/Lippincott Williams & Wilkins.

Sanford, J., Townsend-Rocchiciolli, J., Horigan, A., & Hall, P. (2011). A process of decision making by caregivers of family members with heart failure. *Research and Theory for Nursing Practice: An International Journal, 25,* 55–70.

Siaki, L. A., Loescher, L. J., & Trego, L. L. (2013). Synthesis strategy: Building a culturally sensitive mid-range theory of risk perception using literary, quantitative, and qualitative methods. *Journal of Advanced Nursing, 69,* 726–737.

Spratling, R., & Weaver, S. R. (2012). Theoretical perspective: Resilience in medically fragile adolescents. *Research and Theory for Nursing Practice: An International Journal, 26,* 54–68.

Verran, J. A. (1997). The value of theory-driven (rather than problem-driven) research. *Seminars for Nurse Managers, 5*(4), 169–172.

Wagner, D. L., Bear, M., & Davidson, N. S. (2011). Measuring patient satisfaction with postpartum teaching methods used by nurses within the interaction model of client health behavior. *Research and Theory for Nursing Practice: An International Journal, 25,* 176–190.

8

Quantitative Research Designs for Nursing Practice

Margaret Irwin

Quantitative methods provide an objective means to answer questions and test hypotheses. In a quantitative approach, phenomena are reduced to numerical data for analysis and interpretation. Quantitative methods involve sampling, measurement, analysis, and the overall study design that provides the structure of the research. Statistical analysis of resulting data provides an objective view of the situation. Study implementation involves carrying out study procedures in a particular setting, collecting study data, and data management.

Quantitative methods can be used alone, or in combination with qualitative techniques for a mixed-method approach to analysis. In a mixed-method study design, qualitative results are used to provide additional depth and context to results. Qualitative and quantitative results can also be triangulated to demonstrate whether or not findings from both methods converge to support each other.

This chapter provides an overview of quantitative methods, including defining key variables of interest, measurement, data types, sampling concepts, overall study design, and analysis considerations. Practical aspects in planning and implementing quantitative research in clinical settings are briefly reviewed. Approaches to evaluate clinical as well as statistical significance of quantitative findings are briefly discussed.

STUDY VARIABLES

Every research study begins with the study question. A clear study question forms the foundation for the overall study design and identifies the variables of interest. Variables are the building blocks of a research

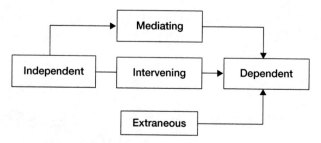

FIGURE 8.1   Types of variables.

study. Suppose, for example, that one is interested in the effect of a patient orientation program on patient's anxiety. The question posed is: Will a more comprehensive orientation program for patients reduce patient anxiety? The variables in this case are the orientation program and anxiety.

There are a number of different types of variables that may influence the subject of research. Interrelationships among possible types of variables are shown in Figure 8.1. As shown here, variables can be *independent, dependent, intervening, mediating,* or *moderating.* Dependent variables may also be termed *outcome* variables. Intervening and extraneous variables may also be termed *confounding* variables. Mediating variables are also termed *moderating* variables. In the previous example, the orientation program would be the *independent* variable. Anxiety would be the *dependent* variable, because the question posed suggests that results in anxiety depend on provision of the orientation program.

Intervening variables are other factors that might directly influence the outcome. Mediating variables are factors that affect the interaction between the independent and dependent variables and facilitate, augment, or reduce the effects of the independent variable. Conversely, moderating variables are factors that influence or create an interactive effect between two other variables. In this scenario, the astute clinician can speculate about other factors that might influence the dependent variable or effectiveness of the orientation program. Anxiety could differ between patients who are undergoing surgery and those who are not. The effectiveness of orientation on anxiety could differ for patients who have an underlying clinical anxiety disorder. These characteristics may affect the dependent variable and confound results obtained and can be seen as intervening variables.

The effect of the orientation program on anxiety may also be mediated by the way in which the orientation program is delivered. Say, for example, the orientation program is provided as a video disc that the patient can view at home prior to initiating treatment. The effectiveness of the program might be mediated by the number of times the patient views it or by whether the patient views it with family members and discusses the information provided with it. The effects of the orientation might be moderated by the patient's mental state. Extraneous variables such as characteristics of the clinical setting or social and family supports might also affect anxiety.

In quantitative methods, sampling and study design are used to control or provide data to explain effects of intervening, extraneous, or mediating variables. Collecting data to measure confounding variables enables analysis to evaluate potential effects on study outcomes. Statistics can then be used to select those factors in a situation that are the most important ones to include in a scientific description of a phenomenon (Marascuilo & Serlin, 1988).

MEASUREMENT

Measurement is the process of assigning numbers to variables. The devices and methods one uses for measurement are referred to as *instrumentation*. There are a variety of methods to obtain data, such as physical measurements; biomedical data; use of questionnaires; and use of patient rating scales, diaries, or responses in structured interviews. Whatever type of instrumentation is used, the characteristics of measurement that determine its quality and utility are *validity, reliability, sensitivity,* and *specificity.*

Validity refers to the degree to which the instrument used is truly a measure of the characteristic of interest. In instrument development, content experts are often used to determine the degree to which the individual items in the instrument represent the objectives of the measure. Two or more experts rate their agreement or disagreement with items on a scale, and the congruence of expert ratings is calculated to create an index. Scales used for this procedure may vary, but the overall index result will fall between −1 and +1. Positive index scores are needed to show validity, and the higher the score, the greater the validity (Waltz, Strickland, & Lenz, 1991). Validity may also be evaluated by comparison of instrument results to results of a known criterion measure, a "gold standard" measure, of the same concept, or to results of another instrument with known validity. The strength of statistical correlation between such measures provides information that can be used to judge validity.

Specific data such as these to determine validity are obtained through psychometric testing. Knowledge of the psychometric properties of an instrument, however, is only one factor to determine the validity of an instrument for a particular clinical application. Additional considerations are the diversity of conditions and types of samples in which the instrument has been tested and used. The degree of similarity between the situations and samples for which the instrument was tested and the situation and patient types in which the instrument may be used is a critical component in determining the validity for the intended application. For example, an instrument that is valid for measurement of functional impairment in the elderly may not be valid for measurement of functional impairment in children.

Reliability is one of three types: *inter-rater, test–retest reliability,* or *internal consistency*. Inter-rater reliability is the degree to which different observers would achieve the same result using the measurement instrument. If different people, using the same tool or making the same observation, would come up with very different results, confidence in the measurement and the resulting accuracy of results would be questionable. The *kappa* statistics can be used to evaluate inter-rater reliability. The value of kappa can be interpreted to represent the proportion of agreement in results among raters that did not occur by chance alone. So a kappa value of 0.65 suggests a 65% agreement between raters. Kappa can range from 0 to 1, and some general interpretations for the strength of agreement have been proposed, such that values greater than 0.4 show at least moderate inter-rater reliability, and values greater than 0.8 are extremely high (Sim & Wright, 2005). These are arbitrary interpretations. In general, it can be said that higher values reflect greater reliability.

Test–retest reliability refers to whether or not the same person using the instrument would get the same result with multiple uses. It is important to differentiate between reliability and expected change over time.

Internal consistency is applicable to measurement instruments such as questionnaires and multiple rating scales. Internal consistency shows the degree to which items on an instrument actually measure a single thing. If internal consistency is high, it suggests that the set of questionnaire items is measuring the same concept or variable. If internal consistency is low, it suggests that individual items within a questionnaire may be measuring different concepts. *Cronbach's alpha* is the statistic used most often to measure internal consistency.

Sensitivity is defined as the number of true positive decisions divided by the number of actual positive cases. It indicates the test ability to identify positive results and the degree to which a measurement method is responsive to changes in the variable of interest. Sensitivity also refers to the magnitude of a change that a measure will detect. The more sensitive a measure, the better it will reflect small changes in interventions that affect the variable being measured and detect positive findings.

Specificity is the degree to which a measurement result is indicative of a single characteristic and can accurately detect negative results.

Mathematically, specificity is the number of negative decisions divided by the number of true negative cases. In clinical settings, a receiver operator curve (ROC) is often used to display sensitivity and specificity (Park, Goo, & Jo, 2004).

In planning research, the objective is to select measurement methods that are specific, sensitive, and provide valid and reliable results. The type of reliability that matters most is related to the study design. In a repeated-measures design, test–retest reliability is important. In a study plan in which multiple observers collect data, it is important to be sure that different people using the same instrument in the same observation would obtain the same result, which means that the tool has good inter-rater reliability.

Availability, practicality, and cost of measurement methods also need to be considered in planning research in the clinical setting. In appraising research for application in the clinical setting, the quality of measurement methods is a factor that contributes to the confidence in overall results. The type of data that are generated with measurements used will also influence the type of analysis that can be done.

UNDERSTANDING DATA

Data are the discrete values that result from measurement of study variables. Quantitative data are one of four types in terms of its numerical scale: *nominal, ordinal, integer,* or *ratio*. These scales indicate a hierarchical structure for the data type, where the ratio scale is the highest scale level.

Nominal scale data assign a "name" to each observation. Gender is an example of a nominal scale variable. Examples of nominal scale variables encountered in the clinical setting are diagnosis-related-group (DRG) designation, diagnosis codes, and procedure codes. Nominal data are the lowest scale level.

Ordinal scales provide numerical data that have an "order." The most common examples of ordinal scale data are Likert-type scales, in which one rates an item on a scale such as (1) "poor," (2) "good," (3) "very good," or (4) "excellent." Responses have an order in relationship to each other, such that "good" is better than "poor," "very good" is better than "good," and so on. However, there is no mathematical relationship in this order. One cannot say that "good" is twice the value of "poor" or that "excellent" is twice the value of "very good." Results from typical patient satisfaction questionnaires used in the clinical setting are examples of ordinal scale data. Ordinal data are above nominal data on the scale hierarchy.

Integer scales provide data in which distances on the numerical scale are equal. The distance between the numbers 1 and 2 is the same as the distance between 2 and 3. The Fahrenheit temperature scale is an example of a typical integer scale. The difference between a temperature of 100°F and 90°F is the same as the difference between a temperature of 90°F and 80°F. One cannot, however say that 100° is exactly twice the temperature of 50°. Integer scales refer to equal distances, not a mathematical relationship. Patient ratings on a standard numerical pain symptom distress scale and patient severity scoring systems are examples of integer scales. Integer data are above ordinal data on the hierarchy of data scales.

Ratio scales provide the same information as integer scales, but in addition, have an absolute zero point. This means that mathematically, on a ratio scale, "20" is exactly twice "10," and "30" is exactly three times "10." Volume, length, weight, and time are examples of ratio scales.

The scale of the measurement has implications for the type of analysis that is most appropriate. The higher the scale level, according to the hierarchy as described above, the broader the range of statistical procedures one can employ. Nonparametric statistics are appropriate when dealing with nominal and ordinal data. Integer and ratio scale data can be analyzed with parametric statistical procedures.

There is some disagreement about the appropriate statistics that one can use with Likert-type, numerical rating scales, and total questionnaire scores. In some instruments, multiple Likert-type responses can be summed to provide total attribute scores or subscale scores. Some argue that resulting data simply order responses, whereas others contend that such scores truly represent the magnitude of the variable being measured, and that items summed for analysis approach the interval scale level. It has been suggested that the statistical analysis used should be driven by the nature of the clinical question, rather than focused on the level of the data (Waltz, Strickland, & Lenz, 1994).

SAMPLING

Given the many factors that can affect the dependent variable, quantitative research is generally designed to control, reduce, or account for as many of these factors as practical. This can be done by establishing study sample inclusion and exclusion criteria, including measurement and analysis of potential confounding variables in the study, and overall study design to reduce threats to validity.

In planning to study the effects of an intervention on patient anxiety, one might exclude patients who have a major anxiety disorder or cognitive impairment to reduce variation in study findings that could be attributed to these variables. Other variables that experience suggests might affect results, such as age, physical symptoms, diagnosis, and so on, can be measured and included in analysis and interpretation of findings. Selecting a homogenous sample of patients for a research study is helpful to reduce effects of confounding variables. However, it should be recognized that studying a very narrowly defined group of patients limits generalizability of findings to other types of patients.

Sampling decisions can also introduce bias into the study, because characteristics of patients included can influence results. Selection of a random sample of patients would be expected to provide a sufficient random distribution of characteristics to reduce such bias; however, random sampling is not often practical in prospective clinical research.

STUDY DESIGN

Quantitative study designs generally fall into one of two categories: descriptive studies or studies to evaluate the effectiveness of an intervention on patient outcomes. The study design is the structure of the research that defines the timing of observations and interventions and strategies used to ensure objectivity.

The study design can be visually represented to show the sequence of observations and interventions in a variety of ways. The X–O model uses an "X" to indicate the intervention, or independent variable, and an "O" to indicate the observation to measure the dependent outcome variable. Examples of the X–O model to illustrate study designs are shown in Figure 8.2.

Design		Representation
Descriptive, repeated measures		O_1 O_2 O_3
Randomized controlled design (no intervention control)	R	O X O O O
Quasi-experimental, single group pretest–posttest design		O X O
Randomized crossover design	R	OX_1 OX_2 O OX_2 OX_1 O

FIGURE 8.2 Example representations of research designs.
O, observation (measurement); R, random assignment to groups; X, intervention (where multiple interventions are used, subscripts show the different interventions).

Descriptive Designs

Descriptive studies provide information about commonalities and differences within a defined group of patients. Descriptive study design is used to identify the incidence or prevalence of conditions, fully describe a phenomenon, and to evaluate the relationships among variables explored as in a *correlation* analysis. Descriptive studies can be seen as exploratory in nature (Beck, 1999). The design may be *retrospective*, with information collected from the records of previous patients or other pre-existing sources of data; *prospective*, with data collected at the present time; or *longitudinal*, with data collection at time points in the future as well.

Correlation designs are used to evaluate relationships or associations among variables. Statistical analysis such as regression and other multivariate techniques can be done to evaluate those variables that may predict or influence results in patient outcomes. Correlation design can be viewed as a type of descriptive design, because it does not involve the attempt to evaluate causality or effects of an intervention.

Designs to Evaluate Effects

There are a variety of research study designs that are used to evaluate the effects of interventions. Each of these designs has strengths and limitations. The goal is to use a design that has few inherent limitations and minimizes potential bias to support internal validity of the study. The study design also needs to be practical in the setting in which it is being implemented. Designs that aim to evaluate effects of interventions include *observational, quasi-experimental* and *experimental*.

Observational Studies

Observational studies are those in which the outcomes of interest are analyzed between groups of patients that received different interventions. In this design, interventions are not controlled and patients are not specifically sampled or assigned to treatments. Patients, interventions, and results are described and statistical analysis of data is used to determine differences in outcomes. This type of design is used when usual clinical care varies, or standard approaches for care have changed over time. Patient outcomes with different concurrent treatments or differences from historical results are compared. Studies identified as *naturalistic* design are a type of observational study. This type of design has several inherent biases and threats to validity and does not provide evidence to determine a cause-and-effect relationship. Comparison to historical control groups introduces the threat of history, and lack of random assignment of patients presents the possibility that factors other than the independent variable created or mediated results found and differences between groups.

In situations in which the independent variable cannot be manipulated, observational studies may be the only option to begin to answer clinical questions about the results of a specific intervention. In this case, it is important to measure and analyze potential intervening and extraneous variables insofar as possible, to begin to rule out other variables that may have produced the results seen. Although a single observational type of study cannot provide evidence of cause and effect, it does provide some evidence that is stronger than case study level evidence, and if multiple observational studies provide the same conclusions, the synthesis of that information provides stronger evidence about efficacy.

Quasi-Experimental Studies

Quasi-experimental designs can be constructed with single or multiple groups, and may involve pretest and post-test or post-test only measurement. The pretest–posttest design is one in which measurement of the dependent variable is done prior to, and then again after an intervention, in the same subject or group. Changes in the dependent variable from pre- to postintervention in each subject are compared. In this design, the individual patient essentially functions as his or her own "control." The difference between pre- and postintervention measurement is analyzed to evaluate the impact of the intervention. In a post-test only design, the intervention is provided and the dependent variable is measured only after the intervention. This design suffers from the same problems as an observational study, and is not particularly informative. In a two-group posttest-only design, the lack of a pretest points to the possibility that any differences between groups may be due to selection bias rather than an intervention effect (Cook & Campbell, 1979).

In quasi-experimental studies, without comparison to a group that did not have the intervention, there is no way to tell whether changes in the outcome would have occurred in any case. An example of this phenomenon is seen with the trajectory of patient anxiety levels in the course of treatment for cancer. A substantial body of research has shown that over time during active antitumor treatment, in the general population of patients with cancer, levels of anxiety tend to decline. If an intervention aimed to reduce anxiety is given to a single group of patients and then anxiety is later measured, it is possible that any decline in anxiety observed would have occurred anyway, without the intervention.

Experimental Designs

Experimental designs involve the use of at least two study groups, one of which is in a control condition, not receiving the experimental intervention. This allows for comparison of outcomes that can overcome the limitation seen in a quasi-experimental design. The critical elements in planning this type of design are the method of patient assignment to groups, and the nature of the control condition.

Patient Assignment to Study Groups

In a *nonrandom* design, patients are assigned to study groups by the researcher, or by patient self-selection of the group in which they want to participate. The key limitation to this approach is the fact that patients in the control or intervention groups may have different characteristics that influence the outcome. This can be addressed to some extent in analysis by examination of the differences between the groups; however, it is likely that the researcher may not have data to compare all of the potential characteristics that function as intervening variables. Another approach is to match patients in an intervention group to those in the control group, either through sample selection or in the analysis of results, based on key characteristics that might influence outcomes. This approach can help reduce unexplained variability; however, it is unlikely that the researcher is able to account for every individual characteristic that might be important. Also, sufficient analysis within subgroups of patients based on these characteristics would generally require a large overall sample size in order to detect statistically and clinically significant differences. Where random assignment is not feasible, a matched control design does provide better evidence than a simple nonrandom group assignment. This type of study design is not a true experimental design, though it may often be labeled as such.

Random assignment of patients to study groups, in a *randomized controlled design* is the generally accepted way to attempt to spread the effect of intervening and extraneous variables across study groups by chance alone. Without random assignment there is a potential for *selection bias*, resulting in selection of particular types of patients to receive particular treatments (The CONSORT Group, 2010). The randomized controlled trial (RCT) is generally viewed as the most valid approach and the only true experimental design. It is important, however, to recognize that not all study questions can be subjected to this approach. Quasi-experimental or observational design is often more practical in the clinical setting.

Control Conditions

The nature of the control condition used in a controlled trial is also important. Studies may use a *placebo* control, *active* control, or *attentional* control as the control condition. In a placebo-controlled trial, individuals in the control group receive an inactive treatment that appears exactly like the intervention being tested. This approach is most often associated with trials of new medications, but is not limited to that type of intervention. In some cases, use of a placebo would be inappropriate, unethical, or impractical. For patients who required medications for a health condition, use of a placebo rather than an active medication would be inappropriate. With interventions that involve invasive procedures, one would not unnecessarily expose patients to risks without any expected benefit, and there may be limited ability to provide an inactive form or "sham" version of the intervention.

In such cases, researchers may use an *active* control group. In this approach, the control group receives a different intervention for the same problem, and outcomes between the two groups are compared. Active controls may be current standard treatments or "usual care" for the problem or a different experimental intervention. Designs with active control conditions may be aimed at testing a new intervention or specifically aimed at comparing the effects of alternate treatments.

One of the recent developments in research design using an active control is a *noninferiority* study design. A noninferiority study design aims to show that an experimental intervention is not less effective than a known treatment. This design requires the investigator to establish a planned margin of effect of the new treatment that is clinically acceptable. The margin is generally determined from the clinically acceptable difference between interventions tested, and the known effect size of the comparison treatment. Statistical analysis is done to test the hypothesis that results are not significantly different from the margin used (U.S. Department of Health and Human Services, 2010). Positive results are interpreted to demonstrate that the experimental intervention is not less effective than the alternative used in the study. One consideration in interpretation of an inferiority design study is whether or not the margin established is clinically acceptable. For example, recent studies in the effectiveness of various antiemetic regimens to prevent nausea and vomiting in patients receiving emetogenic chemotherapy have established a margin of 15% difference in the proportion of patients who obtain complete control of the symptom. It is up to the clinician evaluating these results to judge whether or not that 15% difference is acceptable to say that interventions are essentially equally effective.

Attentional control is a concept that needs to be considered in studies that involve examination of psychosocial, educational, and supportive types of interventions. It can be expected, for many types of patient outcomes, that providing additional attention alone to the patient can result in the patient feeling better. For example, if the researcher is examining the effect of a patient support group or a nursing supportive intervention on patient anxiety, it is likely that giving more attention and spending more time with the patient can reduce anxiety. For valid comparison, the control group should be given similar time and attention as the experimental group. In this area, researchers can provide some kind of "neutral" time and attention to patients as a control condition. A simple example of attentional control use is seen in a study to test the effects of progressive muscle relaxation and guided imagery on pain severity among hospitalized patients with cancer. Patients randomized to the experimental group were given a compact disc (CD) to use for the intervention. Attentional control was provided to the control-group patients by giving them a CD that provided them with general information (Kwekkeboom, Wanta, & Bumpus, 2008).

Other Design Concepts

Crossover Design

A *crossover* design is a type of experimental design used to provide an even stronger basis for comparison between study interventions or conditions. Even with well-controlled randomized designs, it is understood that human experience and outcomes can be affected by a huge number of personal, environment, social, and other factors. In a crossover design, individual patients are exposed to both the control and experimental conditions, and results from each condition in all patients are compared. Usually, subjects are randomly assigned to the sequence in which the intervention or control condition will be provided. One of the major threats in this design is contamination, due to continued effects of either treatment condition. The degree of threat depends on the nature of the intervention. In clinical trials involving medications, patients have a "wash-out" period between study conditions, so that the effects of one medication are no longer present before the patient is exposed to the other medication. With other types of interventions, an appropriate amount of time needed to eliminate intervention effects may not be clear, or may not be possible.

An example of this situation can be seen in a study of the use of self-hypnosis for symptom management in patients with cancer reported by Ebell (2008). In this study, patients were exposed to two research conditions: one involving use of pharmacologic management alone and one in which patients were also taught self-hypnosis to manage pain. Subjects were randomly assigned to the order in which they were treated and then crossed over to the other study condition. The author noted that there appeared to be a carry-over effect of self-hypnosis for those patients who received the self-hypnosis training before they were crossed over to receive only medication. It was likely that patients who had successfully applied self-hypnosis for pain control continued to apply it during the study period in which they were only being actively treated pharmacologically. For these patients, the pharmacologic treatment-only control condition was contaminated by their prior learning (Ebell, 2008).

Longitudinal Design

Longitudinal design involves some duration of follow-up after an intervention to determine longer-term effects over time. It is not clear how long the follow-up needs to be for us to term it a "longitudinal" design, and study follow-up periods can be decades, as seen in some epidemiological research. Depending on the study question, the duration of effect may be of interest, and necessitate some follow-up period for evaluation. In clinical situations or patient problems that last for months or years, the effect of an intervention at a single point in time immediately after an intervention or 2 days later, is not sufficient to address the clinical problem. Measurement of outcomes at subsequent times is used to evaluate duration of effect. Longitudinal studies often involve repeated-measures design. Major problems encountered in longitudinal studies are patient loss to follow-up or subject attrition and the fact that other events can occur between the intervention and the follow-up measurement that are unknown and can affect results.

Duration of Effect

In any design to evaluate the effects of an intervention, the meaningful duration of an effect should also be a consideration in the timing of postintervention measures. In addition to longitudinal designs that evaluate longer term results, one may be interested in knowing shorter term duration of effects. This depends on the nature of the dependent variable of interest. For example, if one wants to know whether provision of therapeutic touch can relieve acute pain, an immediate postintervention measurement can answer that question. However, if one wants to know whether therapeutic touch can relieve a more chronic and lasting symptom, a single immediate postmeasurement provides insufficient information to address the question. In this type of situation, one may consider using a repeated-measures design to see how long an effect lasts.

Repeated-Measures Design

Repeated-measures design refers to measurement of variables multiple times. This approach can be used within any type of descriptive or interventional research. Measurement of dependent variables at multiple points in time enables evaluation of trends and timing of effects. There is no rule to guide the exact timing of repeated measures. Clinical judgment and review of findings from other research in the area can guide this decision.

Design concepts reviewed here can be combined in various ways. Randomized controlled trials often involve pre- and postintervention measurement of dependent variables. Study groups may be included that provide several types of control conditions. Any type of study may be designed to include long-term patient follow-up with a longitudinal approach. Across all types of studies, the design needs to be planned to reduce potential bias and threats to the internal validity of the study. Design features create inherent risks of bias and threats to validity.

SOURCES OF BIAS IN QUANTITATIVE METHODS

Bias is a type of systematic error that can distort findings in quantitative studies (Sica, 2006). There are several typical sources of potential bias in quantitative methods.

- **Selection bias** can be introduced by inclusion of only certain patients in a study. Within specific study inclusion criteria, if only certain patients participate in the study, or patients in one study group drop out, the sample may be biased. The degree to which this is a problem can be addressed by analyzing and describing differences between individuals who do and do not participate in or complete the study, or comparison of the study sample to characteristics of the population at large. This allows appraisal of key patient differences that may influence findings. Another approach that is used to address this type of bias and the related problems of missing data and study attrition is *intent to treat* (ITT) analysis. ITT is most effectively used as a strategy in study design and conduct, rather than just an analytic approach (Gupta, 2011). ITT analysis includes all study subjects regardless of conforming to inclusion criteria, treatments actually received, or withdrawal from the study. This prevents overoptimistic estimates of effectiveness of an intervention. This approach necessitates conducting clinical research to avoid missing data and to continue to follow up as much as possible with individuals who may withdraw. There are a variety of pros and cons for ITT analysis and several approaches in data analysis are used to deal with missing data (Lachin, 2000; Montori & Guyatt, 2001). Although ITT analysis prevents overoptimistic conclusions about effectiveness, it can also underestimate actual effects.
- **Intervention bias** may be introduced in a study in which there are critical differences between individuals who receive an experimental treatment and those who do not. Approaches that are used to address intervention bias are random subject assignment to study groups and matching patients assigned to different study groups on the basis of key variables that are expected to influence outcomes.
- **Measurement bias** can be a problem with the instrumentation used in the research as well as the method of data collection. Investigators are subject to human error and consciously or unconsciously motivated to achieve desired results. These can affect the accuracy of study measurements. Selection of appropriate measurement instruments is important to reduce this potential bias. Keeping data collectors and investigators unaware of patient group assignment in the study through blinding is used to avoid measurement bias introduced by investigators.

THREATS TO VALIDITY

Both research design and implementation affect the validity of the study. Validity can be expressed as the degree of confidence that changes seen in a dependent variable are the result of the independent variable studied, rather than some unknown extraneous variables. In purely descriptive studies, internal validity refers to the accuracy and quality of the study. In studies that are done to evaluate effects of interventions, there are a number of additional specific threats to external and internal validity that have been described (Beck, 1999; Campbell & Stanley, 1966; Cook & Campbell, 1979; Huitt, Hummel, & Kaeck, 1999; Koshar, 2006).

Internal Threats to Validity

Extraneous variables that can reduce internal study validity are outlined below. Although these are discussed as unique issues, it should be recognized that multiple threats can be present, can interact, and can have a cumulative effect on the validity of a given research study. Random assignment to study groups addresses many of these threats, because it allows one to reasonably expect that the distribution of extraneous variables would be similar across groups and has similar effects on outcomes in all study groups. A list of threats to validity, aspects of study design and implementation that are likely to produce the threat, and some approaches to avoid or reduce the threat are shown in Table 8.1.

- **History** is a threat when an observed effect may be due to something other than the intervention and intervening or mediating variables measured between a pretest and posttest. Other unobserved changes may have occurred over time. This threat is more common with longitudinal and repeated-measures designs than those in which data are collected over shorter time periods. History is also a factor in studies using comparison to historical control groups. Measurement and inclusion of potential intervening and mediating variables as covariates in analysis can facilitate interpretation of the role of history in findings.
- **Maturation** results in natural changes over time as subjects become older, wiser, stronger, bored, more or less motivated, and so on. This type of threat is associated with longitudinal designs, particularly those that involve children or individuals with diseases that naturally progress over time. Analysis of potential covariates to illuminate maturation effects can be helpful.

TABLE 8.1 Threats to Internal Validity: Contributing Aspects and Approaches

THREAT	DESIGN ASPECTS	APPROACHES
History	Longitudinal studies Studies using repeated measures Long time period between pre- and postmeasures	Measure potential intervening variables and include in analysis Limit time between pre- and postobservations Random group assignment
Maturation	Longitudinal studies, especially involving children, individuals with conditions that naturally progress	Measure/account for disease progression and other factors Random group assignment
Testing	Repeated measures and pretest–posttest design, especially if the same tool is used repeatedly Test battery administration	Multiple measures and different tool versions Consider mixed-method design Random group assignment
Instrumentation	Biomedical instruments and calibration needs Biological samples—obtaining, storage, and testing Instrument validity, reliability, sensitivity, and specificity	Logical score groupings in analysis to account for floor and ceiling effects Select instruments with known reliability and performance Educate data collectors in instrument use Blinding of data collectors/investigators
Statistical regression	Pretest–posttest design Repeated measures design Sample with extreme high or low scores	Observe changes in extreme scores Random group assignment
Attrition, high dropout rate, mortality	Longitudinal designs Lack of placebo, active or attentional control	Intent to treat design Analyze characteristics of dropouts and compare to remaining sample Plan for attrition in sample size Use appropriate control conditions Minimize participation burden

Contamination/ diffusion of treatment	Studies involving two or more groups in the same location	Plan approaches to minimize study group interactions
	Crossover designs involving patient psychoeducation and behavior-change interventions	Use of attentional control condition
Compensatory rivalry	Two or more group trials with no active or attentional control—comparison to usual care only	Subject blinding
		Placebo, attentional, or active control conditions
Compensatory equalization of treatment	Two or more group trials with no active or attentional control—comparison to usual care only	Blinding of group assignment
		Use of active and attentional control conditions
Selection/sample bias	Nonrandom group assignment	Random group assignment
		Analyze differences between groups in key intervening variables
Lack of intervention fidelity	Multiple intervention providers	Observe or analyze random sample of intervention sessions to assess fidelity
	Complexity and interactive nature of the intervention	Train providers in the intervention
		Clear process and directions

■ **Testing** can be an issue when measurement methods involve the use of patient questionnaires, testing, and self-report measures. Familiarity with a test can enhance performance, because questions and answers may be remembered and "desired" answers can be learned. This is a problem when the same measurement instrument is used multiple times, as in repeated-measures design, or when the measurement itself can cause a change in performance. Effects of testing can also be an issue in studies in which a large battery of questionnaires is administered to patients, where patient fatigue can affect responses. Triangulation of results from several instruments and using alternative forms of a test can address this threat. Use of a mixed-method design can also be employed to confirm quantitative results with qualitative findings.

■ **Instrumentation** is a threat when there is a change in the measurement instrument or scoring by an observer between pre- and post-intervention points. Observer judgment or experience can change over time. With biomedical and technical instrumentation, calibration and instrument reliability should be confirmed. Instrumentation is also an issue with measurement tools that perform differently at the ends of a scale than they do at the midpoint. This situation results in what are termed "floor" or "ceiling" effects in measurement. With ceiling or floor effects, changes in the variable being measured may not be observable if the value is already at the high or the low end of the possible scale. This type of threat is of concern when measurement is done by a single observer, when data are collected in person, and studies in which pretest values are already at extreme high or low values. Selection of valid and reliable instruments with known normative ranges can assist the researcher in determining whether this is a threat in the study.

■ **Statistical regression** is a natural statistical phenomenon in which individuals who have extreme results (either high or low) will have scores that move toward the mean on a repeated test, and the resulting group mean will change. The magnitude of regression depends in part on the test–retest reliability of measurement. The potential for statistical regression is greatest when a study sample demonstrates extreme scores on the instrument used.

■ **Attrition** is a threat when individuals who drop out of a study, or are lost to follow-up, are different from those who remained in the study in ways that influence results. This can create an artifact in results, if study groups are different kinds of people at the posttest time point compared to those who completed a pretest. Attrition is a problem in longitudinal studies and studies that may require substantial effort or impose burden on participants. Obtaining a sample size that accounts for possible attrition should be considered in planning the study. Analysis of key characteristics of those who withdraw versus those who complete the study enables one to determine whether significant differences between those individuals may have influenced results. Attrition also says something about the utility of the intervention. If large numbers of patients drop out of an experimental group, the intervention being tested may not be acceptable to patients, may create too much of a burden to participate, or may be associated with more negative side effects than benefits.

■ **Contamination** occurs if treatment is diffused to subjects in different study groups because participants interact and learn from each other. This can also happen, as previously mentioned, in crossover designs in which subjects who initially receive an education or behavioral intervention continue strategies learned in subsequent observations. This can be a problem with studies involving two or more study groups in the same location. Implementing the study in such a way that groups will not be in contact with each other is one way to avoid this problem.

■ **Compensatory rivalry** is a situation in which subjects in the control group feel neglected or see themselves as underdogs, and are motivated to compete or perform in an attempt to reverse expected effects of an intervention. This is most problematic with study designs in which subjects know they are in the control group and where intact units of staff are assigned to interventions. Blinding study subjects to group assignment and provision of active, placebo, or attentional control conditions can reduce this type of threat.

■ **Compensatory equalization of treatments can occur when** staff or administrators feel that persons who do not receive the intervention are lacking a benefit and compensate for this perceived lack. This threat is most likely in studies in which group assignment is known to others and no placebo, attentional, or active controls are used.

■ **Resentful demoralization of no-treatment groups** can be an issue if individuals who are not receiving what is seen as a more desirable treatment become discouraged and perform at a lower level in retaliation or because they feel dejected. This is a potential threat in study designs in which group assignment is known, and those in which no appropriate control conditions are provided. This may also be more expected in studies involving work or other settings, where individuals may retaliate for lack of a perceived advantage by lowering productivity. Blinding to group assignment and use of appropriate attentional or active control conditions help to address this problem.

■ **Lack of treatment fidelity** occurs when the intervention is not provided in a consistent manner to all study subjects. Treatment fidelity may be an issue when study interventions are provided by several different people, or where the intervention is provided as patient self-care in using or applying a particular approach to manage problems or symptoms. Provider training, provision of clear guidelines, references, and treatment algorithms can enhance performance of the intervention consistently. When the intervention is dependent on patient use, patients reminders can be used, and patient diaries or post-test interviews can be used to assess the patient's adherence to interventions. In clinical drug trials, documentation of protocol violations is used to evaluate treatment fidelity.

External Threats to Validity

External threats to validity refer to the extent to which a given study's findings can be generalized to different people, times, settings, and conditions. This involves potential statistical interactions that may not be readily discernible from specific study data and are best understood through deductive reasoning (Cook & Campbell, 1979). Experience in relevant clinical care and knowledge of the field of study enable judgment of the applicability of findings in larger contexts.

IMPLEMENTING RESEARCH IN THE CLINICAL SETTING

Implementing research involves performing interventions as planned according to the study design and collecting study data. Operationalizing the study in a clinical setting requires a design that is practical as well as wellconstructed to minimize threats to validity. The workability of providing the intervention as planned in the specific setting is an important initial consideration. It is valuable to pilot planned approaches and perform a feasibility study to test the study plan and methods.

Providing the Intervention

The importance of setting was illustrated in a study designed to determine the effectiveness of a brief preoperative hypnosis intervention on severity of postoperative pain (Lew, Kravtiz, Garberoglio, & Williams, 2011). In this study, a 15- to 20-minute hypnosis intervention was provided to surgical outpatients in the surgical holding area. The intervention was complicated by multiple interruptions required in the usual course of preoperative care, a relatively noisy environment, and lack of sufficient privacy. These problems made it difficult to induce a sufficient state in many study participants. The study demonstrated no effect of the intervention. The author noted that the lack of effect was likely due to the inability to provide the intervention appropriately.

If study interventions involve use of specific psychoeducational, supportive, an behavioral interventions, it is important to ensure that the key underlying principles in the approach are used as desired. In addition to general approaches to ensure treatment fidelity, reliability of the intervention can be analyzed by observation of a random sample of interventions directly, or through review of randomly selected video or audiotaped sessions.

Data Collection

Providing health care to individuals generates a wealth of data. Clinical settings maintain computerized data sets for purposes of billing, quality reporting, result reporting, and electronic health records. Clinical practice generates information about individual patient demographic and biomedical information. Specific admission data on patient functional status and other factors are routinely obtained on patient admission to rehabilitation units and home care agencies as required by Medicare and other insurance companies for reimbursement. Hospital administrative and financial data sets contain information such as admission and discharge dates, length of stay, diagnosis codes, and procedure codes. Intensive-care-setting data often include patient severity scores, and emergency departments may generate triage and trauma scores. These data can be used for descriptive analysis and incorporated into interventional studies to provide data about the characteristics of the subjects studied.

Many of the phenomena of interest to nursing are not readily available from existing data sets or incorporated in an easily usable form into electronic medical records. Relevant data must be obtained through review and coding of verbal documentation or directly obtained by patient observation or patient responses on a questionnaire or rating scale. There are many different instruments available to use for patient rating of symptoms, and measurement of attributes such as anxiety, depression, quality of life, and so forth. Internet and literature searches can be used to identify instruments designed to measure a wide variety of patient attributes and symptoms.

Data can also be generated from abstraction and coding of medical record documentation. Suppose one wants to determine whether nurses routinely assess patients for depressive symptoms, and current practice does not include use and documentation of any formal screening tool. Progress notes can be used to collect data from what is documented regarding symptoms of depression. However, to do so, the researcher needs to predefine what documented statements are acceptable as indicators that symptoms have been assessed. One of the challenges in this method is to ensure that all individuals who abstract data interpret verbal documentation in the same way. The investigator would need to decide how documentation would be coded or counted to generate numerical data for use in analysis.

Another challenge with data collection from medical record review comes from the fact that open-ended documentation may not routinely capture information about the variables of interest. Just because a clinician did not ask a patient about his or her experience of fatigue or document that a patient said he or she was fatigued, does not mean that the patient did not experience fatigue. Validity and reliability of abstracted data can be evaluated by auditing a random sample of cases to ensure acceptable interpretation of documentation and data collected.

There also has to be an organized way to collect and manage that information. For this type of data collection, creation of a data-collection tool, or check sheet is essential. A check sheet can be a paper form, or can be set up as a spreadsheet tool for data collection and data entry.

Consideration of practicality and time involved in data collection and data management are important components of planning clinical research. When possible, using existing data and repurposing data for study purposes can address the barrier of time. It is helpful to collaborate with key individuals in an organization to identify what information already exists that can be captured and used to answer study questions. Managers and directors of various clinical departments can identify the type of information that is contained in their systems. Medical record coding professionals can provide insight into how items such as diagnosis and procedure codes can be used to define patient characteristics and outcomes. Infection control and quality professionals can identify the type of information that is available from their work that may already reside in computer systems. Librarians can provide assistance in searching for existing measurement tools and approaches in the area of interest for study. Information systems professionals can assist in efforts to extract data from existing computer systems for analysis.

DATA ANALYSIS

There are two types of statistical analysis—*descriptive* and *inferential*. Descriptive statistics illustrate characteristics within a defined set of data. In contrast, inferential statistics are used to extrapolate findings beyond a single data set to determine the probability that results are applicable beyond the individual sample.

Descriptive Statistics

Descriptive statistics are used whenever the researcher wants to describe the findings within a sample of observations to someone else. Data can be described and communicated more easily if they are organized and summarized. The first step in organizing data for analysis and interpretation is a frequency distribution. Other aspects of describing any set of quantitative results revolve around demonstrating commonalities, differences, and relationships.

The most important characteristics of any distribution of data are the central tendency and the variability (Glass & Hopkins, 1984). The central tendency of the sample in a given attribute is one way to demonstrate what is common in a set of scores—how things look on average. Measures of central tendency are the mean, median, and mode. The mode is the score that occurs most frequently. The median is the 50% percentile of distribution—the point at which one-half of the scores are lower, and one-half of the scores are higher. The mean is the sum of scores divided by the number of scores.

There is no clear answer as to which of these measures is the best. The mean can be used more easily in further statistical analysis, but extreme scores in the distribution will affect it, and it may not be the most accurate representation of the average. The measure that can be used also depends upon the scale of the data gathered. If the data are nominal scale, only the mode is meaningful.

Measures of differences in a set of scores include the range, standard deviation, and variance. The range is the difference between the lowest and highest scores. The standard deviation and variance are calculated from the deviation, or distance, of all scores from the group mean. As such, these provide a view of the overall dispersion of results. The standard deviation is a linear measure. The variance is calculated as the standard deviation squared, providing a more three-dimensional picture of the overall difference in the variable being represented by the data. The standard deviation and variance can be compared between groups to evaluate the magnitude of differences. For example, if one has two samples or two groups with the same mean, but the standard deviation in group 1 is 3, and the standard deviation in group 2 is 6, one can conclude that the variability in group 2 is greater. Just as study design aims to reduce the potential for unexplained variability, analysis attempts to objectively account for the amount of variance found.

There are a number of different measures for assessing relationships and associations among variables. The strategy used depends on the scale and nature of the data. For example, if the researcher is interested in determining if a characteristic is associated with an age, one could calculate a correlation coefficient such as the *Pearson product moment* between the raw values of age and the measure of the characteristic. The relationship between age and some characteristic could also be evaluated with a procedure such as *chi-squared* by using age groups and determining if the average characteristic score, or if the percentage of patients who have the characteristic differs significantly across age groups. Both approaches would yield the same conclusion. There are a variety of correlation statistics that can be used with nominal, ordinal, and integer data.

Inferential Statistics

The term *inferential* comes from the fact that these statistical procedures enable the researcher to draw inferences about populations from sample findings. We are used to talking about whether something is "statistically significant" based on the *p* value of findings, but what does that actually mean? Clear interpretation of meaning necessitates an understanding of basic concepts of error and probability that apply to inferential statistics.

Hypothesis Testing and Error

Inferential statistics use the scientific method, posing a hypothesis that is then tested using probability theory. By convention, one poses a *null hypothesis*, and then calculates the probability of error in concluding that the null hypothesis is false. The underlying principle is that the researcher's theory or proposition is considered false until proven to be true beyond reasonable doubt (Kraemer & Thiemann, 1987). It is useful to have a clear statement of the null hypothesis to clearly interpret the statistical findings. The null hypothesis can be readily derived from the study question. For example, if the study question is: "Is there a relationship between anxiety and pain?" the corresponding null hypothesis would be: "There is *no* relationship between anxiety and pain." To support the researcher's actual theory that there is some relationship between these variables, the researcher has to show that the opposite conclusion, the null hypothesis, is not true.

In probability theory, there are two types of errors in hypothesis testing that can occur, *type I* and *type II*. These are displayed in Figure 8.3. As shown here, a type I error occurs if one concludes that the null hypothesis is false, when it is actually true. In contrast, a type II error occurs if one concludes that the null hypothesis is true, when it is actually false. The probability of a type I error is termed alpha (α), and the probability of a type II error is beta (β). Using the above

Actual situation	Conclusion drawn	
Null hypothesis is true	Null hypothesis is true	Null hypothesis is false Type II error β
Null hypothesis is false	Null hypothesis is true Type I error α	Null hypothesis is false Power $1 - \beta$

FIGURE 8.3   Error types and power.

example, a p value (α) of 0.05 means that the chance of incorrectly concluding that there *is* a relationship between anxiety and pain (making a type I error and incorrectly rejecting the null hypothesis) is 5%. Another way of stating this is that a p value of 0.05 shows that there is a 5% chance that the results occurred by chance alone.

Another approach for hypothesis testing is the use of a *confidence interval* (CI) rather than calculating an actual p value (Savory, 2008; Sim & Reid, 1999). For example, if one obtains a Pearson product-moment correlation coefficient between anxiety and pain of 0.46, and obtains a 95% CI of 0.23 to 0.7, the results obtained are significant at the 0.05 level. If the statistic obtained falls within the CI, and the actual CI does not include 0, the finding is statistically significant, and the null hypothesis can be rejected. In this example the value of 0.46 is within the interval and the CI does not contain 0, so it is significant at the $\alpha = 0.05$ level.

Further interpretation of a CI can be a bit confusing. The CI does not indicate that 95% of the time the correlation coefficient in individuals will be between those values. This CI indicates that there is 95% confidence that the coefficient in the population, rather than an individual or a single sample, would be contained within this range (Savory, 2008). To some extent, one can also say something about the precision of the finding. If the CI is very large, the finding is not very precise.

The actual probability and testing for β (type II error) is not generally done due to the degree of specificity that would be required for the researcher to test the alternative to the null hypothesis. For such testing, it would be necessary to know the possible values of the dependent variable in the theoretical population that underlies the statistical testing. In the real world, this information is not known. To minimize the risk of a type II error, the researcher needs to choose the largest sample size available (Marascuilo & Serlin, 1988).

Power

Another important statistic to consider is *power*. Power indicates the degree of assurance one can have in the statistical conclusions, considering that, even with a low p value and probability of a type I error, there is also still the possibility of a type II error. Statistical power findings give further information about the reliability of conclusions. Power analysis is generally used to determine the sample size that is needed, at a specified level of α, to have confidence in the findings. Usually researchers calculate sample sizes needed to achieve results at least at 80% power. Power at the level of 0.8 indicates that the researcher can expect that 80% of the time the study would yield the correct conclusion in terms of rejecting the null hypothesis. The interpretation of power is shown in Figure 8.3.

Power calculations require that one establishes a critical *effect size* in the dependent variable that one wants to be able to detect, and the probability of making a type I error one will accept. Say, for example, that one is investigating the effect of an intervention on patient self-reported pain severity on a 100-mm visual analogue scale. From reading previous research in this area, and from experience with patients, the researcher identifies that a change in severity of 20 mm is a reasonable reduction in pain. This value can be used as the size of effect that the researcher wants to be able to detect. At the same time, the researcher wants to be able to have 95% confidence that results obtained are not due to chance alone, so α is set at 0.05. These two pieces of information are used to determine the sample size needed to accomplish these goals.

Effect Size

It is important to remember that statistical significance does not necessarily indicate clinical significance, or results that are meaningful for actual clinical practice. There are a number of additional statistics that can be helpful to clinicians in drawing conclusions about potential effects or benefits of interventions. In addition to providing information for power analysis, the concept of effect size can tell us something about how meaningful findings can be in real clinical situations. Effect size is a concept that indicates the magnitude of the relationship observed between variables (Ferguson, 2009). Strength of effect can be evaluated in research results from statistics such as the Pearson product-moment and other correlation coefficients, standard mean difference (SMD), odds ratio (OR), relative risk (RR) ratio, and statistics such as Cohen's *d* and Hedges's *g*.

The Pearson product-moment correlation, designated by *r*, has an effect size between +1 and −1. The correlation coefficient squared (r^2) shows the proportion of the total variance in the dependent variable that is explained by the independent variable. For example, if the correlation between anxiety and severity of pain is 0.4, this says that 16% (0.4^2) of the total variance in pain severity is explained by anxiety. Clinician judgment can be applied to evaluate whether explaining 16% of total variance in pain severity is meaningful or not in the clinical context.

The SMD can be calculated for effect size when results are based on population means and standard deviations. The SMD is calculated as the difference between population means divided by the variance. Cohen's *d* is also based on means and standard deviations as the difference between two population means. It is important to note that effect size measures that use means are not just the average difference between pre- and postresults. In thinking about effect size, both the mean and the variability in results need to be considered together.

Observation*	Treatment group (number of cases)	
	Standard care	New intervention
Event happens/desired outcome occurs	a	b
Event does not happen/desired outcome does not occur	c	d

FIGURE 8.4   Matrix for calculation of odds ratio (OR) and relative risk (RR) ratio.
*The observation can be a positive event, such as improvement in a symptom, or a negative event, such as development of a complication.

OR = (a × d) ÷ (b × c).

RR = [a ÷ (a + b)] ÷ [c ÷ (c + d)].

An OR is used when one of two possible outcomes is evaluated in response to an intervention or exposure to some event. The OR can be constructed with a 2 × 2 or larger table as [OR = (a × d)/ (b × c)] as shown in Figure 8.4. The OR is a practical measure that can be calculated by hand in a clinical setting to determine the odds of a particular event or response for a patient or group of patients. It has been suggested that the information provided by the OR may be easy for patients to understand and might facilitate their participation in treatment decisions based on their odds of treatment success (McHugh, 2009). However, interpreting OR is not completely straightforward. It is the ratio of the odds of success to the odds of failure. An OR of 1 would mean that the odds are the same for both groups. An OR of 4 would mean that one group had four times the *odds* of the results seen compared to the other group, not four times the *likelihood* of having the results seen in another group (Zao, 2007). Making decisions based on OR alone is more akin to betting on horse racing than it is to making risk-based decisions. Testing the statistical significance of an OR can provide more interpretable information (Marascuilo & Serlin, 1988).

Relative risk (RR) ratio is similar to the OR but can be directly interpreted more easily. An RR less than 1 would mean that the result, or event, is less likely to occur, and an RR greater than 1 would mean that the event or outcome is more likely to occur in one group compared to the other. Relative risk is calculated as the incidence of an outcome in one group divided by the incidence of that outcome in another group, as shown in Figure 8.4.

In research reports, it is important that the direction of RR and OR results be clearly stated so that the direction of odds and risk difference are clearly tied to the study groups analyzed. It is also not unusual to find that OR findings are interpreted as if they show the probability of an outcome, which is not the case.

These types of effect size calculations have been used most often in meta-analyses, but they are also now being reported in individual research study reports. For the clinician to evaluate applicability and clinical meaningfulness of study findings, it is important to understand how to interpret these results. These are also calculations that can be readily done in the course of providing care. If such calculations are used in discussion with patients, it is important that unambiguous information can be provided.

DATA MANAGEMENT

Once research data are collected, they need to be stored and prepared for analysis. These processes are generally referred to as *data management*. Data management needs to address how and where raw data will be stored or accessed in study implementation and analysis to protect subject confidentiality, how data will be coded and computerized, how data will be cleaned, and the software that will be used for analysis. Cleaning data is often not given sufficient attention, particularly when data sets extracted from computerized databases are used. It should be remembered that just because data come from a computerized database does not mean it is accurate. Large data sets that are generated from administrative and insurance claims data can contain many errors.

Data cleaning involves identifying errors or extreme values in the data set. Extreme values and potential errors can be identified by looking at frequency distributions to identify aberrant results, and by various data-mining techniques to evaluate the degree to which the data reflect known relationships. For example, an analysis involving the use of hospital administrative data, including length of stay and cost per case, showed that one individual had a length of stay of 2 days and a total cost of $150,000. This cost for such a brief length of stay would be highly unlikely, suggesting that one or both of these values are incorrect. Such findings should be verified, or if not verifiable, treated as missing in data analysis.

There are a variety of statistical software packages that can be used for research analysis, meta-analysis procedures, and power calculations. There are also a number of applications for OR and RR calculation that are freely available on the Internet.

USING CLINICAL RESEARCH

If one understands how to plan and conduct good quality research, one also understands how to appraise research studies to determine applicability in the clinical setting. The same principles of consideration of key variables to reduce unexplained variance, design to avoid bias and threats to validity, instrumentation, and interpretation of statistical results in terms of statistical significance as well as magnitude of effect guide the evaluation of applicability of study findings.

Use of a research planning checklist, such as that shown in Table 8.2 can be used to both plan research and evaluate some aspects

TABLE 8.2   Quantitative Study Design and Planning Checklist

STUDY PLANNING ASPECT	✓
1. The study question and the related null hypothesis are clear.	
2. Independent and variables are clearly identified.	
3. Critical intervening, extraneous, and mediating variables have been identified.	
4. The study sample inclusion and exclusion criteria are defined. Criteria used will reduce potential extraneous variables that can impact the dependent variable.	
5. An appropriate sample size is identified with power analysis.	
6. Published research in the area of interest has been reviewed, and methods and measurement approaches are reviewed.	
7. Measurement methods for all study variables have been identified that are valid and reliable.	
8. Measurement instruments have been developed or obtained, and directions for use and scoring have been reviewed.	
9. Existing data sources that are relevant for study have been identified and steps to obtain these data are in place if relevant.	
10. The type of data generated from measurement is known, and implications for planned statistical analysis are identified.	
11. The overall study design, sequence, and timing of observations and /or interventions, planned. The design has been reviewed for potential threats to internal validity, and steps have been taken to prevent or reduce these threats.	
12. Implementation of the design is planned, including:	
a. An appropriate setting for the conduct of the study	
b. How data will be collected	
c. Who will be involved in data collection	
d. Who will provide interventions, if applicable	
e. Education, training, guidelines, and procedures for data collection and coding have been provided	
f. What steps will be taken to avoid missing data	
13. Methods to ensure intervention fidelity have been identified and are in place, if applicable.	
14. Methods for data storage and computer data entry are planned. Individuals involved in data entry are trained in procedures needed.	
15. Statistical analysis is planned, and appropriate statistical software is available.	

of published research for clinical application. As seen here, planning quantitative research in the clinical setting involves many different factors to produce valid and meaningful results. It can be helpful to have a concrete tool to check off various aspects of study design and implementation, to ensure consideration of appropriate variables, measurement, and consideration of sources of bias and validity threats.

The movement from the idea of research utilization to concepts of evidence-based practice points to the need to use the best quality evidence available, and to the value of combining results from multiple studies to provide such evidence. Given the complexity of providing health care to individuals, as well as the complexity of research design and implementation, it is easy to see how different studies involving the same types of observations can yield conflicting or uncertain results. It is only by considering the full range of findings from a body of work, as well as the quality of research design and conduct, that one can determine the utility of research findings.

SUMMARY

Conducting and using quantitative research involves all aspects of a study, from initially forming a clear research question, through implementation, to analysis and interpretation of results. Understanding variables, the nature of data, bias and validity threats, accurately managing data, and the ability to correctly use and interpret statistics are essential to generating good quality evidence for use in clinical practice.

Collaboration with others is vital in planning and conducting quantitative research. The input of experienced researchers and statisticians facilitates the work of identifying appropriate measurement methods, study design, sample selection, data collection and management approaches, statistical analysis, and accurate interpretation of findings. Collaboration with library science professionals facilitates review of the literature to inform the process and identify measurement instruments. Seeking the input of clinical professionals and others who work in the setting enables determination of both theoretical and practical aspects that need to be considered in implementation and study design. Working with others in the clinical setting can also identify existing data sources that can be used for research purposes.

REFERENCES

Beck, S. (1999). Selecting a design for the study. In M. A. Mateo & K. T. Kirchoff (Eds.), *Using and conducting nursing research in the clinical setting* (2nd ed.). Philadelphia, PA: W.B. Saunders.

Campbell, D. T., & Stanley, J. C. (1966). *Experimental and quasi-experimental designs for research*. Chicago, IL: Rand McNally.

The CONSORT Group. (2013). *Intention to treat analysis.* Retrieved from http://www.consort-statement.org/consort-statement/further-explanations /box6_intention-to-treat-analysis

Cook, T. J., & Campbell, D. T. (1979). *Quasi-experimentation. Design & analysis issues for field settings.* Boston, MA: Houghton Mifflin.

Ebell, H. (2008). The therapist as a traveling companion to the chronically ill: Hypnosis and cancer related symptoms. *Contemporary Hypnosis, 25*(1), 46–56. doi: 10.1002/xh.348

Ferguson, C. J. (2009). An effect size primer: A guide for clinicians and researchers. *Professional Psychology Research and Practice, 40*(5), 532–538. doi: 10.1037/a0015808

Glass, G. V., & Hopkins, K. D. (1984). *Statistical methods in education and psychology* (2nd ed.). Englewood Cliffs, NJ: Prentice-Hall.

Gupta, S. K. (2011). Intention-to-treat concept: A review. *Perspectives in Clinical Research, 2,* 109–112. DOI: 10.4103/2229-3485.83221

Huitt, W., Hummel, J., & Kaeck. D. (1999). *Internal and external validity: General issues.* Retrieved from http://www.edpsycinteractive.org/topics /intro/valdgn.html

Koshar, J. (2006). *Threats to internal validity in quantitative studies.* Retrieved from http://www.sonoma.edu/users/k/koshar/n500a/week09 _intv.html

Kraemer, H. C., & Thiemann, S. (1987). *How many subjects: Statistical power analysis in research.* Newbury Park, CA: Sage.

Kwekkeboom, K. L., Wanta, B., & Bumpus, M. (2008). Individual difference variables and the effects of progressive muscle relaxation and analgesic imagery interventions on cancer pain. *Journal of Pain and Symptom Management, 36,* 604–615. doi: 10.1016/jpainsymman.2007.12.011

Lachin, J. M. (2000). Statistical considerations in the intent-to-treat principle. *Controlled Clinical Trials, 21*(3), 167–189.

Lew, M. W., Kravtiz, K., Garberoglio, C., & Williams, A. C. (2011). Use of preoperative hypnosis to reduce postoperative pain and anesthesia related side effects. *International Journal of Clinical and Experimental Hypnosis, 59,* 406–423. doi: 10.1080/00207144.2011.594737

Marascuilo, L. A., & Serlin, R. C. (1988). *Statistical methods for the social and behavioral sciences.* New York: W.H. Freeman.

Montori, V. M., & Guyatt, G. H. (2001). Intention-to-treat principle. *Canadian Medical Association Journal, 165*(10), 1339–1341.

Park, S. H., Goo, J. M., & Jo, C. (2004). Receiver operating characteristic (ROC) curve: Practical review for radiologists. *Korean Journal of Radiology, 5,* 11–18.

Savory, P. (2008). How do you interpret a confidence interval? *Industrial and management systems Engineering—instructional materials* (Paper 11). Retrieved from http://digitalcommons.unl.edu/imseteach/11

Sica, G. T. (2006). Bias in research studies. *Radiology, 238*(3), 780–789.

Sim, J., & Reid, N. (1999). Statistical inference by confidence intervals: Issues of interpretations and utilization. *Physical Therapy, 79,* 186–195.

Sim, J., & Wright, C. C. (2005). The kappa statistic in reliability studies: Use, interpretation and sample size requirements. *Physical Therapy, 85,* 257–268.

U.S. Department of Health and Human Services Food and Drug Administration Center for Drug Evaluation and Research (CDER) Center for Biologics Evaluation and Research (CBER). (2010). *Guidance for industry. Noninferiority clinical trials.* Retrieved from http://www.fda.gov/downloads /Drugs/GuidanceComplianceRegulatoryInformation/Guidances/UCM202140 .pdf

Waltz, C. F., Strickland, O. L., & Lenz, E. R. (1991). *Measurement in nursing research* (2nd ed.). Philadelphia, PA: FA Davis.

Zao, G. Y. (2007). One relative risk versus two odds ratios: Implications for meta-analyses involving paired and unpaired binary data. *Clinical Trials, 4,* 25–31. Retrieved from http://www.bmj.com/rapid-response/2011/10/27 /use-misuse-and-interpretation-odds-ratios

9

Qualitative Research for Nursing Practice

Beth Rodgers

Qualitative research methods constitute a vital part of nursing knowledge development and provide information that is essential for evidence-based practice. Researchers frequently use methods of this type to address problems relevant to aspects of nursing practice and human existence that cannot be reduced to isolated variables or captured in numerical form. Some of the aspects are critical to what might be considered the holistic aspect of nursing practice—the feelings and subjective experiences of the people with whom nurses interact. To accomplish the goal of using the best evidence available as a basis for nursing practice, nurses must understand the processes involved in this type of research and be able to evaluate the quality of evidence derived from qualitative studies.

When reading reports of qualitative studies, it is immediately apparent that the designs and procedures for qualitative research differ considerably from those of quantitative studies. A question that is often raised when discussing different types of research concerns is whether or not different approaches are sufficiently "scientific" and, therefore, have a legitimate place in the research base of nursing. For many people, the mention of "science" conjures up an image of a laboratory setting or, at least, an environment where the researcher carefully controls the conditions for the investigation by isolating the phenomenon being studied from other elements that might interfere with the results. The researcher, in this view of science, also is presumed to occupy an objective stance, observing the results of the experiment without preconceived ideas or bias. As such, the results are considered to be some form of "Truth" regarding the situation being studied. There is a belief that science, conducted in such a way, provides answers about cause and effect, definitive explanations that serve as "proof" about what happens in certain situations and, in regard to clinical practice, a clear understanding of what is the best thing to do in a particular circumstance. Compared to this idea of science, qualitative research certainly does seem quite unorthodox.

Although society and educational systems, particularly at the early levels where students generally are first introduced to "science," perpetuate this idea of science, it becomes clear with just a little study of research that very little about actual research is consistent with this idea of "science." Finding one absolute, indisputable answer to questions is unreasonable in any context, much less where humans are involved. As humans interact with their environment, they change, the environment changes, and so does the phenomenon being studied. Objectivity, in a complete and unbiased sense, is not a reasonable expectation for any scientist or for any human being, nor is it necessarily desirable in every situation. The mere identification of something as a "problem" involves judgment on the part of the researcher. The researcher's existing biases are integrated throughout the conduct of inquiry and, in fact, often are useful in the research situation as they provide the researcher with important tools for research such as language, concepts, theories, and mechanisms for interacting with human subjects of study. These are all biases in a sense, yet research would not be possible without them. Complete objectivity, therefore, is not possible without dispensing with all that has been learned through both education and development in a social context. Rather than seeing the possibility of one absolute answer or Truth, objectivity, and control as necessary ingredients for science, recent philosophers of science (those who explore what makes science work) provide a contemporary view of science as an attempt to solve problems, to generate solutions that "work," to exercise creativity and innovation in the interest of discovery and development of knowledge, and to link research to a broad interest for the good of society (Rodgers, 2005).

This evolving idea of what constitutes science has fueled a substantial increase in the acceptance and, consequently, the volume of qualitative research being conducted in a variety of disciplines. Qualitative research, although a mainstay of inquiry in the social sciences for nearly a century, has blossomed in acceptance and use in a broad array of disciplines. In nursing, evidence of considerable growth in this area can be seen starting particularly in the 1980s, although there was some discussion of its utility even earlier than that. Quint (1966), for example, produced a seminal work demonstrating the importance of qualitative research in theory development at the dawn of the theory movement in nursing, decades before qualitative research developed any noticeable foothold in nursing. Acceptance of such methods in the research enterprise was slow at first, but in recent decades it has become an essential aspect of nursing's knowledge base, providing valuable information on aspects of human health and illness that are best explored using the capabilities of qualitative methods. The role of qualitative research results in regard to evidence-based practice is still the subject of some debate, although qualitative research appears on "level of evidence" tables with increasing regularity (Melnyk & Fineout-Overholt, 2010), and there is no question that nurses understand the importance of patient experiences in determining the appropriateness of various interventions and practices in health care. It is the relationships that nurses develop with people in the context of health and wellness that differentiate nursing care from other aspects of health and illness work, and those connections with individuals and groups create a strong need for evidence and a scientific base such as is obtained through qualitative research.

WHY QUALITATIVE RESEARCH?

As noted previously, qualitative research is suitable for inquiry that addresses a number of aspects relevant to nursing and provides an important part of the evidence base essential to nursing practice. Qualitative research approaches the study of phenomena in a "natural" setting. Rather than attempt to control elements of the research situation, such as by manipulating variables (for example, an intervention presented in a controlled setting), a qualitative study typically is designed to capture experiences or events as they naturally occur. Qualitative research also excels at capturing people's thoughts and feelings, which are not easily reduced to numbered responses to questions on paper-and-pencil instruments. Qualitative research offers insights important to viewing situations and people holistically and, therefore, is ideal to answer broad questions that warrant in-depth description. Questions for qualitative research often are stated similar to the following:

- What is happening here?
- What is it like for people who experience a particular situation or condition?
- What are the experiences of people with "X" (the phenomenon of interest)?
- What is the meaning of "X" (the phenomenon of interest)?

Answers to such questions meet several significant functions of qualitative research. Qualitative research can be used to provide a deep and rich description of a situation or experience. Qualitative research also helps to provide information about aspects that might be missed with a quantitative study. For example, quantitative research is appropriate for determining whether one intervention is more effective than another in a way that is statistically significant. Such a study, however, will not provide information about what it is like for an individual to live with the intervention. In such a situation, qualitative research makes it possible to capture information that is essential to gaining a complete picture of a situation or experience. Qualitative research also can be very sensitizing, raising awareness of aspects of an experience that might not have been recognized previously. By doing so, nurses are better able to anticipate patient's needs and concerns and understand their perspectives when confronted with a health-related situation. Obviously knowledge of these types is important for nursing practice where nurses need to be able to individualize care and work with psychological, social, and emotional aspects as well as the physiological components of health and illness situations. Qualitative research is ideal for understanding what people think, feel, believe, and live through as they encounter situations related to their health and well-being.

Before continuing, it is important to note that some studies include qualitative data, or data in the form of words, and such data can be an important adjunct to an otherwise quantitatively focused study. For example, a study focused on an educational intervention to promote adherence to a prescribed regimen for treating hypertension could include some important numerical data regarding knowledge, medication use, and diet and exercise changes adopted by the participants. Such numerical data are ideal for making comparisons across groups such as to determine whether the intervention was effective in promoting changes in knowledge and behaviors. A study of this type can be more complete, however, if the researcher also collects data regarding what people thought about the intervention, what they saw as challenges in acting on the information received, and whether they feel capable of continuing with the recommended changes. Such data regarding perceptions and experiences are best collected in a qualitative form based on the words and narratives provided by the participants. In such a situation, the researcher clearly is using qualitative data but the primary focus of the study is on the quantitative testing of effectiveness in regard to the outcomes. This is an important distinction because qualitative studies are conducted and evaluated according to very different guidelines and criteria. The inclusion of qualitative data does not make the study a qualitative one by design. It is necessary to determine the primary focus of the study and use appropriate criteria to guide the design, evaluation, and critique of the inquiry. In general, a study is referred to as "a qualitative study" when the primary focus is on gathering narrative descriptions of experience; those narratives are, of course, expressed in the form of words and the results are presented through words as well. Although there may be some quantitative data in a qualitative study, those data generally are limited to describing the participants. As a general guide, the criteria for conducting or evaluating a qualitative study apply when there are words as data and the majority of the results are reported in the form of words as well. This focus applies to the remainder of this chapter when the reference is made to a "qualitative study."

Numerous examples of specific types of qualitative studies, including different questions and applications, can be found throughout the nursing literature. A worthwhile activity for anyone interested in research of any type is to explore the literature and read reports of completed research that has been conducted using different designs. In qualitative research, this is particularly important as there are multiple types of qualitative studies, each with its own specific question, procedures, and manner of presenting results, as evident in the following section.

TYPES OF QUALITATIVE RESEARCH

As noted above, qualitative research is focused on words as data rather than numbers and the qualitative researcher reports results in the form of words. In spite of this common characteristic among all the qualitative approaches, there are distinct methodologies for qualitative research, each of which has its own unique philosophical underpinnings, history, and procedures for the conduct of a study.

On a very basic level, there is a general type of qualitative research that often appears in the literature. A study might be described as merely "qualitative," "descriptive," "qualitative descriptive," "exploratory," "naturalistic," "field research," or "ethnographic." All of these refer to the collection of data in the form of words (typically through interviews and, occasionally, through observations as well) without any more specific processes involved that are associated with a designated methodology. Qualitative studies can be conducted quite well without being associated with a particular methodology that has specific requirements regarding the question and the collection and analysis of data. Note that "descriptive" research can be quantitative as well, so seeing a study characterized as "descriptive" in a report of research requires a closer look at the nature of the data and the report of results to determine whether it is qualitative or quantitative. The term "ethnographic," similarly can have multiple meanings, referring most generally to research in a natural setting. There is also a distinct methodology known as ethnography, which is discussed below.

More specific methodologies for qualitative research can be found in the literature, however, and, in nursing, some of the more common types of qualitative studies are grounded theory, phenomenology, hermeneutic (most often hermeneutic phenomenology), narrative inquiry, and as noted above, ethnography. *Grounded theory* research was introduced formally in the 1960s based on the work of noted sociologist Anselm Strauss and his colleague Barney Glaser (Glaser & Strauss, 1967). This method is guided by the theoretical viewpoint of symbolic interactionism (Blumer, 1969), although the essential nature of the link to symbolic interactionism has been questioned in recent years. In general, symbolic interactionism holds that people create their sense of self, their reality, societies, and so on, through interaction with other people. How an individual experiences some event or process in life is heavily influenced, if not dependent on, those interactions. In a grounded theory study, the researcher seeks information about the overall "experience" of people in specific situations of interest to the researcher. The researcher conducting an investigation using the methodology of grounded theory will have a research question such as "what is it like to..." or "what is the experience of people with..." The experience that is the focus of research will involve the thoughts, feelings, actions, interactions with others, and interpretations of events associated with the situation being studied as described by the people who are going through that experience.

Grounded theory research has a unique end product in that it is used to construct a substantive theory that provides a detailed depiction of the experience being studied that is derived from (grounded in) the data obtained from participants. This theory is organized around a central idea referred to as the "core variable" (Charmaz, 2006; Glaser, 1978; Glaser & Strauss, 1967), which represents the primary focus of the experience. This core variable represents the "basic sociopsychological process" or BSP, involved in the experience and reflects the symbolic interactionist foundation regarding interaction being important in the shaping of experience. Since Glaser and Strauss pioneered this method in the late 1960s, other variations have been introduced, including a version by Strauss and Corbin (1998). The underlying principles are the same, although the Strauss and Corbin version imposes more structure on the data-analysis process and on the reporting of results. Other adaptations have been created as well, most notably the constructivist orientation provided by Charmaz (2000, 2005, 2006). From the standpoint of the advanced practice nurse who needs to critique and evaluate research for implications for practice, reports of grounded theory studies can be evaluated similarly, keeping in mind the foundations of this approach and the expected outcome of a substantive theory, regardless of the specific variation a researcher used in a study. General criteria for evaluating qualitative studies are discussed later in this chapter.

The qualitative method known as *phenomenology* also is used to study experiences, but is focused on the "meaning" of the "lived experience" of the people in the study. Phenomenology was derived originally from the philosophies of Edmund Husserl (1960) and Maurice Merleau-Ponty (1962/1999), and its origins contributed to the extensive foundation in philosophy that is evident in this method. Based on this foundation, modifications to the method were presented by existentialist philosopher Martin Heidegger, and the method was adapted further as a means of study in psychology. There are numerous unique approaches that are all justifiably referred to as phenomenology, including a variation called *hermeneutic phenomenology* (Plager, 1994) which is fairly common in nursing. All of these approaches have some elements in common, however. Whereas grounded theory is focused on social interaction and processes, phenomenology is a method to study the individual and how the individual ascribes "meaning" to an experience. A significant underpinning of this research method is the idea that humans create their own realities and these realities, in turn, have a strong influence on creating the individual. This idea often is referred to as "co-constitution," capturing the notion that people, and their realities, each have an influence on the construction of each other. Experiences and events have their own essence or what might in common language be referred to as the "facts" of the situation, or what really happened. A person is diagnosed with a chronic illness, for example, and there is solid evidence to support that diagnosis and the fact that it was communicated to the individual. In phenomenology, however, the focus is on the layers of meaning or interpretation that the individual gives to the situation. It is not even necessary that there be "facts" to support the interpretation. As an example, consider an individual who has a family history of a condition associated with cognitive decline. That person might have occasional feelings of being distracted or forgetting to do a particular task and interpret those as a symptom of the impending hereditary decline, even though there is no substantive or documented reason to make that association. The interpretation or meaning the individual assigns to what he or she is experiencing will have a profound influence on the sense of self and the willingness to share the experiences with others. Although all qualitative methods are focused on people's experiences and their own individual realities, the phenomenological researcher typically goes beyond the actual words spoken by an individual to describe the experience in an attempt to interpret these words and identify underlying meaning. For that reason, phenomenology sometimes is referred to as an "interpretive" method (Van Manen, 1990) rather than a "descriptive" one. The product of phenomenological research is a discussion of significant ideas or meaning statements derived through analysis of the participant's words and interpretation of the meanings the experience being studied has for the individual. Phenomenology is a complex and highly variable qualitative method and the sample sizes, analytic approaches, and results will differ depending on the particular orientation employed by the researcher.

Narrative inquiry is another form of qualitative research that is common in nursing. Narrative inquiry (Labov & Waletsky, 1967; Riessman, 1993) is grounded in the premise that people typically construct "stories" about their various life experiences, including stories that form their own identities. These stories represent the individual's way of

weaving together elements of the event into their "story" of their experience. According to Riessman (1993), "the purpose of narrative inquiry
is to see how respondents in interviews impose order on the flow of
experience to make sense of events and actions in their lives" (p. 2).
These stories involve all the typical aspects of a story, including players, supporting players, settings, sequencing of events, and outcomes.
Using the techniques of narrative analysis, the researcher examines
these stories to uncover an underlying narrative that characterizes the
stories associated with an experience (Riley & Hawe, 2005).

The final form of qualitative research that will be discussed here
is ethnography. Ethnography as a specific method (in contrast to the
more generic use of the term "ethnographic" to refer to research that
takes place in a natural setting or "in the field") originated in the discipline of anthropology. Ethnography is focused on the study of culture.
For purposes of this type of research, a culture can comprise any group
or setting in which people share ideology, values, attitudes, customs,
rules, norms, or rituals (Wolf, 2007). In conducting research using the
methodology of ethnography, the researcher typically spends extensive time in the setting being studied. In addition to "getting in," the
process of becoming accepted by the group being studied, a goal in
the early phase of such a study is the identification of "key informants"
or people who are particularly familiar with the setting or experience
and whose perspectives are important for understanding the workings
of the setting. The researcher will observe the group and interactions
among the group, keep extensive notes and talk with individuals in
addition to the key informants whose input is particularly important to
the study. Ethnographies are found much less frequently in the nursing
literature than are examples of the other methods, perhaps because
of the extremely time-intensive nature of the research. In addition,
ethnographies typically are so extensive and detailed that they can be
reported only partially through the usual format of a journal article.

CONDUCTING A QUALITATIVE STUDY

Before attempting the critical evaluation of qualitative studies, it is
necessary to understand how qualitative research is conducted. In
spite of the differences in foundation and development of the various
traditions, the overall procedures for conducting a qualitative study are
quite similar. Those procedures differ considerably from those used in
conducting quantitative studies, and a review of the steps in the process, comparing qualitative and quantitative types of research, can be
helpful in identifying important differences.

It is important to remember that the intent in any type of qualitative research is to capture the individual "realities" of the participants and to provide a detailed description of those realities and the
experiences of the people studied. Therefore, elements of research that

involve ideas such as control, theory or hypothesis testing, reliability, and generalizability, for example, are either inappropriate or take on an entirely different meaning in the context of a qualitative study. To gain an understanding of how qualitative research functions, the steps in conducting a qualitative study are presented along with ideas regarding what to look for in the critique of such research.

Research Problem and Question

As with any type of research, the process of qualitative inquiry begins with identification of a problem and a research question. Problems result when there are new ideas or situations to explore such that little is known about the phenomenon and studies aimed at broad discovery are appropriate. A change in a treatment modality might warrant a study that explores the experiences of people who receive that treatment; staffing patterns for nurses might be explored in regard to the experiences of the nurses who live with that pattern on a regular basis or might lead to exploration of other aspects of the care delivered by the nursing staff. Problems appropriate for qualitative research also exist when there are significant gaps in knowledge. A longstanding procedure might have been studied extensively regarding its effectiveness, yet there may be very little information about what patients think or feel about the treatment and how it affects their daily lives. A problem amenable to qualitative research can be just about anything that can be answered through in-depth discovery and descriptions of the experiences, thoughts, and feelings of people who have encountered the situation being studied.

The questions for qualitative studies appear to be quite similar in spite of the specific tradition of inquiry that underlies the research. There are subtle differences in wording, however, that clue the reader as to the specific tradition being explored. Phenomenology, for example, often involves the phrase "lived experience" or the word "meaning" as a specific focus of the research question for that type of study. Beyond those seemingly minor variations in wording, questions for a qualitative study in general address the broad experience or the thoughts and feelings regarding a life encounter. It is not uncommon for researchers to not provide a specific question statement in their report of qualitative studies; the absence of an actual question is not a weakness in a research report. The purpose of the study and the problem situation that led to the development of the research, however, should be clear to the reader and, ideally, these are presented early in the published report. The question or problem should be one that is appropriate to qualitative inquiry as well. Questions about what "should" be done in a situation or what is "better" are not amenable to any type of research as they call for judgments that go beyond the actual data gained through the study. A researcher can, however, address a question about what people report, what characteristics are identified, how people describe their feelings, and how they live with some situation or experience as a step toward developing conclusions about what is "better" and why that is the case.

Review of Literature

Another step in the research process typically involves a review of the literature. It is a bit misleading to consider this a separate "step" because, as with any type of study, the review of the literature can be very helpful in refining the original problem. The iterative process of reviewing the literature and rethinking the original problem helps the researcher to gain clarity and important perspectives that give direction to the subsequent research. In a quantitative study, the literature review typically provides an important foundation for the research by revealing what is already known about the situation of interest. On this basis, the researcher can determine the appropriate next steps for inquiry and, depending on the type of research, develop a theoretical foundation for the study and possible hypotheses. At this point, qualitative and quantitative studies differ considerably. The qualitative researcher does not intend to build on existing research but typically embarks on an attempt to explore, discover, and describe areas and experiences about which little already is known. In this spirit, the researcher wants to remain as open as is plausible to the many possibilities that can exist in any situation. Using the literature review to frame the study would put some boundaries around what is explored and what might be "seen" in the data that are collected.

Some discussions of qualitative research present the argument that there is no need for any type of literature review prior to embarking on a qualitative study (Glaser & Strauss, 1967). Avoiding contact with existing information is believed to enable the researcher to be more open and unbiased about what might be encountered through the study. Although the idea of being as unbiased as possible is appealing, it is faulty on a couple of levels. First, it is never possible to be completely open and unbiased about anything. The researcher is making judgments from the very beginning of a study by identifying something as a "problem" and by naming phenomena, in other words, by using certain words to label what is being studied. The researcher also inherently possesses some bias due to the researcher's own experience as a human interacting with others and with the knowledge he or she already has accumulated. Diminishing bias in a study is a desirable goal to the extent possible and typically the researcher does not want to skew the study in any particular direction to avoid placing limits on what might be discovered. In qualitative studies, therefore, there often is a literature review though it takes on a different form from that of quantitative studies. The qualitative researcher typically does a thorough literature review prior to the start of the study, but it is oriented toward substantiating that a problem does exist, that qualitative methods are appropriate to address that problem and, in some cases, to gain direction and support for the methods chosen for the study. Rather than provide a foundation for the research, the literature review in a qualitative study enables the researcher to justify the need for the research and the chosen form of qualitative inquiry.

The literature review section that appears relatively early in a report of a qualitative study should be thorough and give good background information about the problem. Because the researcher usually is not building on this existing information to further inquiry in an area, the literature review sometimes is more broad, discussing a wide variety of studies that have been done and often identifying gaps in knowledge rather than focusing on a select few items or articles to provide underpinnings for the research. Ultimately, the researcher uses the literature review to make a clear case for the fact that a researchable problem exists and that it is important to generate information that will fill this gap. As noted before, the appropriateness of qualitative methods to address the problem should be apparent as well.

The use of an initial literature review to substantiate the problem and methods rather than to provide a foundation for the research, as noted above, is not appropriate in a qualitative study. Similarly, in quantitative research, the initial literature review is used to connect the study to previous work, showing how the study presented in a published report relates to other research. In qualitative studies, this connection to existing work is made near the end of the study rather than at the beginning. As themes and patterns are identified in the data obtained during the study, the researcher will conduct an extensive literature review late in the conduct of the study to determine how the ideas that have been discovered relate to extant knowledge. For example, in a study of women's experiences with myocardial infarction (MI; Rodgers, 2007), the researcher returned to the literature to gather information about several aspects of the experience that arose during the study. Although gender roles could be expected to be an issue in this study, the researcher did not anticipate that so many of the participants would refuse to be taken to the hospital by ambulance even when they finally acknowledged that they probably were having a heart attack. This raised questions about the interconnections of age, socioeconomic status, and gender and led to extensive literature review to examine associations among these concepts as a means of connecting the findings from the study with existing knowledge.

When reading published reports of qualitative research, the literature review component needs to be evaluated in regard to the initial phase of substantiating the problem as well as in the discussion section at the end of the report. In this latter section, the researcher discusses the findings of the current study in the context of previous research and theoretical literature. This use of the literature enables additional clarification of the findings of the study as well as a means to connect the findings to what is already known. As a result, there are benefits both to the current research as well as to expanding the knowledge base. The researcher can compare findings to the literature as a step toward expanding and enriching the findings as well as to demonstrate how the research contributes to what has been presented previously in the literature. The elements of a good literature review are appropriate for use in evaluating this component of a qualitative study. Primary sources, evidence of a thorough search, and use of current sources, which would be appropriate in any literature review, are appropriate criteria here as well. The results of the literature review that is done later in the study to expand findings and make connections with existing knowledge are presented in the discussion section of the research report. In this section, the researcher is expected to use relevant literature in discussion of major findings as a means to enhance understanding of the findings and demonstrate a clear connection to prior theory and research.

DESIGN OF QUALITATIVE STUDIES

In qualitative studies, the researcher has a broad problem of interest and specific variables are not identified in advance. As a result, the researcher develops the design for the study based on the problem, the initial literature review, and the purpose—what the researcher intends to accomplish with the study. The typical form of design for a qualitative study is referred to as an *emergent design*—the design actually "emerges" as the study proceeds. In qualitative studies, the researcher is not only free to make changes in the design but, in the course of doing the study actually is expected to make changes in the design to pursue new ideas and areas of inquiry as they are determined to be important. All of the elements of the research design cannot be planned in advance and, in fact, the design usually needs to change in some respects if the researcher is to do a thorough investigation of the phenomenon being studied. This is in stark contrast to how quantitative research typically is conducted. In a quantitative study, the researcher plans every element of the design in advance and then collects data according to the plan. In some instances there may be minor modifications, although if a pilot study is conducted any necessary changes are usually worked out at that time.

A qualitative study functions best when there is a clear starting point and purpose but there is flexibility in the path to complete that objective. New information, things that the researcher could not anticipate, often arise in the course of collecting data from participants.

As new information is obtained through data collection, the astute researcher will realize that there are new avenues to be explored, people with different characteristics that need to be investigated, and new questions to ask in interviews. As an example, consider the study mentioned previously about women and MI. Early in the study it was evident, much to the investigator's surprise, that none of the women interviewed had gone to the hospital by ambulance in spite of their acknowledgment that they probably were having a heart attack at the time. This was an unanticipated finding and certainly something that needed to be explored to provide a meaningful and comprehensive description of the experiences of these women. Merely reporting this to be the case would have been interesting but would have been a lost opportunity for full description. In response to this realization, the investigator made a couple of changes in the study. The investigator began explicitly gathering information from each woman about the actual transportation to receive health care after recognizing she was having an MI. This constituted a change in the interview process. The researcher also added a new site for subject recruitment as those interviewed up to that point in the study had been in a comfortable position economically and the researcher was interested in determining whether this observation persisted in different socioeconomic groups. In one sense, this following of "leads" sometimes is thought of as a form of hypothesis testing, for example, does the mode of transportation to the hospital differ with socioeconomic status, or age, or living situation? The ability to follow a relevant path wherever it may lead in the inquiry is important to achieving the depth and scope of understanding of the situation that is sought in qualitative research and accounts for the need for elements of design to *emerge* in the course of a study. It also is a good example of how what is relevant data may not be evident at the start of a study. Adhering to a predetermined set of variables from the beginning of a study can result in unnecessary restrictions on what is being studied and, consequently, gaps in fully understanding the phenomenon or situation of interest.

Sample Selection

Qualitative researchers often view their research as an interactive process involving the people who are involved in a study. Rather than view them as "subjects" of study, they can be thought of as having an active role in the research; this active role often involves sharing sensitive aspects of their lives and is recognized in researchers commonly referring to them as participants or informants rather than subjects. Participants help to construct the study in a way by offering information about their experiences and this information, in turn, is used by the researcher to determine the appropriate direction of the research. Although some aspects of design can change throughout the conduct of a qualitative study, many elements can be determined in advance. The specific sample typically is not determined in advance and probability samples usually are not appropriate for qualitative research. That does not mean, however, that the researcher simply takes into the study anyone who comes along and is willing to participate. The researcher must establish clear eligibility criteria for selection of participants, and these criteria typically involve competence to provide informed consent to participate, the ability to speak and understand the language of the researcher, and an adequate amount of engagement with the experience being studied. Other factors can be included as appropriate to determine eligibility for a study. Studying the experiences of women with MI, for example, obviously requires that the participants have experienced an MI. Beyond this criterion, the researcher can impose more specific requirements appropriate to the nature of the study. The MI study was focused on women's concurrent experiences rather than on a retrospective account of their situations. Therefore, eligibility criteria included a time frame for the occurrence of the MI relative to data collection. For this study, the participant also could not have had a diagnosis of MI previously as the researcher was interested in each woman's experience of first becoming aware that she had experienced an MI.

Because of the existence of specific criteria for eligibility, the usual sample for a qualitative study is a purposive one; there are relevant and distinct criteria that enable the researcher to purposefully recruit participants who are in the best position to provide data needed for the study. It is not uncommon for qualitative researchers to describe their samples as accidental (or convenience), and that may be an appropriate designation depending on the specificity with which the participants are recruited for the study. Regardless of the specific type of sampling procedure employed, it is important that the qualitative researcher have participants in the study who are willing and capable of describing their experiences with the situation being studied.

Sample size is a concern in any type of research, and qualitative research is no exception. Researchers using quantitative designs have the ability to determine appropriate sample sizes using statistical procedures such as power analysis in many cases. In qualitative research, there is no ability to predict in advance precisely how many participants are needed to produce meaningful results. It is also the case that in qualitative research the amount of data that are generated has bearing on determination of the appropriate sample size. One hour of an audio-recorded interview generally produces as many as 30 pages of single-spaced transcribed text, an incredible amount of data. All of the data in an effectively conducted interview need to be analyzed. As a result, the amount of data available for analysis can be quite large with even a small group of participants. Qualitative research can also consume a lot of time and other resources. These factors in combination contribute to qualitative studies typically having relatively small sample sizes and also contribute to the realization that large samples are not necessary to generate meaningful and credible results due to the volume of data generated. There is no "rule" for what constitutes an adequate sample size in a qualitative study. Rather than counting participants, it is important that the researcher make a strong case that the study involved a considerable volume of data of high quality and that the data were sufficient to provide a cohesive and defensible answer to the research question.

Determination of an adequate sample, therefore, is based on several factors, including the quantity and quality of data generated, the characteristics of the participants, the procedures employed in the study to maximize diversity in the participants and their experiences, and the ability to answer the research question with the data that are generated through the research. In planning to do a qualitative study the researcher can anticipate approximately how many people will be needed in the sample to reach this desired outcome. Because this is not an absolute number, proposals for qualitative research often include a range for the number of participants who will be recruited for the study. Published reports may show sample sizes ranging from 10 to 30 or more. In evaluating these studies, as noted above, there are several factors that need to be considered beyond the actual number of people involved.

A common practice in qualitative research is to use the criterion of "saturation" (Morse, 1991) or "redundancy" (Lincoln & Guba, 1985; Patton, 2001) to determine when the sample size is adequate. Saturation typically is defined as the point at which the researcher is not hearing anything new in the data; in other words, the descriptions provided by participants are sufficiently similar so that there is no need to continue with subject recruitment. For reasons that should be obvious, this can be a very troublesome criterion. First, the researcher is making a fairly bold assumption that talking with additional people will not provide anything new. Second, the failure to obtain new insights through the data collection processes that are being used could be a function of the data collection process itself and not necessarily a reflection of the experiences of the participants. If the researcher is asking leading questions during the interviewing or becomes fixated on certain aspects of the experience, this could lead to a premature sense that there is nothing new being learned through data collection. Finally, the researcher has to avoid the development of bias in interpreting things in a particular way. Such bias could give the false impression that there is nothing new in the data. It is important in qualitative research, as in any study, that the researcher be open to new ideas and insights that arise through data collection and analysis.

Data Collection for Qualitative Research

Any non-numerical data can be used for purposes of qualitative research. This can include notes written when making observations, a review of existing documentation and records such as patient medical records, print media such as books or popular literature, or video recordings. The majority of data collection for qualitative studies occurs through the use of interviews with individuals or in focus groups. Typically interviews are conducted on a face-to-face basis, although telephone and even e-mail or web-based interviews with individuals have been used in qualitative research. Interviews can have any degree of structure, ranging from specific questions that are asked consistently of each participant to an interview that is very openended and nonstructured. The amount of depth and "richness" of the data varies with the degree of structure imposed on data collection: More structure generally leads to less richness and depth, whereas less structure provides greater depth. This may seem counterintuitive at first. In a nonstructured interview, the researcher starts with an overriding question of interest, for example, what is it like for women to learn they have had a heart attack? After starting with a broad opening question, the researcher allows the participant to talk, presenting his or her experience in whatever way is comfortable so that the conversation flows naturally for the participant. This allows the participant to reveal things that are of greatest concern or interest regarding the experience without the researcher providing too much direction or imposing restraint on the conversation. The researcher focuses on listening, delicately guiding the conversation to ensure that relevant aspects are covered and participants provide a thorough account of their experiences, but without abruptly redirecting the interview or otherwise imposing constraints on the conversation. The researcher will have some specific questions that he or she wants to address with each participant, such as symptoms, timeline of events, treatments received, and family history as just a few possibilities. Questions about these aspects of the experience can be incorporated into the interview at appropriate times. The emphasis on listening and facilitating the participants' elaboration about their experiences can be challenging for nurses who are accustomed to collecting information from patients or clients relevant to a health situation. Nurses are very skilled at eliciting specific information and then formulating conclusions and determining the actions that are appropriate. It is easy for the novice qualitative researcher to interject suggestions, make decisions, or prematurely assume understanding of the participant's situations. In an interview for qualitative research, however, the investigator must learn to listen very attentively, returning to significant items in the conversation when appropriate, and gently redirecting when appropriate. Although participants need to be allowed to present their experiences as they perceived them, introducing aspects and ideas they found to be important, the researcher needs to be careful that participants do not ramble completely off topic. If the interview turns into a rambling conversation the participant (not to mention the researcher) can become fatigued and the quality of the interview may be compromised. In addition, people also have busy lives and typically cannot dedicate unlimited time to an interview. The typical in-depth interview lasts about 90 minutes to 2 hours, and the researcher does need to make sure that the interview is sufficiently on track so that the desired information is obtained within a reasonable time frame.

An interesting feature of qualitative research is that some of the data in the study actually come from (or are generated by) the researcher. Data usually are thought of as information that is collected from the people who are being studied, in other words, the subjects of the study. In qualitative studies, however, it is important that the researcher generate some of the data. Such data include notes about the researcher's actions, thought processes, and decisions made throughout the course of the investigation. The researcher also prepares documentation that is helpful to understanding and, later, analyzing the interview data. Notes about the setting or context for an interview as well as observations made during the process of data collection, such as notes about a participant's behaviors or nonverbal communication, are referred to as "field notes." These notes provide insights that are valuable in the analysis of data as they facilitate understanding the situation being studied (Rodgers & Cowles, 1993).

Evaluating the quality of data collection procedures in a qualitative study involves looking at a number of factors related to the subjects as well as the researcher. The researcher must have gathered data from participants who have had the experience being studied, who are able to articulate their experiences, who feel comfortable and unconstrained in sharing their experience, and who have adequate opportunity to share the experiences of interest. Accomplishing this places a considerable burden on the researcher who must develop effective rapport with participants, to ensure confidentiality necessary to protect their identity when discussing matters that can be sensitive to the individual, and to use effective interviewing techniques to obtain comprehensive and clear data that can be analyzed appropriately to answer the research question. In reading a qualitative study, it is important to consider the situation in which the data collection took place, for example, provisions for privacy during the interview; the amount of time allowed for an interview; efforts made by the researcher to establish rapport; and other factors such as gender, culture, ethnicity, language, or age that might affect the researcher–participant relationship; means to ensure accuracy of the data collected such as by audio-recording of interviews; and any other information the researcher provides about strategies used to enhance the quality of the data collected. The researcher also should provide an account of notes that were taken during the data collection session and how these were used to supplement the data collection process and enhance the quality of the data.

Data Analysis in Qualitative Research

Data analysis can be an intimidating process in any study. In qualitative research, the volume of information, along with the lack of any prescribed structure for organizing and analyzing it, can be overwhelming, particularly for investigators new to the process. It is also the case that this process can be the most enjoyable part of the research. This is the part of the research process in which the inquisitive mind, the puzzle solver, the curious and the creative aspects of the nurse are allowed to grow and thrive.

There are many approaches to the analysis of qualitative data with some specific guidelines that are unique to each tradition of research. Grounded theory, for example, involves a process of analysis that leads toward the identification of a "core variable," a central concept that describes the experience being studied, and then categories of information or themes that contribute to that core of the experience. Phenomenology involves a search for "significant statements" and "meaning" in the data, and narrative research focuses on "stories." In spite of these variations, however, all qualitative procedures have in common a similar process of reducing the data to manageable units and then constructing a description of the experience being studied by putting back together the pieces of the data into a coherent whole.

The process of analysis begins with a stage of general data reduction. Typically the researcher will read through the data (assume an interview transcript here for this purpose) identifying statements or parts of statements that carry a unique idea, and will label or "code" those statements using some term that captures the essence of that statement. This process of coding, carried out with all of the data collected in the study (including data generated by the researcher), reduces the large volume of data in the transcripts to smaller segments that then become the focus of further analysis. Working with these codes, the researcher begins to organize the codes into a meaningful structure with common ideas grouped together. The researcher is looking for patterns or recurrent ideas in the data (sometimes called themes), and the data are organized and reorganized into categories until clear patterns or themes can be identified. This process of organizing and categorizing is continued until the researcher can identify the particular themes or categories that account for and reflect the data that have been gathered without leaving any gaps in the resulting cluster of categories (Knafl & Webster, 1988). It is not necessary to account for every element of data in identifying themes or patterns. There will always be more questions, new avenues to explore, ideas of where research is needed, and so on. There should not, however, be major pieces of data that are ignored or left out of this categorizing process or major gaps in the themes that are identified.

The physical management and organization of data are accomplished using a technique that is best described using the metaphor "cut and paste." Historically, researchers would make multiple photocopies of the data (typically the interview transcripts) and cut the transcript into small segments, each segment containing a distinct idea relevant to the focus of the study. The researcher then would paste the segment onto a card (specific cards were developed just for this purpose) and sort those cards according to patterns that were identified in the data. Researchers made various adaptations in this approach to reflect their own style of data organization and analysis: word-processing software could be used, researchers could write or paste the data into large spreadsheet-type formats, or different categories could be identified directly on the transcript pages and coded using unique colors. Since the early 1980s, specific software has been developed for use in qualitative data analysis. Some of the currently popular programs are NVivo (QSR International, 2012) and an earlier version of this software named NUD*IST, ATLAS/ti (Scientific Software Development, 2012), HyperResearch (Researchware, 2011), MAXQDA (VERBI Software, 2013), and others. In reviewing a report of qualitative research, these will be mentioned by the researcher and the nurse reading the report should recognize that these are simply software programs that help with aspects of data management and organization. Software programs do not analyze the data for the researcher, but are very useful in organizing data and facilitating the researcher's cognitive processes of data analysis. The use of software does not enhance the quality of the study, nor does the absence of it detract. Although there are considerable benefits from the use of software by a researcher skilled in the program, the process of analysis ultimately depends on the diligence and cognitive effort of the researcher.

Reporting the Results of a Qualitative Study

The results of a qualitative study are presented in a manner appropriate to the specific method employed. Grounded theory research, for example, produces a type of theoretical construction that presents a substantive description of the experience that was studied. Regardless of the specific approach, results generally consist of a detailed discussion of patterns that were evident in the data collected in the study. Patterns can be organized around a specific concept, such as the core variable in grounded theory research, in a hierarchical manner with themes and subthemes, or as categories of descriptive ideas.

A well-written report of a qualitative study reads like a good story regardless of the specific approach employed in the study. Acknowledging this characteristic of qualitative studies initially may seem to minimize the importance of this type of research. Quite the contrary, however, the fact that a well-written study reads a bit like a good "story" points out the richness of this type of research. A well-written report captures the reader's attention and draws the reader into the experiences presented in the report of the study. The subjects come alive and the reader may begin to feel as if he or she actually knows the participant or at least can relate to his or her experiences. As the researcher is presenting results based on the analysis of the data, quotations using the actual words of the participants provide examples that support the researcher's conclusions. The reader, therefore, does not merely have to rely on the interpretations of the researcher but is presented with evidence that supports these conclusions. Reading these examples not only adds considerable credibility to the findings but also increases the richness and provides detail that is not evident in other types of research. The researcher may use some quantitative data to present demographic information, but it is the words of the participants and the researcher's weaving of these words with detailed analysis that make qualitative research so sensitizing and illustrative of individual experiences.

TRUSTWORTHINESS AND RIGOR

The qualitative study report that is written well gives the reader a strong sense that the results are believable. The voices of the participants seem alive and it is easy to grasp their experiences. Although this can be a valuable observation in assessing the quality of a qualitative study, there are additional criteria that must be considered. In quantitative research, the criteria that are used to evaluate the quality of a study overall are referred to as validity and reliability, and these have been discussed elsewhere in this text. Qualitative studies are carried out to accomplish different purposes and are completed using very different procedures. Consequently, a different set of criteria, referred to using a unique vocabulary, is used to evaluate the varied aspects of a qualitative study.

Noted researchers and methodologists Lincoln and Guba (1985) presented a framework in the mid-1980s that has been accepted widely as offering appropriate criteria to ensure a quality investigation. Similarly, these criteria also can be used to evaluate the quality of studies that have been completed and reported in the literature. To avoid confusion with the criteria of reliability and validity that are used for quantitative research, Lincoln and Guba proposed a broad framework organized around the key concept of "trustworthiness" to evaluate the rigor and overall quality of a study. It is interesting to note that the aspects of research addressed by these criteria could be applied to any type of research, although the terminology here is most commonly used in the context of qualitative research.

The terminology and ideas adopted from Lincoln and Guba (1985) include the essential concerns of "truth value" or credibility, "applicability" or transferability, "consistency" or dependability, and "neutrality" (p. 290). There are some variations of criteria for rigor that have been developed specific to different contexts for qualitative research (Hall & Stevens, 1991; Im, Page, Lin, Tsai, & Cheng, 2004). For general critique purposes, however, the principles explicated by Lincoln and Guba are worth remembering because of the extent to which they reflect the unique strengths of qualitative research. These criteria provide useful general guidelines for evaluating the quality of qualitative studies.

According to Lincoln and Guba (1985), the first criterion, "truth value" addresses an extremely important concern in any research, the concern about whether or not it is reasonable to "believe" or have faith in the results. For qualitative research, this means that there needs to be confidence that the results are an accurate reflection of the participants and the experiences that were studied. There are numerous techniques that qualitative researchers can use to increase the likelihood that results will be "credible." Researchers need, first, to spend sufficient time with participants to be able to fully understand their realities and how they describe their experiences (a technique referred to as "prolonged engagement"). Sufficient contact also is necessary to establish rapport with participants to increase their comfort with the researcher and, consequently, their willingness to share important details. A technique known as triangulation sometimes is used to enhance credibility or trustworthiness. The term "triangulation" is adopted from a process for navigation in which several location points are determined and the intersection of lines drawn from these points is determined. Using simple principles of geometry, it is possible for an individual at sea to pinpoint his or her specific location. When applied to a qualitative study, triangulation means the corroboration of information using multiple sources, multiple methods, different investigators, or even the perspective provided by different theories (Denzin, 1978). In a health-related study, participants' descriptions of their experiences might be triangulated with the accounts of nurses or family members or even with the medical record. It is worth noting, however, that whether or not a participant's description of an experience is factual is not always a concern. People construct their viewpoints and the experiences are shaped by what they believe happened, whether or not such beliefs are based in fact. Someone who experienced major trauma and believes he or she "died" and was brought back to life will, undoubtedly, relate to that experience in a way that is shaped by that belief. Whether or not, clinically, the described events actually took place may be of little consequence. For occasions in which different perspectives or the need to determine actual events are important in the study, triangulation is a very effective technique.

Other techniques also can be used to enhance the trustworthiness of results. A process referred to as "peer debriefing" provides an opportunity for the researcher to talk through aspects of the study with a colleague (peer) who has not invested in the study. This simple act of talking through parts of the study can be helpful in bringing to light some of the thoughts and ideas of the researcher that might not have been recognized otherwise or, in other words, might have stayed hidden in the recesses of the researcher's mind. The peer debriefer asks probing questions, challenges assumptions, encourages exploration and, overall, helps the researcher become aware of any potential misinterpretation, missed clues in the data, and personal value orientation or bias. Complete objectivity in any study is not possible; yet, although it is not possible to be completely devoid of bias in any study, peer debriefing helps the researcher to recognize what bias exists and how it might affect the study. Through this awareness, the researcher can make a conscious effort to limit the influence of bias in the research.

Occasionally researchers will use a technique known as a "member check" to ensure the credibility of findings. In doing a member check, the researcher returns to the participants, or to a subset of participants, and shares findings with them so that they can verify that the researcher correctly understands the views and experiences presented in the interview. A member check can be done at the conclusion of an interview with the interviewer giving the participant a brief summary of the interview for their feedback. It can also be done near the conclusion of a study by taking study results back to some of the participants for their consideration and review. Using this technique, the researcher is able to verify with study participants that the results accurately reflect the experiences that were described to the researcher. In other words, the researcher knows the results are credible because he or she asked the participants themselves to ensure that they are. Member checks are not possible in all studies and research situations. When appropriate, however, they can be a very useful means to ensure that the results of a study are credible or trustworthy.

The second criterion is referred to as "applicability" and addresses an issue similar to generalizability. As noted previously, there is no expectation or desire on the part of qualitative researchers that their results are, in fact, generalizable. Generalizability always has to be considered with great caution and, in qualitative studies, where the emphasis is on depth and richness, it would minimize the role of each unique individual to assume or stipulate that results actually will be generalizable simply by virtue of some feature of how the study was conducted. In contrast, the researcher in a qualitative study acknowledges that the consumer of the research is in the best position to evaluate whether or not results are applicable in other settings. For nurses in practice settings, this means that the nurse is in the best position to determine to what extent results are likely to be useful for clients in the setting in which the nurse works with these individuals. How similar are the contexts and the individuals in the study to those with whom the nurse works? Rather than stipulate that results are generalizable, the obligation of the qualitative researcher is to provide a sufficiently detailed description of the research situation to enable the reader of the research to make the determination whether the results are likely to "transfer" to other settings.

The two remaining criteria for conducting rigorous qualitative inquiry (and for evaluating the rigor of studies that have been reported in the literature) are "consistency" (dependability) and "neutrality" (confirmability). Consistency is similar to the concept of reliability for quantitative studies. In a quantitative study, there is an expectation that repeated use of an instrument will provide comparable results with each administration. In a qualitative study, however, things cannot be expected to be the same with repeated episodes of data collection or with repeated collection of information from different groups. People often change their perspective as they talk about experiences, the act of talking providing an opportunity for reflection with new insights and memories emerging. Similarly, a different investigator might elicit different descriptions from people based on the focus of the interview, whatever cognitive or emotional processing has gone on within the individual, changes in context for data collection, and other factors that can influence what is obtained in a qualitative study. Consequently, it is unreasonable to expect an occurrence comparable to stepping on a bedside scale and receiving the same results each time. What is important, however, is that all aspects of a qualitative study, including the collection of data and the analytic techniques that are employed and the insights generated, are all conducted in a way that is "dependable" or "confirmable." The process must be rigorous and comprehensive and the product must be supported by appropriate data. The question, therefore, is not whether the same results would be obtained if someone else did the research. The appropriate question is whether the results obtained by the researcher who did the study are appropriate, reasonable, and the processes can be traced and documented so that the results are defensible.

Both of these aspects of quality can be assessed using an "audit trail" (Halpern, 1983; Rodgers & Cowles, 1993). Qualitative researchers keep records about all the steps in the process of conducting the study, including procedures, methodological changes that are instituted, insights generated during data analysis, and observational or field notes. These records can be reviewed by other investigators who serve as auditors to ensure that the processes and procedures are carried out in a rigorous manner. All of the steps in the conduct of the study can be retraced and evaluated for quality. Although audits can be conducted on a large-scale basis just as a financial audit of a large company might be conducted, more often a researcher will engage a colleague to serve as a peer reviewer to evaluate aspects of the study on an ongoing basis while the research is being conducted and results are being prepared for dissemination.

SUMMARY

Qualitative research contributes vital information necessary to effective work with human beings. It is valuable in exploring areas about which little is known, in developing theory, and in generating rich and detailed descriptions about the lives of people with whom nurses work. Understanding the human element of health situations, the thoughts, feelings, and perceptions of individuals, is essential to providing sensitive care in a manner appropriate to the people with whom nurses work. This aspect of human experience also contributes essential information for evidence-based practice, illuminating the personal experience associated with various health situations and events. Recognizing the roles and contributions of qualitative research and understanding and critiquing published studies are important abilities for nurses who strive to base their practice on quality evidence relevant to the populations with whom they work.

SUGGESTED ACTIVITIES

1. Discuss with a classmate a clinical problem of interest. Describe how you could approach the problem using a qualitative research question and a quantitative question. What would be the differences in the findings?
2. Write questions that could be used in an interview in a qualitative study of the losses experienced from a chronic illness.

REFERENCES

Blumer, H. (1969). *Symbolic interactionism: Perspective and method.* Englewood Cliffs, NJ: Prentice-Hall.

Charmaz, K. (2000). Grounded theory: Objectivist and constructivist methods. In N. Denzin & Y. Lincoln (Eds.), *Handbook of qualitative research* (2nd ed., pp. 509–535). Thousand Oaks, CA: Sage.

Charmaz, K. (2005). Grounded theory in the 21st century: Applications for advancing social justice studies. In N. Denzin & Y. Lincoln (Eds.), *Handbook of qualitative research* (3rd ed., pp. 507–535). Thousand Oaks, CA: Sage.

Charmaz, K. (2006). *Constructing grounded theory.* London, UK: Sage.

Denzin, N. K. (1978). *Sociological methods.* New York, NY: McGraw-Hill.

Glaser, B. (1978). *Theoretical sensitivity.* Mill Valley, CA: Sociology Press.

Glaser, B., & Strauss, A. (1967). *The discovery of grounded theory.* Chicago, IL: Aldine.

Hall, J. M., & Stevens, P. E. (1991). Rigor in feminist research. *Advances in Nursing Science, 13*(3), 16–29.

Halpern, E. S. (1983). *Auditing naturalistic inquiries: The development and application of a model.* Bloomington, IN: Indiana University. University Microfilms International AAT 8317108.

Husserl, E. (1960). *Cartesian meditations: An introduction to phenomenology* (D. Cairns, trans.). The Hague, Netherlands: Martinus Nijhoff.

Im, E. O., Page, R., Lin, L. C., Tsai, H. M., & Cheng, C. Y. (2004). Rigor in cross-cultural nursing research. *International Journal of Nursing Studies, 41*, 891–899.

Knafl, K. A., & Webster, D. C. (1988). Managing and analyzing qualitative data: A description of tasks, techniques, and materials. *Western Journal of Nursing Research, 10*, 195–210.

Koch, T. (1995). Interpretive approaches in nursing research: The influence of Husserl and Heidegger. *Journal of Advanced Nursing, 21*, 827–836.

Labov, W., & Waletsky, J. (1967). Narrative analysis: Oral versions of personal experience. In J. Helm (Ed.), *Essays on the verbal and visual arts* (pp. 12–44). Seattle, WA: American Ethnological Society.

Lincoln, Y. S., & Guba, E. G. (1985). *Naturalistic inquiry.* Beverly Hills, CA: Sage.

Melnyk, B. M., & Fineout-Overholt, E. (2010). *Evidence-based practice in nursing & healthcare* (2nd ed.). Philadelphia, PA: Lippincott, Williams and Wilkins.

Merleau-Ponty, M. (1999). *The phenomenology of perception.* London: Routledge (Original work published 1962).

Morse, J. M. (1991). Strategies for sampling. In J. M. Morse (Ed.), *Qualitative nursing research: A contemporary dialogue.* Newbury Park, CA: Sage.

Patton, M. Q. (2001). *Qualitative research and evaluation methods* (3rd ed.). Thousand Oaks, CA: Sage.

Plager, K. A. (1994). Hermeneutic phenomenology: A methodology for family health and health promotion study in nursing. In P. Benner (Ed.), *Interpretive phenomenology: Embodiment, caring, and ethics in health and illness* (pp. 65–83). Thousand Oaks, CA: Sage.

QSR International Pty Ltd. (2012). NVivo [Computer software]. Doncaster, Victoria, Australia.

Quint, J. C. (1966). The case for theories generated from empirical data. *Nursing Research, 16*, 109–113.

Researchware. (2011). HyperResearch [Computer software]. Randolph, MA.

Riessman, C. K. (1993). *Narrative analysis.* Newbury Park, CA: Sage.

Riley, T., & Hawe, P. (2005). Researching practice: The methodological case for narrative inquiry. *Health Education Research, 20*, 226–236.

Rodgers, B. L. (1997). Experiences of family members in the nursing home placement of an older adult. *Clinical Nursing Research, 10*, 57–63.

Rodgers, B. L. (2005). *Developing nursing knowledge: Philosophical traditions and influences.* Philadelphia, PA: Lippincott Williams & Wilkins.

Rodgers, B. L. (2007). *Experiences of women with myocardial infarction.* Report to the Wisconsin Women's Health Foundation, Madison, WI.

Rodgers, B. L., & Cowles, K. V. (1993). The qualitative research audit trail: A complex collection of documentation. *Research in Nursing and Health, 16*, 219–226.

Sandelowski, M. (1986). The problem of rigor in qualitative research. *Advances in Nursing Science, 8*(3), 27–37.

Scientific Software Development. (2012). Atlas.ti [Computer software]. Berlin, Germany.

Strauss, A., & Corbin, J. (1998). *Basics of qualitative research: Techniques and procedures for developing grounded theory.* Thousand Oaks, CA: Sage.

Van Manen, M. (1990). *Research lived experience: Human science for an action sensitive pedagogy.* Albany, NY: State University of New York.

VERBI Software. (2013). MAXQDA [Computer software]. Berlin, Germany.

Wolf, Z. R. (2007). Ethnography: The method. In P. L. Munhall (Ed.), *Nursing research: A qualitative perspective* (4th ed., pp. 293–330). Sudbury, MA: Jones and Bartlett.

10

Sampling Methods

Mary D. Bondmass

One of the first and most frequently questions asked in any discussion of sampling is, "*How many subjects do I need in my sample?*" The first and most frequent answer to this question usually is, "*It depends.*" Sampling decisions contribute critically to a study's internal validity (truthfulness or accuracy) and external validity (generalizability or applicability). Asking or answering the question of sample size as the first discussion point about sampling is analogous to the old adage of "putting the cart before the horse," that is, reversing the order of addressing an issue or problem. Although it is extremely important, sampling is about more than just, "*How many subjects do I need for my sample*"; decisions and processes depending on such things as a study's design and a study's data source(s) are related and need to be considered sequentially in planning research. A study's design is its general structure; its data source is the actual sample or more precisely, the individual elements or basic units that make up that sample, keeping in mind that not all elements of a sample are always people (although in health care research, this is often the case). Ethical issues in sampling also need to be considered and part of any discussion and/or decisions on a type or number included in a sample. All of the above are considered in this chapter on sampling methods as an a priori approach to answering, "*How many subjects do I need in my study?*"

This chapter is primarily intended for those who need basic information to critically appraise the sample section of a research article and for those who may be contemplating conducting research or a quality-improvement project; either of whom may need clarification on that "*it depends*" answer that was given above. Prior to addressing the sample-size question, for either of the two intended audiences for this chapter, it is important to understand the logic and basic principles of sampling and some basic concepts related to sampling. This chapter begins with definitions of terms used in the proceeding discussions of the underlying theory and logic of sampling, and sampling methods. The remainder of this chapter provides the reader with a way to answer the question of sample size asked previously; this is accomplished through a recapitulation of central limits theorem as well as of the concept of power and power analysis. Suggested activities are also included at the end of this chapter for you to self-assess your understanding of the content.

TERMINOLOGY

Below and included in the glossary (Exhibit 10.1) are some definitions of terms that will be used throughout this chapter. Many of you have most probably heard these terms before in research discussions, but may not have fully understood them. Moreover, whether you are conducting research or critically appraising the research of others, an understanding of research terminology is foundational for evidence-based practice. The reader is referred back to this section and the Glossary of Terms at any point later in the chapter when a term is used, but the context is not fully understood.

The *theoretical* or *target population* (often simply just referred to as the *population*) is an aggregate of people, groups, objects, or things that meet a designated set of criteria. The population of a particular study is the group of interest that a researcher wishes to make generalizations about. The individual units of a population are referred to as *elements*. Because it is generally impossible to reach an entire population, an accessible population is delineated. An *accessible population* is a subset of the population that is reasonably accessible to a researcher. A *sampling frame* is the listing of people, groups, objects/things, or a procedure developed for drawing a sample from the accessible population. The sampling frame becomes the methodical "how" related to the actual drawing of your sample. Finally, the *sample* consists of those people, groups, or objects that a researcher selects from the accessible population using their sampling frame. Theoretically, a study's actual or true sample usually ends up being a subsample due to non-respondents and attrition; however, for the purpose of a more practical discussion the subsample will simply be referred to here as the study sample. In theory, if error and bias are eliminated or minimized, the study sample should be representative of the population and thereby generalizations can be made about the population from the sample.

As an example, let us say you plan to conduct a study involving an intervention that would decrease salt in the diets of hypertensive African American (AA) women; the desired result of your study is blood pressure control. In your study design, you already

Exhibit 10.1
Glossary of Terms

Cluster sampling refers to a type of sampling method wherein the researcher divides the population into separate groups, called clusters. Then, a simple random sample of clusters is selected from the population. The researcher conducts his or her analysis on data from the sampled clusters. Compared with simple random sampling and stratified sampling, cluster sampling has advantages and disadvantages. For example, given equal sample sizes, cluster sampling usually provides less precision than either simple random sampling or stratified sampling. On the other hand, if travel costs between clusters are high, cluster sampling may be more cost-effective than the other methods.

Convenience sampling is nonprobability sampling, sometimes called an accidental sample, wherein members of the population are chosen based on their relative ease of access. Samples of friends, co-workers, or shoppers at a single mall, are all examples of convenience sampling. Such samples are biased because researchers may unconsciously approach some kinds of respondents and avoid others (Lucas 2012), and respondents who volunteer for a study may differ in unknown but important ways from others (Wiederman 1999).

A *mean* is an average; often the mean is a score of other interval level characteristics that can have an average.

Nonprobability sampling is the process wherein population elements are selected on the basis of their availability, or on a personal judgment or determination that they represent.

A *parameter* is a measurable characteristic of a population, such as a mean or a standard deviation.

Probability sampling is the process wherein all elements in the population have some opportunity of being included in the sample.

Purposive sampling is a nonprobability sampling strategy, sometimes called *judgmental* sampling, in which the researcher chooses the sample based on who he or she thinks would be appropriate for the study.

Quota sampling is nonprobability sampling, sometimes called a strat-based sampling, or ad hoc quotas, wherein a quota is established (say 65% women) and researchers are free to choose any respondent they wish as long as the quota is met.

(continued)

(continued)

Random error or sampling error is the difference between sample estimates and the population parameters.

Randomization refers to the practice of using chance methods (random number tables, flipping a coin, etc.) to assign subjects to treatments.

Representativeness is the quality of a sample having the same distribution of characteristics as the population from which it was drawn (Babbie, 2014).

Sampling bias or nonrepresentative sampling bias is also known as selection bias as this inaccuracy is caused due to not implementing random methods during the selection process, which results in either inadequate or excess representation of some elements in the population.

Sampling design is a combination of the sampling process and the estimation or inferences made to the total group from the sample data (Kirchhoff, 2009).

A *sampling distribution* or finite-sample distribution is the probability distribution of a given statistic based on a random sample. Sampling distributions are important in statistics because they provide a major simplification on the route to statistical inference. More specifically, they allow analytical considerations to be based on the sampling distribution of a statistic, rather than on the joint probability distribution of all the individual sample values (Merberg, 2008).

Simple random sampling refers to any sampling method that has the following properties: (1) the population consists of N objects, (2) the sample consists of n objects, (3) all possible samples of n objects are equally likely to occur. An important benefit of simple random sampling is that it allows researchers to use statistical methods to analyze sample results. For example, given a simple random sample, researchers can use statistical methods to define a confidence interval around a sample mean. Statistical analysis is not appropriate when nonrandom sampling methods are used.

Snowball sampling is a nonprobability sampling method, sometimes called network sampling, in which the first respondent refers a friend. The friend also refers a friend, and so on. Such samples are biased because they give people with more social connections an unknown but higher chance of selection (Berg 2006).

The *standard deviation* is a numerical value used to indicate how widely individuals in a group vary. If individual observations vary greatly from the group mean, the standard deviation is big; and vice versa. It is important to distinguish between the standard deviation of a population and the standard deviation of a sample. They have a different notation, and are computed differently. The standard deviation of a population is denoted by σ, and the standard deviation of a sample, by s.

The *standard error* is a measure of the variability of a statistic. It is an estimate of the standard deviation of a sampling distribution. The standard error depends on three factors: (1) the number of observations in the population, (2) the number of observations in the sample, and (3) the way that the random sample is chosen.

The *standard error of the mean*, also called the standard deviation of the mean, is a method used to estimate the standard deviation of a sampling distribution.

A *statistic* is a characteristic of a sample. Generally, a statistic is used to estimate the value of a population parameter.

Statistics is a discipline that allows researchers to evaluate conclusions derived from sample data.

Stratified sampling refers to a type of sampling method, wherein the researcher divides the population into separate groups called strata. Then, a probability sample (often a simple random sample) is drawn from each group. Stratified sampling has several advantages over simple random sampling. For example, by using stratified sampling, it may be possible to reduce the sample size required to achieve a given precision, or it may be possible to increase the precision with the same sample size.

With *systematic random sampling*, a list of every member of the population is created. From the list, one randomly selects the first sample element from the first k elements on the population list. Thereafter, we select every kth element on the list.

This method is different from simple random sampling since every possible sample of n elements is not equally likely.

A *variable* in statistics has two defining characteristics: (1) it is an attribute that describes a person, place, thing, or idea and (2) the value of the variable can "vary" from one entity to another.

Note: All the above definitions, except where otherwise noted, are taken directly from *STAT TRAK Statistics and Probability Dictionary* (an accredited university sponsored website) http://stattrek.com/statistics /dictionary.aspx have in mind that your *target population* will be AA women with hypertension, but this could include millions of women and clearly there is no way to intervene and collect data on this entire population. You will need to limit your subject search to those hypertensive AA women whom you can reasonably access yet still have them belong to, and be representative of, your original *target population*. Your *accessible population* may depend heavily on the logistics of where you plan to carry out your study. For the purposes of this example, let us say you work at an urban medical center in Chicago wherein many hypertensive AA women are treated. You therefore may define your *accessible population* as hypertensive AA women attending a particular clinic(s) in Chicago. Finally, your *sample* is the number of consenting subjects or participants selected (randomly or otherwise) from your *accessible population* to be actually included in your study. The study sample, in theory, then serves as a surrogate or proxy representative of your originally targeted population of hypertensive AA women. Figure 10.1 graphically depicts the relationship between the

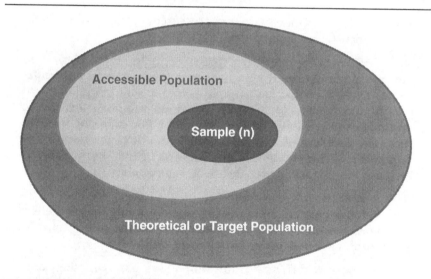

FIGURE 10.1   Relationship between theoretical and accessible populations and samples. A sample is drawn from the accessible population, that is derived from somewhere within the theoretical or target population. The sample always has a number associated with it represented often as a lower or uppercase *N*. At times the lowercase "*n*" will refer to groups within a sample and the uppercase "*N*" to the total sample. However generally within a well-written article, the reader can easily surmise which value the author(s) is referring to without further explanation be it a lower- or uppercase value. The uppercase *N* has also been used to represent the number of cases in the sampling frame.

theoretical/target and accessible population and the study sample and the Glossary of Terms (Exhibit 10.1) contains multiple other useful research terms.

SAMPLING THEORY AND LOGIC

The definition of sampling has not changed over the decades; older and more recent references can be found that define sampling similarly as the process of selecting a subset of observations from an entire population, such that the characteristics of the subset (e.g., the sample) will be representative enough to draw conclusions or make inferences about the population (Babbie, 2012; Henry, 1990; Kish, 1965).

The Central Limit Theorem (CLT), originally credited to Simon-Pierre Laplace in the early 1800s, provides the theoretical foundation for sampling and probability theory. The CLT basically states that given certain conditions, the mean of a sufficiently large number of independent random variables will be approximately normally distributed (Rice, 1995). Simply put, the CLT tells us that if we take the mean of multiple samples and plot the frequencies of the means, we will get a normal distribution (e.g., a bell curve).

The logic of sampling then is rather simple; it is efficient and accurate. The efficiency of sampling relates to gaining information about a large group from a small group; that is, your population of interest (large group) can be studied via a sample (small group), thereby obtaining the information that is sought at an acceptable cost. Accuracy is assumed because of the CLT, but only when sampling errors are minimized (Babbie, 201).

Random error, also called sampling error is incidental and is related to expected fluctuations among samples from a given population and/or unpredictable fluctuations in the readings of a measurement apparatus, or in the experimenter's interpretation of the instrumental reading. Considering that all measurements are prone to random error, precision in any instrumentation used and human attention to making precise measurements with those instruments would be a way to decrease random error (Taylor, 1999). Conversely, nonrandom error (e.g., conscious or unconscious bias), should be avoided or minimized to decrease the likelihood of erroneous conclusions.

A small sampling distribution could be constructed to demonstrate sampling error, but in theory, there are infinite numbers of sampling distributions that could be created, so we never really see a true sampling distribution. Sampling error can be calculated even though we never actually see the sampling distribution; the calculation is based on the standard deviation of the sample (standard error of the mean [*SEM*]). The standard deviation of the sampling distribution of the mean is called the standard error; the standard error is called sampling error (Babbie, 2012). Rather than try to reteach the whole of sampling theory here, when reading a research article, keep the following two statistics "pearls" in mind related to error:

- The greater the sample's standard deviation, the greater the standard error (and the sampling error).
- The standard error is also related to the sample size; therefore, the greater your sample size, the smaller the standard error (because the greater the sample size, the closer your sample is to the actual population itself).

Another way of looking at this last point is, when you know that values are likely to be different, increase your sample size. This last point should be useful regardless of whether you are conducting the research or critically appraising a study.

Using the previous example of the study related to hypertensive AA women, if you were to include only 15 women in the study sample, the standard error would theoretically be much larger than if your sample included 150 hypertensive AA women. The likelihood of 150 versus 15 subjects being representative of the target population increases with the sample size and therefore decreases the standard error.

PROBABILITY AND NONPROBABILITY SAMPLING

There are two classifications of sampling methods; probability and nonprobability sampling. Each method can have a number of different sample types within the respective classification. Although probability sampling could theoretically be used in both quantitative and qualitative research, nonprobability sampling is more frequently seen in qualitative research.

Probability Sampling

Probability samples are those samples selected using some component of probability theory, typically involving some sort of randomization feature such as the two different concepts of random selection or random assignment. Although addressing the general concept of randomization, I am always reminded of a quote that I learned in my very first statistic course and I feel compelled to share at this point in the chapter; it is intended to provide comic relief to what some might consider a very dry subject thus far and to make a point. *"If you don't believe in random sampling, the next time you have a blood test tell the doctor to take it all"* (unknown author). I have seen this quote attributed to several people including the former presidential candidate Thomas E. Dewey, a U.S. Census deputy, and Confucius. Although I doubt it is the latter, or any of the former for that matter, I will leave the credit to an unknown author, and ask the reader to just take a moment here to reflect on the underlying meaning of the quote.

In probability samples, the elements of population theoretically have an equal chance of being included in a particular sample. Although some may argue the blood test example above could be interpreted as convenience sampling, I contend it is a random sample and representative of the whole population of blood components in the donor's blood vessels. When research demands precise, statistical descriptions of large populations, probability sampling is used. Generally, all large-scale survey research and clinical trials use probability sampling methods. The fundamental premise of probability sampling is to provide useful descriptions of the total population, and therefore a sample from that population must basically demonstrate the same variation as in that population. This is not as straightforward as it may appear; if you recall the above discussion on error, you can probably imagine the multiple ways that either random or nonrandom error can affect the ability of a probability sample to perform as expected, that is, to be a representative sample of the population. The major advantage of probability sampling is fairness; the major disadvantage is the possibility of flaws to the randomness model. Some common probability samples include *simple random, stratified, cluster,* and *systemic samples.* As a self-assessment of your understanding of probability samples, design a sampling method for each of the common probability sample types listed here using the hypothetical study of hypertensive AA women from above. See the Glossary of Terms for description of each of the probability sample types to assist you in this learning activity.

Nonprobability Sampling

When nonprobability sampling methods are used, every element in the population does not have an equal chance of being in a study sample; therefore nonprobability samples are less likely than probability samples to be representative of the population. Moreover, nonprobability samples may be more predisposed to error. There are advantages, however, to nonprobability sampling, primarily the ease of implementation, and with control strategies, nonprobability methods can produce credible samples. Also keep in mind that the purpose and design of a particular study using nonprobability methods might not be to demonstrate population representativeness. Many qualitative studies are not interested in representativeness of a population, but rather in simply describing in depth the lived experience of individual elements of a population or other qualitative strategies. The four common types of nonprobability sampling include purposive (judgmental), snowball (network), quota (strata-based), and convenience (accidental) samples; the latter of the four is the most commonly used. See the Glossary of Terms (Exhibit 10.1) for a description of each of the nonprobability sample types.

RELATED CONCEPTS

Sample Size

At the beginning of this chapter, the question was posed as to "*How many subjects do I need in my sample?*" The answer was given as "*it depends,*" and this last portion of the chapter discusses why. The number of subjects or participants in a study is part of the overall design process as well as the sampling plan and should be determined prior to beginning any research, recognizing that there are advantages to both large and small sample sizes. Aside from methodological design issues and conclusion validity, a priori determination of sample size may have both economical and ethical considerations. Research is a costly enterprise, the more the subjects recruited, and ultimately retained in a sample, the more the money that your research will generally cost in dollars and institution and human resources. Moreover, the researcher has an ethical responsibility to the subjects of human and even animal research not to expose them to any more procedural processes and/ or pain and/or inconvenience than needed; larger is not necessarily better and may be unethical when statistical significance can be demonstrated by a predetermined and possibly smaller sample size than an arbitrary larger number that just "seems large enough."

Despite the importance of sample-size determinations, there is no universally agreed upon method for this within the health care professions; however, nurses who lead or participate in research teams as well as nurses who critically appraise research for practice require a basic understanding of the factors involved in sample-size determination. Study and population characteristics, measurement issues, effect size, and practical issues are all factors affecting sample-size determination. Generally, more complex studies, with multiple variables and relationships being explored, require larger samples. Although there are others, two relatively simple methods of sample-size determination will be presented here, including the "Rule of 30" with its basis in CLT and statistical power and power analysis.

"Rule of 30"

As noted, the more complex the study, as defined by the number of variables and number of groups examined, the larger a sample may need to be. The CLT is the theoretical basis for the "Rule of 30." According to the previously mathematically proven CLT, the mean of a randomly generated sample of 30 or more elements approximates the population mean for any characteristic (Hinkle, Wierma, & Jurs, 2003). This rule is described by Hinkle et al. (2003) as a minimum of 30 elements for each variable of interest in a sample. Additionally, if subgroups are being compared (e.g., perhaps gender or racial differences), each group needs to be representative of the total sample; generally this means at least 30 elements also in each subgroup. Attrition rates need to be estimated; these rates can often be estimated from reports of similar studies and need to be added to the number derived from the "Rule of 30" calculation.

Using the previous study example related to hypertensive AA women, let us say you wanted to use the "Rule of 30" to determine your study's sample size. Unfortunately, it is not just simply planning to have a sample size of 30 subjects; one must also consider the number of variables to be studied and the number of groups that the researcher plans to use in the study. It was noted in the previous example that the dependent or outcome variable of interest was blood pressure control. How the researcher defines or operationalizes blood pressure control (i.e., if you are interested in both systolic and diastolic values, then you have two dependent variables) and the actual study design (i.e.. if you plan a one-group pre/post design or a multiple-group comparative design) also influences the "Rule of 30." Therefore if you chose to use both systolic and diastolic blood pressures as outcome variables and you planned a two-group (control and intervention) comparative design, according to the "Rule of 30," you would need 120 subjects in the final sample (30 per variable and 30 per group). An experienced researcher might also inflate this "Rule of 30" sample size of 120 to accommodate for attrition or dropout of subjects during the study period.

Statistical Power and Power Analysis

Statistical power is the probability of a statistical test finding a significant difference, if such a difference indeed exists; it is the probability of rejecting the null hypothesis when it is false (Cohen, 1997). Simply put, it is the probability of not committing a Type II error, or false-negative rate (β); as the power increases the likelihood of making a false-negative decision related to your study's results decreases. Power is statistically represented as $1-\beta$, and 0.80 is generally accepted as adequate statistical power for a study (Cohen, 1997). Others have opined that statistical power is analogous to the sensitivity of a diagnostic test, and one may mentally substitute the word "sensitivity" for the word "power" to assist in understanding the concept (Browner & Newman, 1987; Eng, 2003).

Power is affected by four major factors, including the significance criterion (α), the magnitude of the effect (effect size), the sample size, and the study design. Two clinical pearls related to power and power analysis are as follows: as the effect size increases, you may be able to decrease your sample size, because if the effect of the intervention is large, it should be detected easily in a smaller sample; conversely, if you have a small effect size, you would need to increase your sample size to be able to detect that effect.

Power analysis can be used to calculate the minimum sample size required so that it is reasonably likely to detect an effect of a given size. Power analysis can also be used to calculate the minimum effect size that is likely to be detected in a study using a given sample size. Cohen (1997) presents power tables in his text, which some may find very useful and, if you are so inclined, you can find the actual statistical calculations there also. More and more publishers now encourage researchers to calculate and publish the effect size for each variable in their study, so that others can be more exact in their own power analysis calculation when using a similar intervention or treatment. However, if you do not choose to calculate by hand your own power and/or effect size (not sure why you would want to), there are open (free) online power calculators that can decrease work and stress levels for the average health care practitioner tasked with determining sample size for a study or quality-improvement project. The best online power analysis tool I have found, available for both Mac and Windows, is called G*Power3 and it is available from the Department of Experimental Psychology Heinrich-Heine-University in Düsseldorf, Germany. Much of the website is in German, but instructions are also in English. The G*Power3 website is http://www.psycho.uni-duesseldorf.de/abteilungen/aap/gpower3.

Once again using the previous hypothetical study of an intervention to decrease salt intake in hypertensive AA women, let us assume you plan to have two groups of randomly assigned participants (subjects) to receive or not receive (i.e., a control group) your intervention. For this example, your outcome or dependent variable is systolic blood pressure only; a literature search indicates that interventions similar to yours have demonstrated small (0.20) to medium (0.50) effect sizes (Cohen, 1997). In designing your study, you want to determine how many participants will reasonably be needed (power of 0.80) to demonstrate statistical difference between the intervention and control groups, given a certain effect size. The following three points are examples of the results of a priori power analyses to make this determination. Because the effect size is not definitive, you choose to do a power analysis using multiple effect sizes to cover the range or from small to medium. The reader is asked to pay particular attention to the sample-size requirement (to achieve 0.80 power) when the effect size changes. What does this tell you about the desired effect size?

- Using a two-tailed independent t-test, with an alpha error probability of 0.05, and a medium effect size of 0.50, 64 participants per group ($N = 128$) would be needed to achieve 0.80 power to detect statistical differences between the groups, if such differences exist.

- Using a two-tailed independent *t*-test, with an alpha error probability of 0.05, and an effect size of 0.35, 130 participants per group (*N* = 260) would be needed to achieve 0.80 power to detect statistical differences between the groups, if such differences exist.
- Using a two-tailed independent *t*-test, with an alpha error probability of 0.05, and a small effect size of 0.20, 394 participants per group (*N* = 788) would be needed to achieve 0.80 power to detect statistical differences between the groups, if such differences exist.

See Exhibit 10.2 for G*Power3's five different types of statistical power analysis offered.

Exhibit 10.2
G*Power3: Five Types of Statistical Power Analysis

- A priori (sample size *N* is computed as a function of power level 1-β, significance level α, and the to-be-detected population effect size)
- Compromise (both α and 1-β are computed as functions of effect size, *N*, and an error probability ratio q = β/α)
- Criterion (α and the associated decision criterion are computed as a function of 1-β, the effect size, and *N*)
- Posthoc (1-β is computed as a function of α, the population effect size, and *N*)
- Sensitivity (population effect size is computed as a function of α, 1-β, and *N*)

Source: Faul, Erdfelder, Buchner, & Lang (2009); Faul, Erdfelder, Lang & Buchner (2007).

SUMMARY

In summary, sampling is the process of selecting a subset of observations from an entire population, such that the characteristics of the subset (e.g., the sample) will be representative enough to draw conclusions or make inferences about the population. Sampling decisions contribute critically to a study's internal and external validity and need to be made thoughtfully and judiciously. Decisions and processes depending on such things as a study's design and a study's data source(s) are related and need to be considered sequentially in planning research. Economical and ethical issues in sampling also need to be considered and should be part of any discussion and/or decisions on a type or number included in a sample. Choosing between probability and nonprobability sampling and the type of sample within each category are the key to the validity of a study's conclusions. Finally, determination of the sample size can be made easier and is likely to be more accurate when one has an understanding of the basic logic and principles related to sampling and by using established strategies such as the CLT theory with the "Rule of 30" strategy and applications like G*Power3, the validated, open-access power-analysis tool.

The reader is reminded that this chapter discusses the theory and a small section of the mathematics of sampling and is not inclusive of all the concepts that clinicians and/or researchers need to be cognizant of. Simply finding statistical differences does not always correlate with clinical significance or relevance. It is very satisfying when an intervention is found to be both clinically and statistically significant, but this is not always the case and the advanced practice nurse should be able to discern the difference. Additionally, statistical significance does not "prove" that the results demonstrated are generalizable to the target population (see Chapter 1), but may only be suggestive of this at best. Multiple studies and rigorous systematic reviews presenting synthesizing results are also needed for a researched intervention to become part of evidence-based practice.

SUGGESTED ACTIVITIES

You are interested in differences related to three variables, including systolic blood pressure, HgbA$_1$C levels, and weight, for African American Type II diabetic patients seen at your clinic. You want to determine whether there are differences in patient outcomes after 3 months of treatment by a family nurse practitioner (NP) compared to the family medical doctor (MD). You are also interested in three variables, but in two groups of patients to see whether the provider has an effect.

Complete the following exercises:

1. What type of sampling method and sample type would you use?
2. Using the "Rule of 30," determine sample size needed for your study.
3. For the same patients described above, but this time using G*Power3, determine the sample size needed per group to have 0.80 power, with a 0.25 effect size, alpha of 0.05, and using a *t*-test for mean independent samples.
4. Repeat No. 3 keeping everything the same but change the effect size to 0.50. What happens to the sample size? Why? Try an effect size of 0.10. Now what happens to the sample size?

Although No. 3 and No. 4 may seem beyond the scope of this chapter, following the instruction on the G*Power3 website and the information given in this exercise, you may surprise yourself and any colleagues you may be working with, by conducting this quality-improvement study.

REFERENCES

Babbie, E. R. (2012). *The practice of social research* (13th ed.). Belmont, CA: Wadsworth.

Browner, W. S., & Newman, T. B. (1987). Are all significant *P* values created equal? The analogy between diagnostic tests and clinical research. *Journal of the American Medical Association, 257*(18), 2459–2463.

Coyne, I. T. (1997). Sampling in qualitative research. Purposeful and theoretical sampling: Merging on clear boundaries? *Journal of Advanced Nursing, 26*(3), 623–630.

Eng, J. (2003). Sample size estimation: How many individuals should be studied? *Radiology, 227,* 309–313. doi: 10.1148/radiol.2272012051

Henry, B. T. (1990). *Practical sampling.* Newbury Park, CA: Sage.

Hinkle, D. E., Wiersma, W., & Jurs, S. G. (2003). *Applied Statistics for the Behavioral Sciences* (pp. 145–146). Concord, CA: Houghton Mifflin.

Kish, L. (1965). *Survey sampling.* New York, NY: John Wiley.

Rice, J. (1995). *Mathematical statistics and data analysis* (2nd ed.). Pacific Grove, CA: Duxbury Press.

Taylor, J. R. (1999). *An introduction to error analysis: The study of uncertainties in physical measurements* (p. 94). Mill Valley, CA: University Science Books.

11

Designing Questionnaires and Data Collection Forms

Karin T. Kirchhoff

The most common tool used in data collection is the questionnaire. Because its use is so common, most individuals assume that the construction of questionnaires is easy. Those who have filled out poorly constructed questionnaires know that something is wrong but may not be aware of which rules in questionnaire construction were violated. This chapter details one approach to designing questionnaires that has been used for national and local surveys with good response rates. Comments about ease of completion are included. Although all of these suggestions may not work in one questionnaire, they can be used as guidelines for general use, with violations only for good reasons. At the same time, the seeming simplicity of a majority of these suggestions does not account for their value. When read, they may seem simple, but if they are used to critique questionnaires received in the mail, their significance will become apparent.

The purposes of questionnaire construction are many and varied. The content in this chapter can be applied to the simplest data collection purpose or to the most elegant study. Questionnaires can be used for research, quality assurance, administrative decision making, or collection of data about patients' preferences. Most situations require the development of a form specific to the topic under investigation; in other cases, there may be a standardized form available or a compilation of forms used for specific types of studies. Frank-Stromborg and Olsen (2004) have compiled a volume of instruments that can be used in clinical health care research.

This content of this chapter applies to questionnaires developed for telephone interviews, face-to-face interviews, or mailed surveys. Emphasis is placed on mailed questionnaires because the researcher is not available to answer a respondent's questions. In telephone interviews and face-to-face interviews, more information is able to be obtained by the respondent if needed. For those methods, lines should be drawn on the tool to lead the eye to specific tasks and the next section. In face-to-face interviews, lists or visual aids can be shown to the respondent, but this option is not readily available in telephone interviews unless the questionnaire is mailed ahead of time. In deciding whether to use mailed questionnaires or telephone interviews, it is important to consider sample characteristics and how they influence the respondent's interactions with the questions.

GENERAL CONSIDERATIONS

Let us address some general considerations about the items included in the questionnaire and the type of data generated from them. Item types should be interesting to the intended audience; otherwise the intended respondent will not even begin to answer questions. Individual items should not be embarrassing or threatening to the respondent; if they are, special care is needed to facilitate a response. The respondent's task should be easy to complete; he or she should be asked to circle an item or check a box, rather than write out an answer. The cover letter, introduction, and tone of the questions should convey respect for the respondents and for their privacy and be written in a conversational tone.

The amount and type of data needed should be carefully planned and the intended analysis should be determined before the questionnaire is finalized. Many investigators fail to make decisions about the difference between necessary and "interesting" data. The "interesting" information unnecessarily lengthens the questionnaire and may actually prevent the completion because of the number of pages or the estimated length of time necessary. The novice may wallow in the data and then find that the "interesting" data may not even enter into the final analysis. Such data should not have been collected. It is a waste of the respondents' and the investigators' time.

The use of "dummy" tables is helpful in ensuring that all needed data are collected (see Exhibit 11.1 for an example). In the "dummy" table, the title, the column (e.g., Employment status), and the row labels (e.g., yes/no) can be determined. In the cells, the proposed data (e.g., the number or percentage of the whole) can be reviewed to see whether the correct information was collected and at the correct level of measurement (see Chapter 13). For example, if age is collected by category (21–30, 31–40, and 41–50), the options can form the rows of a table. However, if the actual age is not collected, the data are *not* able to be used later to determine whether there is a correlation between age and an attitude score or to calculate the average age of the respondents. When actual ages have not been obtained, the individual is only able to be placed in a category of ages. On the other hand, by asking age in years, the researcher can calculate correlations and also compute the average age of the sample. Ages can be put into categories later if this is desirable. If the researcher does not assess the planned analysis ahead of time, some necessary data may not be collected, compromising the final report. Further discussion on level of measurement of data is provided in Chapter 13 on analyzing quantitative data.

Exhibit 11.1
Dummy Table Example

Employment Status	Desiring Child Care	
	Yes	No
Part time	# or %	# or %
Full time	# or %	# or %

The major reason for taking the time to properly design a questionnaire is to reduce respondent burden, which then helps to increase the response rate. The goal of a well-designed questionnaire is to engage the respondent in the process, make the respondent feel that the task is important, and encourage the respondent to complete the task readily and easily. Most of the following information is intended to achieve this goal.

APPEARANCE

Format

The initial appearance of the questionnaire is important. How the items are laid out and the overall format contributes to the appearance. The black-to-white ratio is critical. White should clearly predominate. When there is too much print on a page, the respondent feels that the task is difficult or even overwhelming, even if the questionnaire is only a few pages long. The crowding of black on the page, especially by reduction techniques used in photocopying, does not fool respondents into thinking that the task is any less time consuming than it is, just because the questionnaire does not contain a lot of pages. It is more important to attend to the appearance than to the number of pages. The complexity of a questionnaire is not determined simply by the number of pages. The ease of the tasks and the spacing between items are more critical concerns. Obviously, the number of pages is *a* factor, but it is not *the* factor. Many investigators think that if they reduce a five-page questionnaire to a three-page questionnaire by reducing the print size, they make it less overwhelming to respondents, but the respondents may think differently and respond accordingly.

The cover letter and the questionnaire need to look "official." People are not motivated to respond if the questionnaire looks like it was produced on a printer low on toner. Some software packages can give a very official appearance with little effort. Use of institutional letterhead for the cover letter lends an official nature to the survey.

The size of the page is also important. The default size of 8.5 × 11" is not the only possibility. If the questionnaire is to be printed professionally, many sizes are available. One option is to use a centerfold approach, creating the appearance of a booklet. How the questionnaire will be mailed is one consideration that will affect the researcher's decision on what size of paper to use. The size of the envelope may be another limiting factor.

Color and Quality of Paper

Although white or near-white paper may give the best appearance, the researcher may choose another color for several reasons. For instance, when potential respondents need to be separated by groups, the use of different colors for each group will make the task easier. Using a color other than white also makes it less likely that the questionnaire will get lost on the respondent's desk. The use of dark colors should be avoided since black print on them is hard to read. The weight of the paper can give the impression of cheapness if it is too light; on the other hand, a heavy paper may increase the cost of postage. Physically feel the paper stock before printing questionnaires, and weigh the number of pages required along with the envelope and the return envelope to determine if a slight reduction in weight will avoid the need for additional postage.

Spacing

Spacing throughout the questionnaire is important. Spacing between questions should be greater than the spacing between the lines of each question, allowing the respondent to quickly read each question. Also, the spacing between response options should be sufficient to make it easy to determine which option was selected, especially if the task of the respondent is to circle a number. When material is single spaced, it can be difficult to determine which number was circled. Following these suggestions enhances the overall black-to-white ratio, as well.

Respondent Code

Another consideration is the place for a respondent code number. Usually an underscore line is placed at the upper-right corner on the first page. Although code numbers are essential if follow-up is anticipated, respondents are sometimes troubled by these numbers and either erase or obliterate them. This concern is particularly true when respondents fear an administrator's reaction to their answers or worry about lack of privacy. An explanation for the use of a code number in the cover letter may alleviate this concern but may not be sufficient if any of the information is at all revealing. When no respondent code is used, it is not possible to follow up on the nonrespondents because they cannot be separated from those who have responded. Not using a code number means that everyone will need to get a second and third contact, increasing costs of the study.

When respondent codes are not used on questionnaires, different colors of paper can be used to represent separate subgroups. In this instance, response rates can still be determined for the entire sample, as well as for each subgroup. Selective follow-up without code numbers can be done on everyone in the subgroup with a low response rate if funds and time permit.

Typeface

The typeface should be chosen carefully for readability and appearance. Script typeface should be avoided. The size of the typeface should be selected with the reader in mind. For example, if the questionnaire is to be read by the elderly, the typeface should be larger than would be required for a middle-aged adult. A good test is to have a few persons close to the intended respondents in age answer the planned questionnaire and describe the ease of completion.

SECTIONS OF THE QUESTIONNAIRE

Questionnaires are structured with several components. These include the title, directions for the respondents, questions to be answered, transition statement(s) when sections change, and a closing statement. The title should relate to the content of the questionnaire. Many times beginners will label it "Questionnaire" but that is like naming a baby "baby." Directions for completing the questions follow the title. For example, the direction may be that the respondent is to select the best possible option and circle a response code. The implication here is that there is only one option per question and that all options selected require a circle around a number or letter by that option. Directions would be different if they were to select as many as apply. Specific directions may be required for each section of the questionnaire, and these should be explained in a conversational manner. Items should be as similar as possible to facilitate completion and reduce respondent burden. The closing statement should thank the respondent for the time and effort taken to complete the tasks. Questions to be asked of respondents are addressed next.

An item consists of a question (or request for information) and possible response options. First, we discuss information about the questions; we then address response options.

Questions

Type of Questions

The choice between open-ended and closed-ended questions depends on several factors. The *nature of the question to be answered* by the data is one factor. Are feelings to be obtained, or facts? Feelings, especially if detail is needed, are best obtained in the respondent's own words. Therefore, open-ended questions would be the choice. Facts are more easily categorized. When detail is not required, closed-ended items should be used. If the desired outcome is a set of statements from respondents, open-ended questions should be chosen. If a quick count of responses in different categories is desired, closed-ended items will make the task easier.

Another issue in choosing between open- and closed-ended questions is *how much is known about the possible responses*. If all options are known, they can be provided in a list and the respondents can choose among them. If only some information is available, open-ended questions might be used. In instances when most of the options are known and the format calls for closed-ended responses, the use of "Other (please specify)_____" gives respondents a chance to answer if their response does not match the provided responses.

One of the most important factors in selecting between the two types of questions is the *sample size*. When dealing with a small number of questionnaires (fewer than 30), the researcher can use either option. With larger surveys (e.g., an entire hospital or institution or a national survey), closed-ended questions are preferable. They can be more readily summarized.

There are tradeoffs with either choice. Richness of responses and freedom of expression are lost with closed-ended questions. Ease of analysis and time are lost when open-ended questions are used unnecessarily. The investigator's burden is different with each. The time spent on designing the closed-ended items can be significant, but their analysis is relatively quick. Open-ended items are quicker to design but may take significantly longer to analyze. Where the time is spent—up front in design or later in analysis—may be an additional factor in the researcher's decision making.

Wording of the Questions

The researcher should select the words used carefully, avoiding slang, abbreviations, and words that have several meanings. When using terms that may not be familiar to the respondent, the researcher should provide a definition. One should try to avoid abbreviations altogether if possible. If that is not possible, it is a good idea to spell out the abbreviation the first time it is used and perhaps later if the second use is separated from the initial use.

The clarity of the questions and of potential responses should be ensured before the questionnaire is printed. The best way to do this is to pretest the questionnaire on several people who are similar to the intended respondents. Their responses will draw out any additional meanings or potentially confusing items. These individuals should be interviewed to assess any problems they had with completing the questionnaire, to determine what they thought the questions meant, and how difficult they found it to complete the questionnaire. It is helpful to time these pretests, because that information can then be included in the cover letter to help the final respondents estimate how long it will take them to complete the questionnaire.

Guidelines for Well-Written Questions

1. Use a conversational tone. The tone of the questions and of the entire questionnaire should be as if the respondent were present. For example, the question:

Sex   M____
     F ____

should be expressed as:

What is your sex? Is it

Male?   1
or Female?   2

Using the word *gender* instead of *sex* in this question may be preferable because it avoids some strange responses.

2. Avoid leading questions that suggest the expected response. An example is:

Problem: Most mothers ensure that their infants receive immunizations as infants. Has your child been immunized?

Yes   1
No   2

Revision: Has your child been immunized?

Yes   1
No   2

3. Avoid double-barreled questions that ask two questions at the same time. An example is:

Problem: Do you prefer learning about your illness in a group format, or would you rather use written material?

Yes   1
No   2

Revision: Do you prefer a group format for learning about your
         illness?

Yes   1
No   2

Do you prefer written materials for learning about your illness?

Yes   1
No   2

4. Try to state questions simply and directly without being too wordy.
   For some questions, the respondent wonders, "What was the question?" after reading wordy sections. A direct approach is more likely
   to yield the desired information.

5. Avoid double negatives.

   Problem: Should the nurse not be responsible for case management?

   Yes   1
   No   2

   Revision: Who should be responsible for case management?
   The physician   1
   The nurse   2
   An administrator   3
   Other (please specify) 4

6. Do not assume that the respondent has too much knowledge.

   Problem: Are you in favor of care for walk-ins in the clinic?

   Yes   1
   No   2

   Revision: In the clinic, walk-ins will be seen in short appointments
            on the same day they call in with questions, rather than
            being scheduled for appointments later in the week. There
            will be a block of 1-hour appointments in both the morn-
            ing and the afternoon left open for them.

   Are you in favor of walk-ins in the clinic?
   Yes   1
   No   2

Response Options

Responses are developed for closed-ended questions. The designer
of the questionnaire needs to have an idea about what the common
options could be. Some options are dichotomous such as "yes" and
"no." Some are more complex. When not all options are known, there
should be an open-ended opportunity for the respondent to give an
answer. Different types of options have common mistakes that are
made in their use. These are detailed next.

Guidelines for Writing Response Options

There are also guidelines for the use of the response options. The most common ones are listed here.

1. Do not make response options *too* vague or *too* specific.
   Problem (too vague): How often do you call in sick?

Never	1
Rarely	2
Occasionally	3
Regularly	4

   Revision: How often did you call in sick in the past 6 months?

Not at all	1
1–2 times	2
3–4 times	3
more than 4 times	4

   Problem (too vague): Which state are you from? _____

   Revision: In which state do you live? _____

   In which state do you work? _____

   Problem (too specific): How many total books did you read last year? _____

   Revision: How many books did you read last year?

None	1
1–3	2
4–6	3
More than 7	4

2. The categories should be mutually exclusive, that is, there should be no overlap. This can become a problem when ranges are given. For example:

   Problem: How old are you?

20–30 years	1
30–40 years	2
40–50 years	3
50 or more years old	4

   The person who is 30 years of age does not know whether to circle a "1" or a "2."

   Revision: How old are you?

20–29 years	1
30–39 years	2
40–49 years	3
50 or more years old	4

3. The categories must be inclusive and exhaustive.

In the previous example, only if all the respondents contacted were at least 20 years old would the categories be inclusive of all respondents. The last response, "50 or more years old," exhausts the upper age limit. The only caution in the use of such a range is that such a grouping loses detail. If only a few respondents are expected to fall into this category, then it may be adequate.

4. The order of options given is from *smaller* to *larger* or from *negative* to *positive*.

As an example: values for "not at all" are scored with "0" or "1" and the maximum value is scored as "5." In the analysis and explanation of the findings, it is easy to explain that higher numbers mean more of something. A mean satisfaction score that is higher than another mean satisfaction score would then be a more desirable finding.

The revised example in the next problem illustrates the correct order. If the coding were reversed, a higher score would mean less agreement (or more disagreement).

5. The balance of the options should be parallel.

Problem: Do you agree that nurses should receive a higher salary?

Extremely strongly disagree	1
Very strongly disagree	2
Strongly disagree	3
Agree	4
Strongly agree	5

Revision: Do you agree that nurses should receive a higher salary?

Strongly disagree	1
Disagree	2
Agree	3
Strongly agree	4

To further clarify point 4, if the order of the options were reversed, a high mean on this question would signify less agreement. That could be very confusing to those who review the data in the write-up of the findings.

6. Limit the number of different types of response options chosen for use in the same questionnaire.

Common response options are:

approve–disapprove
agree–disagree (*alone* or with *strongly* in front of each for two additional options)
better–about the same–worse
very good–good–poor–very poor

A neutral middle can be provided if needed, such as "uncertain." Whenever possible, the use of the same response options across questions is preferred. The respondent's task becomes more difficult when it is necessary to adjust to multiple types of options. The respondent feels required to constantly "change gears," and the burden is increased.

7. The number of response options per question should be minimized. The usual recommendation is to have four or five possible responses. If a neutral middle response is desired, then five responses should be used, with the third or middle response being the neutral one. If there is an even number of responses, the respondent is forced to choose one side or the other (such as in the revision in point 5) and may find this frustrating. The respondent may feel that neither agreement nor disagreement is the right answer for him or her. Undecided respondents should be given a neutral choice that reflects their position, which avoids a negative emotional response that might result in the respondent deciding to not answer the item or, worse, not to return the questionnaire. On the other hand, if decisions need to be made on the basis of the degree of agreement obtained, the surveyor may wish to force the respondent to choose a side. This type of forced choice should be used judiciously.

    When more details or spread of ratings are desired, responses can include six or seven options per question. When more than seven options are offered, the task of discriminating among them becomes difficult for the respondent, perhaps even meaningless.

8. The responses should match the question.
    If the question is about how satisfied the patient is with the services, the options should not be "agree/disagree." Although this suggestion is obvious, it is easily violated if one is not careful.

Ordering of the Questions

At the end of this chapter is a questionnaire (Appendix 11.A), which was used to survey intensive care unit (ICU) nurses at several ICUs (Kirchhoff, Conradt, & Anumandla, 2003). The respondents were asked what type of information they use to prepare families for withdrawal of life support. In this case, researchers were interested in the words or phrases used, so the question was left open ended.

    Opening questions are critical questions and should be related to the main topic and the title of the questionnaire. These questions serve to engage the responder to begin the task. Responders will be confused unless they are prepared for the flow of questions. This is one of many reasons that demographic questions should not be first.

Questions of similar format should be grouped together. For example, if there are several clusters of "agree–disagree" questions, these should be grouped, unless there is some reason not to do so. Possible reasons for not grouping them include a major shift in content or a particular task that is required.

When the respondent task changes, or when a major change in topic occurs, a transitional sentence or paragraph should precede the change. In the sample questionnaire, each section asks for different information.

In the sample questionnaire, the desired respondents were ICU nurses identified by a member of the organization. If there were no local person involved in providing respondents for the study, it would have been good to establish at the outset whether the nurses were eligible for the study. The first question could be a filter question asking whether the nurse provides care to ICU patients, thereby eliminating someone who works in the ICU solely in an educator role.

If all respondents answer all questions, the logistics of the questionnaire are simple to set up. In some instances, some respondents might not answer every question, requiring a skip option. Skip patterns can become confusing; the directions should be placed close to the response option. People read from left to right; this principle is used when the response to be read precedes the response options. In the same way, the skip directions are given immediately before the option requiring an answer.

Another factor to consider in the ordering of questions is the chronology of events. If this is an issue in the questionnaire under construction, the order of questions may be partially dictated by chronology. For example, if information about the health of a child is to be obtained, the first questions should pertain to the child's birth, and later questions should focus on infancy and childhood.

Sensitive questions should be placed near the middle of the questionnaire, at a point where some rapport with the respondent has been developed. If they appear too early, this intrusion can lead some respondents to decide not to complete the entire questionnaire. On the other hand, if sensitive questions are placed too close to the end, the respondent may feel an abrupt ending in a difficult conversation. If the entire topic of the questionnaire is sensitive, the reader will be informed by reading Lee (1993), who wrote about researching sensitive topics.

Demographic questions should always appear at the end. They are the least interesting to the respondent and will be completed only if the respondent feels that a commitment has been made to finish the task. In the sample questionnaire provided, the planned analysis concerns only what nurses do with families. No analysis is planned about differences among the nurses relative to age groups or levels of experience or about whether preparation varied according to these demographics. These data were therefore not collected.

Clinical Data Collection Forms

There are a few additional comments to be made about tools used for recording clinical data or chart information in contrast to tools used for asking questions. Data collection forms are used in clinical studies to record observations or in quality-improvement activities to record compliance with standards. Most of the previous comments still apply.

In order to reduce the amount of writing, units of measurements should be written out where information is to be entered (e.g., _____mmHg). The use of checks or circles to complete a selection when the options are known will also reduce the amount of writing required.

When data are to be collected from various sections of a chart or in a series of steps, the data-entry spaces should be placed in the order in which they occur, whether the data are on paper or screens. For example, if the order sheet is first in the paper chart, followed by progress notes, nursing notes, and graphs, the data collection should be ordered in that manner. When screens need to be navigated, the order of appearance should be taken into account.

The instructions about pretesting apply to data collection forms, as well. By pretesting on a real chart or an electronic record, one can determine whether the order has been reversed and whether placement of items is optimal. When the order of data collection is not preserved, there is a greater tendency to skip entry, resulting in missing data.

FOLLOWING THE DEVELOPMENT OF THE QUESTIONNAIRE

Many questionnaires are analyzed by simply counting the number of respondents for each category of response. If more complex analysis is desired, whoever is assisting with the data analysis should have some input into the process of how the data are collected. If consultation on the proposed analysis is needed, the consultant should review the questionnaire before the questionnaire is printed. Revisions may be necessary solely for analytic reasons.

Once the questionnaire has been developed, it should be pretested on subjects who are similar to the respondents who will be used. No matter how simple it seems, the pretest usually reveals areas for improvement. It is also helpful to debrief the subjects to find out what they thought about each question and the reason for the answers given. Additional areas for revision may become evident.

Distribution of Questionnaires

Plans for obtaining an adequate response rate should be made. Some researchers recommend that one obtain at least a 50% response rate; others might suggest at least a 70% response rate. Different groups of respondents have different usual response rates. Nurses have a higher usual rate than do the recently bereaved, for example, who have had low rates (Kirchhoff & Kehl, 2008). Factors to be considered in achieving the desired return rate include (1) how the questionnaire is to be distributed and returned, and (2) how the researchers will be able to track and contact nonresponders. Personal delivery, along with immediate collection of the completed questionnaire, results in the highest return rate. Mailed questionnaires should include a cover letter and a return stamped and self-addressed envelope. Follow-up on mailed questionnaires requires that the researcher keep track of code numbers, checking off those returned and sending an additional mailing(s) to those who have not yet responded.

Mailed questionnaires with a cover letter and a return envelope have been the most used method historically. Obtaining an address for a respondent can pose difficulties. Mailing to the person at work when the topic is work related can be easier than mailing to a home address. Mailing to a job category at an institution, when the desired respondent is not known, adds another level of complexity—how to get the questionnaire to, for example, the APRN in Cardiology. Using a generic address may lead to the intended person if there is one.

Other methods of distribution take advantage of the Internet. The researcher can send an e-mail to the desired respondent with a link to a survey posted on SurveyMonkey® or another such service. At present the charges are free for 10 questions per survey and 100 responses per survey and monthly fees for more. E-mails are sometimes easier to find on institutional websites. Although web-based surveys are cheaper to administer than those that use regular mail and returns are faster, they also have lower response rates than mailed surveys. There is also the issue of higher rates of nondelivery to e-mail addresses than to postal addresses (McDonald & Adam, 2003). Sending a postcard as a surface mail notification before sending an e-mail increases the Internet response, bringing it closer to the response for the postal method, but an e-mail-only method of delivery yields the lowest rate (Kaplowitz, Hadlock, & Levine, 2004).

Follow-up plans for all methods include developing a timeline for one or more additional contacts or telephone calls. When tracking returns, the investigator can plot the cumulative returns by day. When the return line plateaus, it signals that it is a good time to start the next wave of follow-up, whether by phone, e-mail, or regular mail. A cogent follow-up letter explaining the need for replies from all study respondents is helpful.

Phone follow-up has the additional advantage of permitting the respondent to clarify his or her reasons for not responding. The first mailing might not have been received, for example, especially in a complex organization. Questions that are answered in the phone call may permit the respondent to reply.

CODING THE RESULTS

This section considers issues in coding quantitative data resulting from surveys. Directions for coding qualitative data are found in Chapter 9, on qualitative designs.

The plans for analysis need to be made according to the amount of data, the intended level of analysis, and the method planned. If there will be a large data set or if a complicated analysis is anticipated, computer entry of the data is a necessity. With smaller data sets and when simple counts are planned, a manual system might be faster, although more errors are possible this way.

Entry of the data into the computer can be done in several ways. All of the responses can be entered onto a Scantron sheet with response bubbles. Although this method is easy for the investigator, it is cumbersome for the respondent, who has to be sure that the response is placed on the right numbered line. If the questionnaire is complicated and/or multiple sources of data are used, it may be easier to enter responses into an Excel spreadsheet or an Access database. These products facilitate the calculation of descriptive statistics that may be sufficient for analytic purposes without the researchers having to export the data to a statistical program.

If the questionnaire is precoded and simple, the numbers circled by the respondent may be directly entered into the appropriate Excel column. In this case, each subject will be a row and each answer will be found in one column. One should plan to check for errors, especially if a high degree of accuracy is needed.

TeleForm v10 is a software package consisting of several functions:

- Form Designer: Design forms/surveys optimized for automated computer recognition
- Reader: A service that waits for incoming forms whether from scanned papers, e-mail, fax, or other means
- Verifier: A program an operator can open to view processed forms, and if needed, make decisions on character recognition that could not be read with the specified confidence level
- AutoMerge Publisher: Print forms with unique IDs, barcodes, or any number of data premerged onto the form at the time of printing

This expensive software is available from Cardiff and is probably available only in larger survey centers or major industries. If scanned questionnaires are planned rather than faxes, the need for a scanner that has an automated data feeder will add to the costs of the initial setup. For subsequent surveys, costs of data entry, time required, and error rates are all reduced with this system. Another option to consider is Qualtrics Research Suite, an enterprise online survey software solution that collects, analyzes, and acts on relevant data.

The first run of the data should include a count of all the values for each variable. That allows numbers out of the expected range, illegal values, to be detected. For example, a yes-or-no question that was coded "1" and "2" would not have response numbers from "3" to "8." A "9" might be a legitimate value if the convention of inserting a "9" where there are missing data was followed. If illegal values are found, the ID number for the questionnaire containing the incorrect value needs to be determined. Then the original questionnaire for that subject should be reviewed to look for the correct value, and the spreadsheet should be corrected. This process, called data cleaning, should be done before any meaningful statistics are calculated.

SUMMARY

Multiple decisions about questionnaire design, the questions to be asked, and the responses that are anticipated influence the quantity and the accuracy of the data that will be collected. The response rate will partially determine the value of the results to the intended audience. Development of well-designed data collection forms is vital in collecting accurate evidence for practice.

SUGGESTED ACTIVITIES

1. Select a topic that allows both open-ended and closed-ended responses. Develop three to four questions in each format. Discuss with a partner the advantages and disadvantages of each format.
2. Select a quality-improvement topic from your clinical setting. Describe how you would design a tool to collect data, the process you would use to collect the data, and how you would feed back the results to those involved.

REFERENCES

Frank-Stromborg, M., & Olsen, S. J. (2004). *Instruments for clinical health-care research* (3rd ed.). Sudbury, MA: Jones & Bartlett.

Kaplowitz, M., Hadlock, T., & Levine, R. (2004). A comparison of web and email surveys. *Public Opinion Quarterly, 68*(1), 94–101.

Kirchhoff, K. T., Conradt, K. L., & Anumandla, P. R. (2003). ICU nurses' preparation of families for death of patients following withdrawal of ventilator support. *Applied Nursing Research, 16*(2), 85–92.

Kirchhoff, K. T., & Kehl, K. A. (2008). Recruiting participants in end-of-life research. *American Journal of Hospice and Palliative Care, 24*(6), 515–521.

Lee, R. M. (1993). *Doing research on sensitive topics.* Newbury Park, CA: Sage.

McDonald, H., & Adam, S. (2003). A comparison of online and postal data collection methods in marketing research. *Marketing Intelligence & Planning, 21*(2), 85–95.

ADDITIONAL READING

Dillman, D. A. (1978). *Mail and telephone surveys: The total design method.* New York: John Wiley.

Fowler, F. J. (1988). *Survey research methods.* Newbury Park, CA: Sage.

Harris, L. E., Weinberger, M., & Tierney, W. M. (1997). Assessing inner-city patients' hospital experiences: A controlled trial of telephone interviews versus mailed surveys. *Medical Care, 35*(1), 70–76.

Jagger, J. (1982). Data collection instruments: Sidestepping the pitfalls. *Nurse Educator, 7*(3), 25–28.

Payne, S. L. (1951). *The art of asking questions.* Princeton, NJ: Princeton University Press.

Spilker, B., & Schoenfelder, J. (1991). *Data collection forms in clinical trials.* New York, NY: Raven Press.

Sudman, S., & Bradburn, N. M. (1982). Asking questions: A practical guide to questionnaire design. San Francisco, CA: Jossey-Bass.

Warwick, D. P., & Linninger, C. A. (1975). *The sample survey: Theory and practice.* New York: McGraw-Hill.

APPENDIX 11.A

FAMILY EXPERIENCE DOCUMENT

In the ICU, families may choose to be with their loved one following withdrawal of equipment, resulting in the patient's death. Hence, families witness their loved one progress toward death. This form aims to collect information from you, to help us formulate a message for families to prepare them for this experience ahead of time. As a nurse, please describe your various objective findings and observations, based on your experience, by completing the following sections.

A. **Physical Sensations/Observations:** (What you see, hear, smell, and feel [on touch] in a withdrawn dying patient.) Complete as many sections as possible.

1. Respiratory:

_____

_____

2. Skin:

_____

_____

3. Neurological:

_____

_____

4. Musculoskeletal:

_____

_____

5. Sense organs: (eyes, ears, nose, tongue, and their functions)

_____

_____

6. Gastrointestinal:

_____

_____

7. Genito-urinary:

_____

_____

8. Others:

_____

_____

_____

_____

B. Temporal Characteristics: (Duration and sequence of events from withdrawal of equipment to death of the patient.)

_____

_____

_____

_____

_____

_____

C. Environmental Features: (The kind of environment the withdrawn patient is in; like the characteristics of the ICU cubicle or unit in which the patient is in, transfer of the patient to a different unit after withdrawal of equipment, the people in the cubicle or unit, the activities taking place, etc.)

_____

_____

_____

_____

_____

_____

D. Cause of Sensations, Experiences: (What are the immediate causes and processes of the physical sensations/observations that you have identified?)

_____

_____

_____

_____

_____

_____

_____

_____

E. Other information that you think is important to be included in the **family intervention** preparing families for the death of their loved one.

_____

_____

_____

_____

_____

Thanks for your time!!

12

Physiological Data Collection Methods

Susan K. Frazier

Evidence-based practice is the clinical application of research findings that have been synthesized, replicated in appropriate populations of patients, evaluated for scientific rigor, and found to be effective. The intent of evidence-based practice is to optimize patient outcomes. Thus, it is essential that clinicians are skillful in the critique and evaluation of research studies to determine their scientific soundness and appropriateness for application to clinical practice. Biomedical instruments are commonly used to collect data about physiological status; biological functions and processes; and the consequences of disorders, injuries, and malfunctions; thus, an important component of the evaluation of those studies is appraisal of these instruments and their ability to accurately quantify the desired physiological measure.

Clinicians use biomedical instrumentation daily in practice to acquire data about patient condition and to monitor patient progress. However, biomedical instruments used in the clinical setting and in research studies must be evaluated to ensure that the values generated are an accurate reflection of reality. Study findings may be called into question if the biomedical instrument that was used was not appropriate, sensitive, or did not provide accurate or reliable data. Reports of studies must include information demonstrating the appropriateness, accuracy, and reliability of these measures. Thus, a clear understanding of the principles of biomedical instrumentation, physiological variables that can be measured, and the characteristics of biomedical instrumentation used to evaluate biomedical instruments are vital.

Biomedical instruments extend human senses by measuring changes in physiological variables and amplifying and displaying these, so that they can be heard or visualized. Many physiological changes are minute and not detectable with our senses alone. For example, the electrocardiogram monitors millivolt changes in electrical activity occurring in cardiac myocytes, amplifies the signal to volts, and displays the signal audibly as a sound, or visually as a waveform on a screen or a printout from a computer.

CLASSIFICATION OF BIOMEDICAL INSTRUMENTS

Biomedical instruments are classified as in vivo and in vitro. In vivo means "within the living"; thus, in vivo instruments are applied directly within or on a living organism. In vitro means "in the glass"; this indicates that living cells or tissues are studied in test tubes or Petri dishes after removal from the body. A cardiac monitor is an example of an in vivo instrument, as the sensing electrodes are applied directly to the individual. In vitro instruments measure intracellular activity in cells located outside of the body. For example, cytotoxicity testing evaluates the ability of a compound like a new drug to produce alterations in cellular function and apoptosis, or cell death (Eisenbrand et al., 2002). Blood samples removed from an individual can also be analyzed for electrolyte concentrations or evaluated for specific DNA sequences to diagnose a genetic disease using a polymerase chain reaction technique.

In vivo instruments can be categorized as invasive or noninvasive. Invasive instruments require that a body cavity be entered or the skin broken for measures to be made. The introduction of an arterial catheter connected to a pressure transducer to monitor arterial blood pressure is an example of invasive biomedical instrumentation. A noninvasive biomedical instrument uses the skin surface to apply the sensing device. A 12-lead electrocardiograph (ECG) and a bedside cardiac monitor are examples of noninvasive biomedical instruments.

The selection of an invasive or noninvasive instrument is a central consideration in clinical practice and research. The use of noninvasive instruments is often preferred because they are associated with fewer risks. Another important consideration is the potential type and number of mechanical issues associated with the instrument and measurement technique. For example, invasive intracranial pressure monitoring instruments connected to a catheter placed in a ventricle in the brain may be invalid because they are misplaced in as many as 12% of cases (Saladino, White, Wijdicks, & Lanzino, 2009), may become infected in up to 18% of cases (Camacho et al., 2011), or may become obstructed by thrombus or brain tissue in as many as 25% of placements (Arif et al., 2012). However, noninvasive instruments used to measure intracranial pressure that include transcranial Doppler ultrasonography, tympanic membrane displacement measures, magnetic resonance imaging, and optic nerve sheath diameter measurement are less sensitive, less accurate, and are unable to be used in 10% to 60% of patients because of anatomical variations (Raboel, Bartek, Andresen, Bellander, & Romneri, 2012). Thus, the invasive measures may be preferable.

Prior to selection of a biomedical instrument, another consideration is the frequency of data collection required, either continuous or
intermittent. Intermittent or cross-sectional measures provide a measure at only one point in time, and important alterations in a variable
may be missed. For example, intermittent, indirect measures of arterial
blood pressure may be obtained using an automated oscillating blood
pressure cuff; frequency of measures can be altered by reprogramming
the instrument. However, continuous measurement of arterial blood
pressure with an intra-arterial catheter connected to a transducer provides a continuous direct measure of intra-arterial pressure with greater
responsiveness to rapid alterations in blood pressure that could be
lifethreatening. Thus, the frequency of data capture must be considered.

Although in vitro biomedical instrumentation does not pose direct
risks to an individual in clinical practice or research, there must be
consideration for the sample required for the measurement. For example, samples can include blood, tissue, urine, saliva, sputum, bone mar-
row, vaginal secretions, fecal material, or gastric contents. Sampling
techniques may be associated with complications like bleeding, hema-
toma formation, pain, infection, and disability for a period of time.
The burden to the individual clearly will vary depending on the type
of sample needed, and the instrument that provides the most accurate
measurement with the least burden to the individual should be the
first choice.

In vitro measures may also be categorized as direct or indirect
measures. For example, a direct measurement of catecholamine concentration can be performed using blood or plasma, whereas an indirect measure could evaluate the breakdown products of catecholamines
in urine. Elevated carbon monoxide (CO) levels secondary to cigarette
smoking can be directly measured in blood using a CO-oximeter, and
indirectly measured in exhaled air using an ecolyzer.

CATEGORIES OF PHYSIOLOGICAL VARIABLES DETECTED
BY BIOMEDICAL INSTRUMENTS

Physiological variables are commonly measured in hospitals, clinics,
and community and home settings to evaluate health status, diagnose
diseases, determine efficacy of therapeutic regimens, and provide metrics for goal setting. Monitoring of physiological variables is a vital component of comprehensive nursing care, particularly during acute illness
and injury, and provides a wealth of quantitative data that can also be
used in nursing research. However, to ensure accuracy of physiological data through the use of biomedical instruments, the components of
the organism–instrument system, the subject, stimulus, and biomedical
instrument, must be understood. A variety of physiological variables
can be measured using biomedical instrumentation (Table 12.1).

TABLE 12.1   Categories of Variables That Can Be Detected by Biomedical Instruments

MEASURED VARIABLE	EXAMPLES OF MEASURES	CLASSIFICATION OF MEASURE
Electrical potential	Brain—electroencephalogram	In vivo
	Heart—electrocardiogram	
	Muscle—electromyogram	
Pressure waves	Arterial—systolic, diastolic, mean pressures	In vivo
	Veins—central venous pressure	
	Pulmonary—intra-airway, intrapleural pressures	
	Esophagus—esophageal pressure	
	Bladder—intra-abdominal pressure	
	Uterus—force of uterine contraction	
Mechanical waves	Cardiac—heart sounds	In vivo
	Acoustic—sound	
Temperature	Surface—skin temperature	In vivo
	Core—pulmonary artery temperature, rectal	
	Other—tympanic and oral	
Gases	Pulmonary gas—inhaled or exhaled oxygen, carbon dioxide, nitrogen, carbon monoxide	In vivo
	Arterial and venous blood—partial pressure of oxygen, carbon dioxide, carbon monoxide	In vitro
Cellular products	Hormones—insulin, thyroid hormones	In vitro
	Proteins—albumin	
	Enzymes—creatine kinase MB, alkaline phosphatase	
	Cytokines—tumor necrosis factor-α (TNF-α)	
	Nucleic acids—DNA, RNA (ribonucleic acid)	

COMPONENTS OF THE ORGANISM–INSTRUMENT SYSTEM

The components of the organism–instrument system include the subject, the stimulus, the sensing equipment, the signal conditioning equipment, the display equipment, and the recording and data-processing equipment (Figure 12.1). The principles of each component of the system will be discussed separately because each component requires evaluation to ensure that the data obtained are an authentic reflection of reality. However, these components must function together as a system to produce high-quality, accurate, and reliable data.

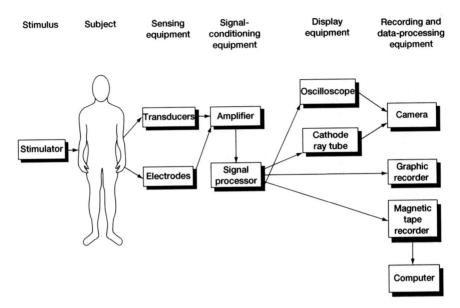

FIGURE 12.1   Schema of the organism–instrument system.
From Polit and Hungler (1987).

Subject

The subject of the system is the individual, either healthy or ill, from whom data will be obtained. The majority of nursing science studies focus on humans who have specific demographic and clinical characteristics. Individuals included in nursing research studies may be healthy or have an acute or chronic health condition. A number of nursing science studies also test interventions intended to improve health outcomes in a group of individuals with selected characteristics. The demographic and clinical characteristics of the individuals included in a study will be dependent on the research purpose and specific aims of the study. For example, a study with the purpose of testing a cognitive-behavioral intervention to reduce depressive symptoms in women with breast cancer would require the establishment of a specific group of inclusion and exclusion criteria, like age range and comorbid conditions that should be included and excluded. Clinical characteristics might include the type of tumor and the stage on entry into the study. However, other demographic and clinical characteristics are often important to fully characterize those included in the study, and to evaluate whether other variables may influence the outcomes of interest. For example, the type of payment used by an individual for health care could influence the choice and the length of treatment, which could in turn, influence survival and quality of life. Thus, careful attention to the selection of demographic and clinical variables is essential.

There are research purposes and specific aims that cannot be studied in humans because of the need for invasive in vivo measures that would be inappropriate in humans, and the high potential for serious adverse reactions and risks. These studies typically are performed in animal models, in vitro cell cultures, or with computer models. Animals included in such studies are selected for their similarities to human function in relevant organ or cellular systems. The numbers of animals used for research have been decreasing in recent years, and the 3Rs, replacement, refinement and reduction, are encouraged in scientific inquiry (Festing & Wilkinson, 2007). Replacement is the use of other equally effective models when available, refinement refers to modification of study design and measures to eliminate discomfort and decrease required numbers of animals, and reduction is a decrease in the number of animals needed for a study because of the use of more sensitive measures and more powerful statistical tests.

Stimulus

The specific aims of a research study will determine the variables that should be measured. Once the variables to be measured are identified, an experimental stimulus may be identified. The stimulus could be a nursing care procedure like endotracheal suctioning or position change, which alters the physiological variables to be measured. Other stimuli might include minute electric shocks to elicit an electromyogram (EMG), auditory stimuli like intensive care noise or environmental noise, tactile stimulation by touching skin, visual stimulation with a flashing light, or a mechanical stimulus like the application of pressure to a body area; any of these stimuli could generate alterations in heart rate, cardiac rhythm, blood pressure, and intracranial pressure. In these examples, a stimulus elicits a response in physiological variables, which is then measured by biomedical instrumentation. In an experimental study, the stimulus can be altered by changing its duration, intensity, or frequency. For example, the effect of environmental noise in an intensive care unit lasting for 5, 10, or 15 minutes (duration) can be measured at 20 and 50 decibels (intensity) every 30 minutes (frequency) in a number of physiological variables.

Sensing Equipment

Sensing equipment is required to detect alterations in a physiological variable. Transducers and recording electrodes are types of sensing equipment that are commonly used in research and clinical practice for the measurement of physiological variables. Transducers sense a non-electrical signal and convert it to an electrical signal, whereas electrodes sense an electrical signal.

Transducers

A transducer is a device that converts one form of energy into an electrical signal, measures physiological phenomena like pressure, temperature, or partial pressure of gases, and simultaneously produces an electrical signal in volts proportional to the change in the variable. Conversion to volts is required because a biomedical instrument is an electronic device that will only respond to changes in electrical output.

There are a number of different types of transducers. A pressure transducer senses displacement produced by a pressure wave, as with cardiac contraction. The transducer is most often placed outside the individual, and connected to an arterial or venous blood vessel by a catheter and specialized pressurized tubing filled with fluid. The transducer contains a fluid-filled dome that covers the surface of the sensing diaphragm on the transducer. As the pressure within the blood vessel varies with pulsatile blood flow, the sensing diaphragm is displaced alternately inward and outward. The sensing diaphragm in the transducer is connected by a wire to a bonded or semiconductor strain gauge. When this wire is stretched, the electrical resistance increases; conversely, when the wire is allowed to contract, resistance decreases. As the pressure fluctuates in the blood vessel, the pressure change is transmitted to the sensing diaphragm, which bows inward and outward, changing the resistance in the wire. According to Ohm's Law, which states that voltage = current × resistance, as the resistance in the wire increases and decreases, and the current remains constant, the voltage varies proportionally. Using this law, the transducer converts sensed pressure changes into voltage, which then can be measured by a biomedical instrument.

Temperature is often measured with a resistance thermometer or thermistor, another type of transducer. A thermistor is a wire whose resistance increases and decreases as temperature increases and decreases. With a thermistor, changes in temperature are converted to voltage using Ohm's Law and measured with a biomedical instrument. A thermistor can measure skin surface temperature, oral or rectal temperature, and core body temperature with a pulmonary artery catheter.

Another type of transducer is found in an arterial blood gas analyzer, which contains electrodes for oxygen, carbon dioxide, and pH; these electrodes are biochemical transducers that convert the detected concentration of gas pressure or the concentration of hydrogen ions to an electrical signal, both of which are detectable using biomedical instruments.

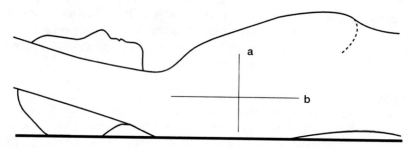

FIGURE 12.2   The reference plane.

There are a number of considerations when using a transducer to collect physiological data to ensure accuracy and reliability. Pressures are measured using specific reference planes, like the right atrium of the heart for cardiovascular pressures. The right atrium is located at a fixed point along the midaxillary line at the fourth intercostal space (Figure 12.2). This point is identified while the individual is in a supine position. The pressure transducer balancing port is positioned so that it is perfectly horizontal to the right atrium of the individual using a level (Bisnaire & Robinson, 1999). Leveling a transducer using the appropriate reference point is vital; for each inch (2.5 cm) of difference between the balancing port and the right atrium, the blood pressure varies 2 mmHg (Magder, 2007; Rice, Fernandez, Jarog, & Jensen, 2000). If the position of the individual is changed, then the transducer must be releveled.

The reference point for intracranial pressure measurement is the level of the ventricles of the brain, which is in line with the foramen of Monro (Thompson, 2011). In the supine position, the foramen is level with the tragus of the ear or the outer canthus of the eye; in the lateral position, the foramen is level with the midsagittal line between the eyebrows. Position change again requires releveling for accurate measurement (Bridges, Woods, Brengelmann, Mitchell, & Laurent-Bopp, 2000).

After the appropriate level of the pressure transducer is achieved, it must then be balanced and zeroed by opening the balancing port and exposing the sensing diaphragm to atmospheric pressure. This procedure establishes the strain gauge at zero voltage with respect to atmospheric pressure. Balancing and zeroing the transducer are critical to the degree of sensitivity required to measure pressure. In the transducer, four strain gauges, or resistances, are mounted to a sensing diaphragm; these resistances are connected to form a Wheatstone bridge circuit (Figure 12.3). The strain gauges are connected so that as pressure increases, two stretch and two contract; the sensitivity of the transducer is then increased by fourfold. When the balancing port is exposed to atmospheric pressure, the strain gauges are balanced or

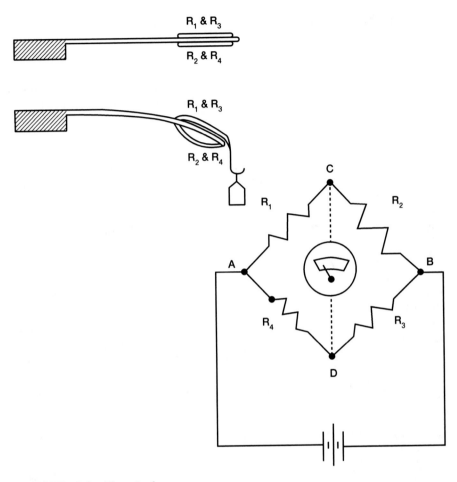

FIGURE 12.3   The strain gauge.

equal, and the voltage output is set at zero. When the balancing port is closed and the arterial catheter is connected to the pressure transducer, the actual pressure changes occurring in the blood vessel cause the sensing diaphragm to move inward and outward, which changes the resistance in the wires and the voltage output. Transducers that are not zeroed may systematically add or subtract from the actual values, and introduce an error into each measure made.

Particularly for research studies, a pressure transducer must also be calibrated against a column of mercury (Hg) or water (H_2O), depending on the range of pressures to be measured. Known values of pressure in increments of 50 to 250 mmHg for arterial pressure, 5 to 50 mmHg for pulmonary arterial pressure, or 5 to 25 cm H_2O for central venous or intracranial pressure are applied to the transducer to determine whether the output is linear. Linearity refers to the extent to which an input change is directly proportional to an output change. Thus, for every 1 mmHg change in pressure there is a 1 mmHg change in the measurement; this linear response must be consistent through the range of possible pressures. This procedure verifies that changes in blood pressure are proportional to the voltage output. To ensure the accuracy and reliability of research data, the transducer should be calibrated before, during, and after data collection.

The same principles of balancing, zeroing, and calibrating apply to temperature and biochemical transducers. To be zeroed, an oxygen electrode of a blood gas analyzer is exposed to a solution with no oxygen, and then is calibrated against a solution with a known oxygen concentration. Most blood gas analyzers automatically calibrate the electrodes regularly to ensure the accuracy and reliability of the data.

Recording Electrodes

Recording electrodes sense naturally occurring electrical signals, most often from the heart (electrocardiogram), the brain (electroencephalogram), and muscles (electromyogram). Natural electrical signals occur because of ion currents produced when positive and negative ion cellular concentrations change, as during a cardiac action potential (Schmukler, 1992). There are three types of electrodes: surface electrodes, indwelling macroelectrodes, and microelectrodes. Surface electrodes are most commonly used in clinical practice and in research with humans. An example of indwelling macroelectrodes is a needle electrode, where a needle is placed in subdermal tissue. Microelectrodes are often placed in a single cell outside of the body to measure ionic currents directly at the cellular level.

Surface electrodes are placed on the skin surface to record the sum of electrical potentials. For example, each cardiac myocyte has an electrical action potential that stimulates contraction; the surface electrodes capture the sum of all action potentials during cardiac contraction, which produces the typical PQRST waveform. Surface electrodes have a floating silver–silver chloride (Ag/AgCl) button at the top of a hollow column filled with gel. The floating electrode is used to reduce movement artifact by eliminating direct contact between the metal in the recording electrode and the skin. Skin contact is maintained through a bridge of electrolyte jelly or cream applied in direct contact with the skin surface. The electrolyte material reduces impedance, or the opposition to current flow, produced by surface oils and the outer horny layer of the skin. Practice standards recommend skin preparation prior to surface-electrode placement, which includes shaving the electrode sites, removing skin oil, and light abrasion with a dry cloth to remove skin debris to maximize conduction and improve signal acquisition (Drew et al., 2004).

Signal Conditioning Equipment

Signals produced by a transducer or detected by electrodes are usually measured in millivolts, and must be amplified to volts to drive the display unit. Display units may be an oscilloscope, a computer, or a graphic recorder. Most display units require an input voltage of 5 to 10 volts (Enderle & Bronzino, 2012). Amplification of the signal is often referred to as "increasing the gain." Once a signal has been amplified, the frequency of the signal in cycles per second is modified to eliminate noise or artifact. An example of artifact is the muscle movement seen on an electrocardiogram; another example is 60-cycle (Hz) noise from environmental electrical interference. Electronic filters are another component of the signal-conditioning equipment that controls noise or artifact by rejecting the unwanted signals. Artifact can also be separated, diluted, or omitted by adjusting the sensitivity control on a biomedical instrument.

Display Equipment

Once a physiological signal has been modified and amplified by signal-conditioning equipment, the display equipment converts the electrical signals into visual or auditory output that our senses can detect and evaluate.

Cathode Ray Oscilloscope and Computers

A cathode ray oscilloscope displays physiological data on a phosphor screen. An oscilloscope is actually a voltmeter with a rapid response time, which is ideal for the capture of cardiac and hemodynamic waveforms. A beam of electrons produced by an electron gun has little inertia and is, therefore, capable of rapid motion and response to minute changes. Horizontal and vertical plates dictate whether the beam on the screen appears in the vertical or the horizontal plane. The rapidly changing output voltages from transducers or electrodes cause the beam of electrons to be displaced proportionally to the change, and this forms the shape of a waveform. This display is typically a graph of voltage change by time. Many instruments can alter the time axis.

In the clinical setting, cathode ray oscilloscopes have been replaced by computers and computer screens that display the voltage change or waveforms by time, and often display multiple measured variables. Heart rate, cardiac rhythm, blood pressures, respiratory rate, and oxygen saturation are common physiological variables that may be displayed continuously and simultaneously on a computer screen. These data are automatically stored, and can be retrieved to evaluate trends over time, and to compare changes in physiological variables at different points in time. Computers with specialized software can be used to acquire, store, and analyze a wide variety of research data. However, the rate of data acquisition should be sufficient to ensure that accurate values of physiological data are captured. Software systems also typically convert analog signals into digital values that can be transported into a data spreadsheet.

Graphic Recorders

A permanent recording of the physiological data can be made by using a graphic recorder. The two basic types of graphic recorders are the curvilinear and the rectilinear recorders. A curvilinear recorder comprises a display system in which pens move in an arc and produce a display on curvilinear paper. Curvilinear recorders are relatively inexpensive and are useful for graphic data display, but are self-limiting due to the arc of the pen. Thus, it is not possible to obtain an exact data value using this type of recorder. In the clinical setting, graphic recorders are typically of the curvilinear variety. A rectilinear recorder comprises a system in which the pens move in a linear mode and produce a display that can be used to determine an exact value. These recorders are considerably more expensive than curvilinear models, but are more useful for the collection of research data where precision is vital.

In addition to the type of recorder, the method of producing the graph must be considered. Typically, recording pens use ink to produce graphs on the surface of recording paper. Thermal array recorders use a heat stylus pen and heat-sensitive paper to display the data. Unfortunately, a thermal graph fades with time and the data will become useless; thus, another method for saving the data must be used.

CHARACTERISTICS OF BIOMEDICAL INSTRUMENTS

Biomedical instruments have specifications that demonstrate their ability to measure the variable of interest. These specifications are important in the decision-making process before use. The important characteristics of an instrument include the range, the frequency response, specificity, stability, linear response, and the signal-to-noise ratio.

Range

The range of an instrument is the complete set of values that an instrument can measure. For example, a scale may measure from 0 to 100 g, a cardiac monitor 1 to 250 beats per minute, and a centigrade thermometer 0°C to 60°C. It is critical that the instruments chosen to record research data have the capability to measure physiological phenomena in the ranges needed. The range of an instrument can be determined from the instrument specifications in the equipment manual. Generally, the manual also provides information about the reliability of the instrument within the range specified.

Frequency Response

The frequency response of an instrument is the capacity of the instrument to respond equally well to rapid and slow components of a signal. For example, measuring the action potential of a neuron requires equipment with a fast response time, because the total time for an action potential occurs in milliseconds. As a result, to display this type of physiological phenomenon, an oscilloscope or computer is required. A graphic recorder cannot be used to measure a neural action potential because the frequency response is too slow. The inertia of the pen as it moves across the graph paper results in a slow response time.

Sensitivity

Sensitivity of an instrument is the degree of change in the physiological variable that the instrument can detect. For example, one instrument might weigh material within one tenth of a gram (0.1 g); another instrument might weigh the same material within one hundredth of a gram (0.01 g). Obviously, the equipment that weighs the material within one hundredth of a gram is more sensitive. The instrument chosen for a study should have the degree of sensitivity that responds to the research purpose.

Stability

Stability of an instrument is the ability to maintain calibration over a given time interval. Over time, biomedical instruments frequently suffer gradual loss of calibration; this is referred to as calibration drift. It is important that a biomedical instrument maintain calibration, because the reliability of the data is dependent on an accurate measure. The specifications describe the stability of the instrument over time, and indicate the manufacturer recommendation for recalibration frequency. Because loss of calibration, or drift, is common among biomedical instruments, it is important to evaluate the calibration before, during, and after an experiment to ensure the reliability of the data collected.

Linearity

Linearity of an instrument is the extent to which an input change is directly proportional to an output change. For instance, for every 1 degree of actual change in temperature, there is a 1-degree change recorded by the thermometer. Linearity should be evaluated for the entire range of the instrument.

Signal-to-Noise Ratio

Signal-to-noise ratio of an instrument is the relationship between the signal strength and the amount of noise or artifact detected. The higher the signal-to-noise ratio, the fewer the artifacts and the clearer the signal obtained.

CHARACTERISTICS OF THE MEASUREMENTS OBTAINED BY USING BIOMEDICAL INSTRUMENTS

Measurement of physiological data using biomedical instruments is fundamental to many nursing science studies. However, not every instrument functions equally well for all circumstances, and inattention to any one component of the organism–equipment system may result in the collection of data that are not an accurate reflection of reality. Thus, there are basic characteristics of the data collected that must be considered for every physiological variable. These features include the validity, accuracy, and precision or reliability.

Validity is the extent to which the biomedical instrument measures the actual variable of interest, and accuracy is the degree to which the measured value reflects the actual value. For example, the validity of cardiac output measure taken with bioimpedance can be evaluated by inspection of the waveform obtained by the instrument, and the validity and degree of accuracy by comparison with a "gold standard" measure like the Fick equation or a thermodilution measure. Reliability refers to the accuracy of the measure over time. When using new measures and new biomedical instruments, validity, accuracy, and reliability should be evaluated using a gold-standard measure and reported. This evaluation can be accomplished by calculation of the bias and precision of the measure. The bias is the mean difference between the two measures taken simultaneously using two methods, and the precision is the standard deviation of the differences. The smaller the value of the bias, the lesser the difference there is between the two measures; the smaller the value of the precision, the more reliable these measures are over time (Bland & Altman, 1986).

USING BIOMEDICAL INSTRUMENTATION FOR RESEARCH PURPOSES

A number of clinical biomedical instruments are used to evaluate patient status. An increasing number of studies use physiological values from these instruments as research data. However, several considerations require examination prior to use of these data for research. The use of bedside pulse oximetry as a data collection instrument is evaluated as an illustrative example considering the characteristics of biomedical instrumentation. Any biomedical instrument used to obtain physiological data for research purposes must be thoroughly evaluated prior to selection and use for research purposes.

Oxygen Saturation

Oxygen is transported to metabolically active tissues either combined with hemoglobin or dissolved in plasma. Arterial blood gas evaluation of the partial pressure of oxygen (PaO_2) provides a measure of the partial pressure of oxygen dissolved in plasma; however, the PaO_2 represents only about 2% of the total oxygen transported. The primary means for oxygen transport is the binding of oxygen molecules with hemoglobin molecules to form saturated hemoglobin or oxyhemoglobin (HbO_2). Clinically, oxygen saturation can be measured by obtaining an invasive arterial blood gas sample, and determined in vitro using a CO-oximeter. An alternative noninvasive measure of oxygen saturation can be determined by pulse oximetry (SpO_2). A clear understanding of the instrumentation and technique of these two measurement techniques is vital to ensure that the data obtained with a pulse oximeter are an accurate reflection of reality.

Measurement of Oxygen Saturation

Measurement of hemoglobin saturation may be either a fractional or a functional measurement. A fractional measurement of hemoglobin saturation is performed by a CO-oximeter, which is typically associated with a blood gas analyzer, and is obtained by analysis of a blood sample. The CO-oximeter uses four or more wavelengths of light to determine the proportion of each type of hemoglobin in the sample. Total hemoglobin includes hemoglobin bound to oxygen molecules or oxyhemoglobin (HbO_2), hemoglobin available for binding with oxygen or desaturated hemoglobin (deoxyHb), and hemoglobin that is not capable of binding with oxygen, either carboxyhemoglobin (HbCO) or methemoglobin (Hbmet). The fractional oxygen saturation is the ratio of oxygen-saturated hemoglobin or oxyhemoglobin (HbO_2) to the *total* number of hemoglobin molecules. Thus, the status of total hemoglobin is evaluated with a fractional measurement (Table 12.2).

Measurement of hemoglobin saturation by pulse oximetry integrates elements of optical plethysmography with spectrophotometry. Optical plethysmography generates waveforms from pulsatile blood as the blood moves past sophisticated light-absorbance instrumentation. The presence of pulsatile blood differentiates the arterial bed from the

TABLE 12.2   Normal Values of Fractional and Functional Hemoglobin Saturation

VARIABLE	TYPE OF MEASURE	NORMAL RANGE OF VALUES
Oxyhemoglobin	Fractional	Arterial 94%–100%
		Venous 40%–70%
	Functional	95%–100%
Deoxyhemoglobin	Fractional	0%–3%
Carboxyhemoglobin	Fractional	Nonsmoker < 2%
		Light smoker 4%–5%
		Heavy smoker 6%–8%
		Newborn 10%–12%
Methemoglobin	Fractional	0.4%–1%

venous, to ensure that the saturation measurement is arterial in origin. Concurrently, spectrophotometry yields quantitative calculations of hemoglobin saturation based on the absorption of multiple wavelengths of light by the hemoglobin molecules. In a pulse oximeter, two light-emitting diodes (LEDs) expose the hemoglobin molecules to two wavelengths of light: a red light (~660 nm) and an infrared light (~920 nm). The oxygen-binding status of hemoglobin molecules determines the absorption of the different wavelengths of light by the hemoglobin molecules. Hemoglobin can be saturated with oxygen, reduced or deoxygenated, bound to carbon monoxide, carboxyhemoglobin, or oxidized with iron atoms, methemoglobin. A photodetector placed in opposition to the LEDs measures the degree of absorption of the red and infrared light by the hemoglobin molecule. Saturated hemoglobin absorbs a greater degree of infrared light, whereas reduced hemoglobin absorbs a greater degree of red light. Thus, the calculation of hemoglobin saturation by the pulse oximeter is based on the relative amounts of red and infrared light transmitted through the pulsatile blood to the photodetector.

A pulse oximeter provides a functional measurement of hemoglobin saturation. A functional measurement is the ratio of oxygen saturated hemoglobin to the total amount of hemoglobin *available for binding* to oxygen. This type of measurement does not include evaluation of hemoglobin that is not available for binding with oxygen (carboxyhemoglobin and methemoglobin). For comparison purposes, a fractional saturation value can be converted to a functional value using the following equation:

Functional SaO_2 = (Fractional SaO_2/100) – (%HbCO + %Hbmet) × 100

Newer pulse-oximetry technology has been developed that uses eight wavelengths of light and is capable of making noninvasive fractional measures of carboxyhemoglobin and methemoglobin.

The primary use is rapid detection of carbon monoxide poisoning. Compared with CO-oximetry values, this technology has a reported bias and precision for carboxyhemoglobin of 0.1% and 2.5%, respectively; thus, compared with gold standard measures, pulse-oximetry measures will be between –6% and 4%. For example, an actual measure of carboxyhemoglobin of 10% could be displayed using the noninvasive technique as a value between 4% and 14% (Zaouter & Zavorsky, 2012).

Validity of Oxygen-Saturation Measurement by Pulse Oximetry

The fractional measurement of oxygen saturation by a CO-oximeter using four or more wavelengths of light is the gold-standard measure of oxygen saturation. A number of studies have compared the functional values obtained by pulse oximetry with simultaneous fractional measurement of oxygen saturation by CO-oximeter. In the range of 70% to 100% oxygen saturation, there is a strong correlation between these values (range of correlation coefficients, $r = 0.92$ to 0.98). Within this range of values, pulse oximetry has been demonstrated to accurately reflect *functional* hemoglobin saturation. However, when oxygen-saturation values are less than 70%, pulse oximetry may provide a falsely high value, because of the calculation algorithm used in this biomedical instrument (Avant, Lowe, & Torres, 1997).

SpO_2 may be a clinically useful indicator of oxygen transport; however, both the clinician and the researcher must remember that the use of a functional measurement of oxygen saturation does not reflect tissue oxygen delivery. Thus, a high SpO_2 value from pulse oximetry does not necessarily indicate adequate tissue oxygen delivery. Shifts in the oxyhemoglobin dissociation curve caused by hypothermia, alkalosis, or a decrease in 2,3-DPG can significantly alter tissue oxygen delivery, even though the functional oxygen saturation value appears normal, as these situations reduce the release of oxygen from hemoglobin at the cellular level.

Accuracy of Pulse Oximetry

Certain clinical and technical phenomena may reduce the accuracy of saturation values obtained by pulse oximetry (Batchelder & Raley, 2007) (see Table 12.3). Weak arterial pulsation produced by shock states, hypothermia with shunting of blood flow from the periphery, or increased systemic vascular resistance may result in significantly reduced or absent light absorption detection by the sensor. An oximeter is not capable of calculating an SpO_2 value if pulsatile flow is not detected. Venous pulsation, as a result of right ventricular failure or a partial obstruction to venous outflow, also reduces the accuracy of SpO_2 values. In the presence of both arterial and venous pulsatile flow,

TABLE 12.3 Clinical and Technical Factors That Reduce the Accuracy of SpO$_2$ Values

Individual Factors	Inadequate pulsatile arterial blood flow—hypotension, hypothermia, increased systemic vascular resistance
	Pulsatile venous blood flow—right ventricular failure
	Elevated levels of dysfunctional hemoglobin—carboxyhemoglobin, methemoglobin
	Anemia
	Presence of systemic dyes in the blood
	Hyperlipidemia
Technical Factors	Motion artifact
	Ambient light interference
	Optical shunt
	Optical cross-talk
	Electrical interference

the SpO$_2$ value may be a composite value derived from light absorbance from both arterial and venous hemoglobin. In this instance, the SpO$_2$ value provided will be lower than actual arterial saturation.

Abnormalities in the blood may also produce inaccurate values of oxygen saturation. Anemia may reduce the accuracy of pulse-oximetry values, particularly as SpO$_2$ values decrease. The cause for this inaccuracy is not well understood, but may be secondary to the scattering of light in the plasma, which produces a shift in the degree of red light absorbed (Hannhart, Haberer, Saunier, & Laxenaire, 1991). In addition, the presence of a significant portion of hemoglobin that is unavailable for oxygen binding, like carboxyhemoglobin and methemoglobin, also reduces the accuracy of pulse-oximetry measurements. For example, at a carbon monoxide partial pressure of only 0.1 mmHg, hemoglobin is 50% saturated with carbon monoxide. However, a functional measurement of saturation by the pulse oximeter may indicate very high oxygen saturation, as the remaining 50% of hemoglobin may be fully saturated with oxygen. This saturation value is further misleading, because the presence of high levels of carboxyhemoglobin increases the affinity of hemoglobin for oxygen and reduces oxygen unloading at the tissues, depriving metabolically active tissue of necessary oxygen.

Concentrations of certain substances in the arterial blood have been suggested to influence the accuracy of pulse oximetry (Schnapp & Cohen, 1990). The effect of high levels of bilirubin on the accuracy of pulse oximetry is described inconsistently in the research literature. The majority of studies that compare SaO$_2$ with SpO$_2$ in the presence of hyperbilirubinemia (bilirubin up to 46.3 mg/dL) suggest that high bilirubin levels do not interfere with the accuracy of SpO$_2$ when saturation is greater than 90%. Use of systemic dyes has also been demonstrated to affect the accuracy of pulse-oximetry measurement. Indigo carmine, indocyanine green, and methylene blue absorb light at wavelengths similar to those used by the pulse oximeter (660 nm), and alter the accuracy of SpO$_2$ values. Elevated lipid levels either from endogenous lipids or administration of exogenous lipid solutions, in conjunction with total parenteral nutrition, may produce an artificially lower SpO$_2$ value. The presence of fingernail polish has not been demonstrated to influence the accuracy of SpO$_2$ (Rodden, Spicer, Diaz, & Stever, 2007). There is some evidence that accuracy of pulse oximetry is reduced at low saturations in individuals with highly pigmented skin, with errors up to 10% (Feiner, Severinghaus, & Bicker, 2007).

In addition to clinical factors, technical factors may also reduce the accuracy of pulse-oximetry values (Schnapp & Cohen, 1990). Motion artifact may be interpreted by the photodetector as arterial pulsation. High-intensity, high-quantity ambient light like that found with heat lamps, surgical lights, and fluorescent lights may reduce the accuracy of SpO$_2$ values. The ambient light may be detected by the pulse-oximetry photodetector, and the photodetector receives information from both the LEDs and the ambient light source. The SpO$_2$ value is then a composite value and is likely inaccurate. An optical shunt may occur when some of the light from the LEDs is transmitted to the photodetector without passing through a pulsatile vascular bed. The degree of red and infrared light received by the photodetector is again a composite of light exposed to hemoglobin and light not exposed to pulsatile blood; thus, the SpO$_2$ value is inaccurate. Optical cross-talk may occur when the pulse-oximetry sensor is placed in proximity to another instrument also using red and/or infrared light. In this instance, the light emitted by the secondary instrument may be received by the pulse-oximetry photodetector. The SpO$_2$ will again be a composite value that will be inaccurate. Excessive signal noise, in the form of electrical interference, may be received and may interfere with signal acquisition. Signal processing may be disrupted by significant electrical interference, with resultant delayed values that may be inaccurate.

Bias is a statistical indicator of the accuracy of a measurement and is determined by calculating the mean difference between SaO$_2$ and SpO$_2$. The greater the calculated bias, the less accurate the measurement technique in comparison with a gold-standard value. Bias for pulse oximetry values is reported to vary depending on the degree of hypoxemia; so, as oxygen saturation decreases, bias increases. Bias for pulse-oximetry measures is reported to range from less than 0.5% to as much as 10%. Thus, the measured values could be seriously inaccurate, particularly at critical values.

Pulse-oximetry values in general are reported to have a margin of error or bias of ±2% of the actual SaO$_2$ value. This degree of error provides a wide range of potential values if SpO$_2$ values are normally distributed. The investigator must determine whether measures with this degree of potential error provide sufficiently accurate data to address the research objectives.

Precision and Reliability of Oxygen Saturation by Pulse Oximetry

Pulse oximetry can detect a 1% change in oxygen saturation. However, the speed of response by the pulse oximeter is reported to diminish as actual SaO_2 values decrease. A statistical measure of the reproducibility of pulse-oximetry measures is precision. This value is obtained by calculating the standard deviation of the bias measurement. The precision measure is analogous to the scatter of data points in measures made over time. Precision measures for pulse oximetry are reported to be 2% to 4% (Perkins, McAuley, Giles, Routledge, & Gao, 2003).

Pulse-oximetry measures are reported to be generally consistent over time (Hannhart, Haberer, Saunier, & Laxenaire, 1991). A majority of studies that evaluated reliability of pulse oximetry performed these studies with relationship to consistency of measurement over time using different probe types (reusable or disposable, finger, ear, and nose). The development of motion artifact appears to be the primary influence on the reliability of pulse-oximetry measures. However, other threats to accuracy also influence the reliability of this type of measurement.

Guidelines to Increase the Utility of Pulse Oximetry for Research Purposes

If SpO_2 values are to be used as research data, the investigator must ensure that these data are valid, precise, and reliable. Recently, Milner and Mathews (2012) evaluated 847 pulse-oximeter sensors used in 27 hospitals, and found that 11% of these contained electrical malfunctions that reduced accuracy, 23% of the oximeters emitted light spectra different from that reported by the manufacturer, and 31% of the oximeters were not functioning as expected. None of the inpatient facilities had a procedure or the equipment available for evaluation and calibration of these oximeters. Dugani et al. (2011) found that the use of an oximeter tester could identify faulty electronics and demonstrate the degree of error in SpO_2 measurements, but only 65% of biomedical engineers responding to a survey self-reported accuracy testing of pulse oximeters in their facility. These data indicate that the accuracy of clinical values of SpO_2 may be questionable in many facilities. The following guidelines improve the likelihood that these data will be useful. However, the investigator must determine whether SpO_2 will actually provide the data required to answer the research questions or test research hypotheses.

▪ Select a pulse oximeter with indicators of pulsatile signal strength and ability to observe a pulse waveform to ensure that adequate, appropriate signal quality is available.

▪ Ensure that probe type and probe position are optimal to detect arterial pulsation without technical interference from ambient light, optical shunt, or cross-talk.

▪ Assess the association between the apical heart rate and the heart rate detected by the pulse oximeter. These values should be the same.

▪ Evaluate the individual for the presence of dysfunctional hemoglobin, hyperbilirubinemia, hyperlipidemia, and anemia prior to data collection to ensure that these factors are not influencing SpO_2 values.

▪ Stabilize the probe so that motion artifact is not a significant confounding factor.

▪ Analyze the relationship between SpO_2 and SaO_2 obtained by CO-oximetry regularly. These values should be highly correlated with minimal bias. Calculate the bias and precision to evaluate the accuracy and repeatability of the data.

▪ Perform instrument calibration and accuracy testing prior to each experimental use of the biomedical instrument, and evaluate the equipment using a known standard concentration.

SUMMARY

When evaluating and critiquing the appropriateness of research studies to implement evidence-based practice in the clinical setting, knowledge about biomedical instrumentation is essential to determine the validity, accuracy, and reliability of the physiological data acquired. The components of the organism–instrument system include the subject, the stimulus, the sensing equipment, the signal conditioning equipment, the display equipment, and the recording and data-processing equipment. Consideration must be given to the ability of any biomedical instrument to provide valid, precise, and reliable data to ensure that the conclusions derived from research studies are from rigorous measures, and are meaningful and useful.

SUGGESTED ACTIVITIES

1. Select a research article in which biomedical instrumentation was used to collect physiological data. Review and critique the article. Evaluate whether the data collected using the instrumentation were valid, accurate, and reliable. Determine whether the results of the reviewed study are appropriate to apply to clinical practice.

2. Select a physiological variable, such as carbon dioxide. Search the literature to determine different methods to measure carbon dioxide, including measurement from blood (blood gases in vitro) or in vivo measures of tissue carbon dioxide ($TcPCO_2$) or exhaled carbon dioxide ($ETCO_2$). Design a study to measure carbon dioxide in a human research subject and provide the rationale for the choice on the basis of the method of measurement and human subject concerns (direct versus indirect method and in vivo versus in vitro method). Compare and contrast the validity, reliability, and accuracy of these methods.

REFERENCES

Arif, S. H., Bhat, A. R., Wani, M. A., Raina, T., Ramzan, A., Kirmani, A., Hussain, Z., Tabassum, R., Baba, A., & Bari, S. (2012). Infective and non-infective complications of external ventricular drainage. *JK-Practitioner, 17*(1–3), 27–32.

Avant, M., Lowe, N., & Torres, A. (1997). A comparison of accuracy and signal consistency of two reusable pulse oximeter probes in critically ill children. *Respiratory Care, 42*(7), 698–704.

Batchelder, P. B., & Raley, D. M. (2007). Maximizing the laboratory setting for testing devices and understanding statistical output in pulse oximetry. *Anesthesia & Analgesia, 105*(6), S85–S94.

Bisnaire, D., & Robinson, L. (1999). Accuracy of leveling hemodynamic transducer systems. *Canadian Association of Critical Care Nurses, 10*, 16–19.

Bland, J. M., & Altman, D. G. (1986). Statistical methods for assessing agreement between two methods of clinical measurement. *Lancet, 1*, 307–310.

Bridges, E. J., Woods, S. L., Brengelmann, G. L., Mitchell, P., & Laurent-Bopp, D. (2000). Effect of the 30° lateral recumbent position on pulmonary artery and pulmonary artery wedge pressures in critically ill adult cardiac surgery patients. *American Journal of Critical Care, 9*, 262–275.

Camacho, E. F., Boszczowski, I., Basso, M., Jeng, B. C., Freire, M. P., & Guimarães, T., Teixeira, M. J., & Costa, S. F. (2011). Infection rate and risk factors associated with infections related to external ventricular drain. *Infection, 39*(1), 47–51.

Drew, B. J., Califf, R. M., Funk, M., Kaufman, E. S., Krucoff, M. W., & Laks, M. M., Macfarlane, P. W., Sommargren, C., Swiryn, S., & Van Hare, G. F. (2004). Practice standards for electrocardiographic monitoring in hospital settings. *Circulation, 111*, 2721–2746.

Dugani, S., Hodzovic, I., Sindhakar, S., Nadra, A., Dunstan, C., & Wilkes, A. R., Mecklenburgh, J. (2011). Evaluation of a pulse oximeter sensor tester. *Journal of Clinical Monitoring and Computing, 25*(3), 163–170.

Eisenbrand, G., Pool-Zobel, B., Baker, V., Balls, M., Blaauboer, B. J., Boobis, A., Carere, A., Kevekordes, S., Lhuguenot, J. C., Pieters, R., & Kleiner, J. (2002). Methods of in vitro toxicology. *Food and Chemical Toxicology, 40*, 193–236.

Enderle, J., & Bronzino, J. (2012). *Introduction to biomedical engineering* (3rd ed.). New York, NY: Elsevier.

Feiner, J. R., Severinghaus, J. W., & Bicker, P. E. (2007). Dark skin decreases the accuracy of pulse oximeters at low oxygen saturation: The effects of oximeter probe type and gender. *Anesthesia and Analgesia, 105*(6 Suppl.), S18–S23.

Festing, S., & Wilkinson, R. (2007). The ethics of animal research. *EMBO Reports, 8*(6), 526–530.

Hannhart, B., Haberer, J. P., Saunier, C., & Laxenaire, M. C. (1991). Accuracy and precision of fourteen pulse oximeters. *European Respiratory Journal, 4*(1), 115–119.

Magder, S. (2007). Invasive hemodynamic monitoring: Technical issues. *Critical Care Clinics, 23*, 401–414.

Milner, Q. J., & Mathews, G. R. (2012). An assessment of the accuracy of pulse oximeters. *Anaesthesia, 67*(40), 396–401.

Perkins, G. D., McAuley, D. F., Giles, S., Routledge, H., & Gao, F. (2003). Do changes in pulse oximeter oxygen saturation predict equivalent changes in arterial oxygen saturation? *Critical Care, 7*(4), R67.

Polit, D. F., & Hungler, B. P. (1987). *Nursing research: Principles and methods* (3rd ed.). Philadelphia, PA: Lippincott.

Raboel, P. H., Bartek, J., Andresen, M., Bellander, B. M., & Romneri, B. (2012). Intracranial pressure monitoring: Invasive versus non-invasive methods. A review. *Critical Care Research and Practice.* Retrieved from http://www.ncbi.nlm.nih.gov/pmc/articles/PMC3376474

Rice, W. P., Fernandez, E. G., Jarog, D., & Jensen, A. (2000). A comparison of hydrostatic leveling methods in invasive pressure monitoring. *Critical Care Nurse, 20*, 20–30.

Rodden, A. M., Spicer, L., Diaz, V. A., & Stever, T. E. (2007). Does fingernail polish affect pulse oximeter readings? *Intensive and Critical Care Nursing, 23*(1), 51–55.

Saladino, A., White, J. B., Wijdicks, E. F. M., & Lanzino, G. (2009). Malplacement of ventricular catheters by neurosurgeons: A single institution experience. *Neurocritical Care, 10*(2), 248–252.

Schmukler, R. (1992). A brief history of bioelectrodes. *Annals of Biomedical Engineering, 20*(3), 265–268.

Schnapp, L. M., & Cohen, N. H. (1990). Pulse oximetry. Uses and abuses. *Chest, 98*(5), 1244–1250.

Thompson, H. J. (2011). *Care of the patient undergoing intracranial pressure monitoring/external ventricular drainage or lumbar drainage.* AACN Clinical Practice Guideline Series, AACN, CA: Aliso Viejo.

Zaouter, C., & Zavorsky, G. S. (2012). The measurement of carboxyhemoglobin and methemoglobin using a non-invasive pulse CO-oximeter. *Respiratory Physiology and Neurobiology, 182*(2–3), 88–92.

13

Psychosocial Data Collection Methods

Carol Glod

Psychosocial measures are instruments that researchers and advanced practice nurses (APNs) use to measure variables related to psychological, emotional, behavioral, and related areas in a study. In general, instruments focus on certain topics or content domains such as depression or anxiety. Psychosocial data collection methods are important to guide the use of evidence in nursing practice. They are often used for approved research studies; however, increasingly these tools are used to evaluate patients clinically or to assess treatment response.

Where do the instruments exist, and how does a researcher or APN locate them? One place to start is with other established researchers in the field. Another source is relevant articles located and reviewed in preparation for the study. An examination of the methods and instruments section of earlier studies often gives a detailed account of which measures were used and some of their key characteristics. Because most published manuscripts do not include the actual scales, the reference list should contain a citation for the original instrument. Permission to use a new or original scale may have to be requested from the author(s). Finally, libraries and Internet sources contain compilations of standardized instruments that can be obtained by searching for keywords that reflect the concept under study. There are also books that include primarily tools for measuring concepts (Frank-Stromborg & Olsen, 2004). Some instruments are copyrighted and can be purchased for a fee. The fee may be a one-time purchase fee or a per-copy or per-use fee. To purchase some instruments, one may have to have certain credentials, such as a PhD. A variety of well-established scales of different types exist to measure concepts such as depression and anxiety and to answer different research questions.

These concepts may be measured using interviews, whether structured or semistructured, or questionnaires that are administered by the researcher and/or completed by the participant. Other methods, such as observation and checklists, may be used along with standardized tests to collect data on behaviors to validate observations. For example, a study that examines the sleep of hospitalized cancer patients may include nursing observations and an established patient self-report scale.

SELECTION OF INSTRUMENTS

The selection of a measurement tool for psychosocial variables depends on the research question, variables of interest, age of participant, and other factors. A general rule is that the research question dictates the broader method to be used, whether a qualitative, quantitative, or mixed method. Having a research question and key variables that are well defined helps to direct the selection of a method. Before considering various established instruments, the researcher should think about several important questions, including the study purpose, characteristics of the sample, the concept or content to be measured, and practical considerations. For the measure to be suitable, it should have established *reliability* and *validity* (see Exhibit 13.1).

Exhibit 13.1
Factors to Consider When Selecting an Instrument

Does the instrument measure the concept being examined?
What are the psychometric properties of the instrument?

Reliability
   Stability
   Equivalence
   Homogeneity
Validity
   Content validity
   Criterion-related validity
   Construct validity
Is the instrument feasible?
   Instrument availability
   Costs of data collection tools
   Nature of the study sample

Source: Mateo and Kirchhoff (1999).

INSTRUMENT DEVELOPMENT

Occasionally, an investigator who is interested in a certain concept or area of study may find that there are no available scales or instruments that reflect that specific research problem. Creating new scales or questionnaires can be tempting; however, their development requires a deliberate and systematic approach. Beginning researchers may think it is a simple process to create a new scale for psychosocial variables; however, there are several steps involved. An initial step often is to bring together a group of experts in the field; these may be patients who experience a certain diagnosis or response to a problem or experienced nurses who know the topic well and can serve as content experts. For example, a nurse researcher interested in immigrant mothers' health practices with their children may bring together 6 or 8 representative mothers to generate potential items for a questionnaire during a meeting that lasts from 1 to 2 hours. Next, content experts should review the draft questions, which should also be pretested, revised, and tested for validity and reliability. Overall, the creation of a new instrument requires extensive time and effort but is appropriate when existing measures are unavailable or inadequate for the purpose. It is generally more feasible to use existing scales. Then results can be compared across samples.

Reliability and Validity

Reliability and *validity* are two important and essential concepts that relate to each potential instrument that the investigator is considering. They have specific definitions in research and can be easily confused. *Validity* refers to whether the instrument actually measures what it is supposed to measure. For example, if the nurse is interested in measuring acute stress, the instrument should measure the concept of stress and not related ones, such as anxiety or depression. There are different types of validity, detailed later in this chapter. *Reliability* refers to whether the tool conveys consistent and reproducible data, for example, from one participant to another or from one point in time to another. Several types of reliability exist, as well. For a scale to be valid, it must be reliable.

Validity

Validity is the degree to which a tool measures what it is supposed to measure (Mateo & Kirchhoff, 1999). There are three types of validity: content, criterion-related, and construct.

  Content validity relates to an instrument's adequacy in covering all concepts pertaining to the phenomena being studied. If the purpose of the tool is to learn whether the patient is anxious before taking an examination, the questions should include a list of behaviors that anxious people report when they are experiencing anxiety. Content experts are vital in the development of valid and reliable tools (Mateo & Kirchhoff, 1999). Generally, "content experts," colleagues with expertise and experience in the area, are identified. Ways to identify experts include publications in refereed journals, research in the phenomenon of interest, clinical expertise, and familiarity with the dimensions being measured. It is important that an instrument be reviewed for content by persons who possess characteristics and experiences similar to those of the participants in a study.

Criterion-related validity, which can be either predictive or concurrent, measures the extent to which a tool is related to other criteria (Mateo & Kirchhoff, 1999). Predictive validity is the adequacy of the tool to estimate the individual performance or behavior in the future. For example, if a tool is developed to measure clinical competence of nurses, persons who respond to the tool can be followed over time to see if this score correlates with other measures of competence, such as performance appraisals, commendations, or other indications of competence. If results indicate that there is a high correlation coefficient (0.90), it means that the clinical competence scale can be used to predict future performance appraisals. Concurrent validity is the ability of a tool to compare the respondent's status at a given time to a criterion (Mateo & Kirchhoff, 1999). For example, when a patient is asked to complete a questionnaire to determine the presence of anxiety, results of the test can be compared to the same patient's ratings on an established measure of anxiety administered at the same time.

Construct validity is concerned with the ability of the instrument to adequately measure the underlying concept (Mateo & Kirchhoff, 1999). With this type of validity, the researcher's concern relates to whether the scores represent the degree to which a person possesses a trait. Because construct validity is a judgment based on a number of studies, it takes time to establish this type of validity. These studies compare results in groups that should be similar (convergent validity) or different (divergent validity). Scores on the anxiety tool should be lower among those who are receiving a massage and higher among those taking a final exam.

Reliability

Reliability is a basic characteristic of an instrument when it is used for collecting accurate, stable, and usable research data (Mateo & Kirchhoff, 1999). The reliability of a tool is the degree of consistency in scores achieved by subjects across repeated measurements. The comparison is usually reported as a *reliability coefficient*. The reliability coefficient is determined by the proportion of true variability (attributed to true differences among respondents) to the total obtained variability (attributed to the result of true differences among respondents and differences related to other factors). Reliability coefficients normally range between 0 and 1.00; the higher the value, the greater the reliability. In general, coefficients greater than 0.70 are considered appropriate; however, in some circumstances this will vary. The researcher takes a chance that data across repeated administrations will not be consistent when instruments with reliability estimates of 0.60 or lower are used (Mateo & Kirchhoff, 1999).

Three aspects should be considered when determining the reliability of instruments: (1) stability, (2) equivalence, and (3) homogeneity (Burns & Grove, 2005; Mateo & Kirchhoff, 1999). The *stability* of a tool refers to its ability to consistently measure the phenomenon being studied; this is determined through test–retest reliability. The tool is administered to the same person or persons on two separate occasions. Scores of the two sets of data are then compared, and the correlation is derived. The recommended interval between testing times is 2 to 4 weeks (Burns & Grove, 2005; Mateo & Kirchhoff, 1999). The time that must lapse between the two points of measurement is important; it should be long enough so that respondents do not remember their answers on the first test, yet not so long that change in the respondents can take place. The length of time between points is dependent on and influenced by the nature of the phenomenon under investigation. Interpretation of the test–retest correlation coefficient should be done with caution, because it might not represent the stability of the instrument; rather, it might indicate that change has occurred in those being assessed. For example, change can occur among nurses being evaluated with regard to their attitudes toward work schedules; for instance, persons who responded to the first test may have since gained seniority and now be working their preferred shifts. In this case, the second test might yield a more positive result, and the correlation coefficient obtained when the two sets of scores are compared would represent a change in the respondents rather than being an accurate measure of the stability of the tool (Mateo & Kirchhoff, 1999).

Equivalence should be determined when two versions of the same tool are used to measure a concept (alternate forms) or when two or more persons are asked to rate the same event or the behavior of another person (interrater reliability; Mateo & Kirchhoff, 1999). In alternate-form reliability, two versions of the same instrument are developed and administered. The scores obtained from the two tools should be similar. It is helpful for the researcher to know whether a published instrument has alternate forms; when there are, a decision must be made about which form to use. For example, the Beck Depression Inventory (BDI) has a long and a short form (Beck & Steer, 1993). The researcher might decide to use the short form to test patients with short attention spans or low energy levels. Establishing interrater reliability is important when two or more observers are used for collecting data. Considerations relating to this type of reliability have already been discussed.

The *homogeneity* of an instrument is determined most commonly by calculating a Cronbach's alpha coefficient. This test is found in a number of statistical packages. This test is a way of determining whether each item on an instrument measures the same thing. A "high" value of alpha helps to provide evidence, when combined with literature and background, that the items in the scale measure a certain construct. A reliability coefficient of 0.70 or higher is generally considered "acceptable" in most psychosocial research. Internal consistency reliability estimates are also calculated by using the Kuder–Richardson formula, described in measurement textbooks.

When more than one concept is measured in an instrument, Cronbach's alpha is computed on the subscales, rather than the whole scale. If the scale does not attempt to measure a single concept or has subscales that measure several concepts, this test is not useful.

TYPES AND CHARACTERISTICS OF INSTRUMENTS

In general, there are several common types of measures or instruments available to measure the selected concept under investigation. Researchers use *semistructured* or *structured* interviews with detailed questions that either guide (semistructured) the interviewer or outline a specific set of questions. The principal investigator or study staff follows the order of questions during an interview with the participant. Another option is *self-report scales* that are given to the research subject to complete; examples include scales such as the BDI. Self-report instruments differ from clinician- and nurse-rated ones on the basis of who actually completes them.

Other scales may contain *open-ended* or *closed* questions. Open-ended questions allow more exploration and the opportunity for freer responses, without restraint or limitation. For example, in qualitative research, the researcher frequently asks open-ended questions, such as "what is your experience with . . ." or "tell me about. . ." Open-ended responses allow participants to answer in their own words. Closed-ended questions, although more common, direct respondents to choose an answer from a predetermined list of possible alternatives. As a result, the participants may be pointed in certain directions that may not be appropriate or that lack uniqueness. Many of the scales used in psychosocial research have *ordinal* items, with numbers assigned to different categories that reflect increasing order, such as 0 = none, 1 = slight, 2 = mild, 3 = moderate, and 4 = severe.

Visual Analog Scales

The Visual Analog Scale (VAS) uses a 100-mm line with "anchors" at either end to explore the participant's opinion about a specific concept along a continuum. Respondents place an X on the line to mark where they stand on the continuum. For example, questions on pain prompt the respondents to describe their experience of pain at the corresponding point on the line, which has anchors of "none" and "very much"; a mark made 80 mm from the end would signify 80% understanding. Convenient and simple, the VAS is an attractive means of rating continuous measurement.

Whether structured, detailed, or open-ended, every scale has advantages as well as limitations. There are several things to consider for psychosocial tools. Many of the instruments result in a certain rating (e.g., a numerical score that indicates a moderate level of depression). These rating scales attempt to measure the underlying concept (depression) efficiently and comprehensively and to attach to it a number that then is interpreted to represent a certain range (a given score indicates a given level of depression). The researcher cannot assume that a certain score or level of score on an established scale indicates the presence of a disorder. For example, the researcher cannot assume that a total score on a depression scale means that the participant actually should be diagnosed with depression. Some people assume, incorrectly, that a scale score that results in a certain degree or severity of symptoms produces a diagnosis. These instruments are in reality only part of an evaluation for a disorder.

There are several general types of instruments that measure psychological symptoms or overall functioning. Each uses either *continuous* or *categorical* responses. Continuous variables or items usually have quantifiable intervals or values, such as weight or blood pressure. In general, categorical items contain forced and mutually exclusive choices, such as *strongly agree, agree, disagree,* and *strongly disagree,* in contrast to continuous items, which literally contain a blended continuum of responses without specific choices. When there are two possible choices or values, such as gender, the categorical variable is termed *dichotomous.* For psychological or psychosocial ratings, the focus is generally on self-report (or parent report for children) or clinician-rated symptoms. Although these scales are most typically used for research purposes, they can also be used in clinical situations to aid in diagnostic evaluation or to help to monitor treatment response or symptoms over time. The instruments focus on particular symptoms or concepts such as anxiety, depression, suicide, mania, suicide risk, or attention problems. Examples of commonly used instruments, along with their purpose and a general overview of their characteristics, are described.

Clinical Global Impressions Scale

Clinical Global Impressions (CGI) is a categorical scale used for rating change from baseline over the duration of a clinical trial (Guy, 1976).

The CGI consists of three global scales formatted for use with similar scoring. The scales assess global improvement, severity of illness, and efficacy index. Clinical Global Impressions-Improvement (CGI-I) is a clinician-administered scale commonly used in studies of adults and children to assess posttreatment ratings at the discretion of the researcher.

The CGI-I consists of one item ranked 0 to 7 that compares patient condition at admission to the project to the patient's condition at a later time (Guy, 1976). The seven levels of improvement include 0 = not assessed, 1 = very much improved, 2 = much improved, 3 = minimally improved, 4 = no change, 5 = minimally worse, 6 = much worse, and 7 = very much worse. They are most commonly rated by the clinician and the patient. Investigators looking for at least moderate improvement on a global generic scale usually expect an improvement score of 50% or more (Bobes, 1998). Previous studies of commonly used antidepressants have used the proportion of CGI-I responders, defined as patients assigned a CGI-I score of 2 or lower by clinicians ("very much" or "much" improved).

The Mini Mental State Examination

Several versions of the Mini Mental State Examination (MMSE) have been developed and used since its original development (Folstein, Folstein, & McHugh, 1975). Widely used as a screening instrument for cognitive impairment, the MMSE is an easy tool used to assess changes in cognitive function, often with older adults and as a screening for dementia. This is a common instrument that nurses use to identify changes in mental status such as orientation, registration, attention and calculation, word recall, and language and visuospatial ability. It contains 11 questions and takes about 10 minutes to administer. The maximum score is 30; scores less than 24 may indicate cognitive impairment, whereas scores from 10 to 19 may reflect moderate levels of cognitive impairment. Educational level, age, and other factors may also influence the score. Similar to other available instruments, the MMSE is not a diagnostic tool for Alzheimer's disease or other forms of dementia and does not substitute for a mental status exam. Since its creation in 1975, the MMSE has been validated and extensively used in both clinical practice and research (Crum et al., 1993).

Since its introduction, the MMSE has been revised to address problematic items and adjust tasks to difficulty level. Although raw scores remain the same, the most recent version, the MMSE-2: Standard Version, has comparable scores to the MMSE. In addition, there are two other versions. The MMSE-2: Brief Version is used for quick clinical or research screening. The MMSE-2: Expanded Version includes additional tasks related to memory and processing and is more sensitive to different dementia symptoms and aging effects. Versions are available in many different languages for application to different patient populations. The original MMSE is free; however, the current official versions are copyrighted and are ordered through Psychological Assessment Resources (PAR) (www.parinc.com).

Brief Psychiatric Rating Scale

The Brief Psychiatric Rating Scale (BPRS) is one of the most frequently used clinician-rated measures. It has existed for more than 40 years (Overall & Gorham, 1962, 1976). It consists of 18 items rated on a 7-point severity scale and is used for general overall assessment of broad psychiatric symptoms. The BPRS takes about 20 minutes to complete. Its scoring results in an overall total score as well as scores on five major factors: anxious depression, thinking disturbance, withdrawal–retardation, hostile suspiciousness, and tension–excitement. More specific, yet similar scales that measure positive and negative symptoms of major mental illnesses (such as the Positive and Negative Symptoms Scale [PANSS]) are derived partly from the BPRS and have well-established validity and reliability. Discriminant validity of the items and subscales separated three homogeneous psychiatric diagnoses in patients (Lachar et al., 2001). The ratings of each individual item were compared for different raters. Using large samples of psychiatric patients in multiple studies, individual BPRS item interrater reliability estimates ranged from 0.54 to 0.92 (median = 0.785), with the majority of values (10 of 18) demonstrating very good agreement (greater than 0.74; Lachar et al., 2001). Interrater reliability agreement was $r = 0.57$ for total scores and ranged from $r = 0.60$ to 0.84 for the factor subscales.

The CAGE Questionnaire

Alcohol and substance abuse are increasingly prevalent in traditional nursing settings and with younger populations, including college students. Screening for potential alcohol problems is important in all settings, particularly health care settings. Alcohol abuse and alcoholism may be hidden for years and thus nurses are in a prime position to detect potential serious situations. A variety of instruments are available, but the CAGE is one short, simple, easy-to-use tool to assess patients on admission or during treatment (Ewing, 1984). The CAGE detects alcohol problems over the course of a person's lifetime. It is easy to remember and has been shown to be effective in detecting a range of alcohol problems (Ewing, 1984). It includes four simple questions:

C Have you ever felt you should *cut down* on your drinking?

A Have people *annoyed* you by criticizing your drinking?

G Have you ever felt bad or *guilty* about your drinking?

E *Eye opener:* Have you ever had a drink first thing in the morning to steady your nerves or to get rid of a hangover?

Two positive answers indicate a positive test. Once detected on a screening tool such as this, a more complete evaluation is frequently recommended. Several hundred instruments also exist that delve into more information and can detect serious alcohol abuse or dependence, and can be found at www.niaaa.nih.gov/publications/AssessingAlcohol /factsheets.htm.

Child Behavior Checklist

The Child Behavior Checklist (CBCL) is a 118-item standardized measure that rates general behavior for children aged 4 to 18, drawing on hundreds of studies of children (Achenbach, 1991). Parents (and/ or guardians) complete questions about children's social competence and behavioral or emotional problems, reflecting either the child's current behavior or behaviors that have occurred over the past 6 months. Items are rated from 0 to 2, with 0 = not true; 1 = somewhat or sometimes true; 2 = very true or often true. The 20 social competence items reflect the child's amount and quality of participation in sports, hobbies, games, activities, organizations, jobs and chores, and friendships; how well the child gets along with others and plays and works by himself or herself; and school performance (Achenbach, 1991). Two open-ended questions are included as well.

The CBCL has well-established reliability and construct validity. Intraclass correlations for individual items equal 0.90 "between item scores obtained from mothers filling out the CBCL at 1-week intervals, mothers and fathers filling out the CBCL on their clinically-referred children, and three different interviewers obtaining CBCLs from parents of demographically matched triads of children" (Achenbach, 1991). Good stability of the scale exists for both behavior problems and social competencies over time, with correlations of 0.84 and 0.97, respectively. Test–retest reliability of mothers' ratings is generally 0.89.

Zung Self-Rating Depression Scale

The Zung Self-Rating Depression Scale is a 20-question self-report depression scale (Zung, 1965; see Exhibit 13.2). Using a Likert scale,

Exhibit 13.2

Zung Self-Rating Depression Scale

For each item below, please place a check mark (✓) in the column that best describes how often you felt or behaved this way during the past several days.

Place check mark (✓) in correct column.	A little of the time	Some of the time	A good part of the time	Most of the time
1. I feel down-hearted and blue.				
2. Morning is when I feel the best.				
3. I have crying spells or feel like it.				
4. I have trouble sleeping at night.				
5. I eat as much as I used to.				
6. I still enjoy sex.				
7. I notice that I am losing weight.				
8. I have trouble with constipation.				
9. My heart beats faster than usual.				
10. I get tired for no reason.				
11. My mind is as clear as it used to be.				
12. I find it easy to do the things I used to.				
13. I am restless and can't keep still.				
14. I feel hopeful about the future.				
15. I am more irritable than usual.				
16. I find it easy to make decisions.				
17. I feel that I am useful and needed.				
18. My life is pretty full.				
19. I feel that others would be better off if I were dead.				
20. I still enjoy the things I used to do.				

(continued)

(continued)

The Zung Self-Rating Depression Scale (Zung, 1965) was designed by W. W. Zung to assess the level of depression for patients diagnosed with depressive disorder.

The Zung Self-Rating Depression Scale is a short self-administered survey to quantify the depressed status of a patient. There are 20 items on the scale that rate the four common characteristics of depression: the pervasive effect, the physiological equivalents, other disturbances, and psychomotor activities.

There are 10 positively worded and 10 negatively worded questions. Each question is scored on a scale of 1 to 4 (a little of the time; some of the time; good part of the time; most of the time).

The scores range from 25 to 100.

- 25–49: Normal Range
- 50–59: Mildly Depressed
- 60–69: Moderately Depressed
- 70 and above: Severely Depressed

Source: Zung (1965).

answers are scored on a 1 to 4 scale, with 1 representing minimal or none of the time, and 4 severe or most of the time. The 20 questions reflect common symptoms experienced in depression, including those on mood, appetite, and sleep; difficulty with completing tasks, making decisions, and reasoning; physical symptoms and suicidal thoughts. Questions are asked in either positive or negative format, for example, "I notice that I am losing weight" (negative); "I eat as much as I used to" (positive). Based on the answers, each item is summed to obtain a raw score. Using the Index Score, total scores less than 50 indicate normal functioning, whereas scores from 50 to 59 indicate mild depressive symptoms. Scores from 60 to 69 are consistent with moderate levels, whereas those equal to or above 70 indicate severe or extreme levels of depression.

The Zung is easy to administer and available, with established validity and reliability (Biggs, Wylie, & Ziegler, 1978). It is a well-established tool to measure clinical severity of depression. Similar to other instruments, it can be used to help assess patient-reported symptoms at baseline and to aid in evaluation of treatment effect over time. It is important to remember that the Zung is not a diagnostic instrument, and thus cannot be used to establish the presence of clinical disorders such as major depression.

Hamilton Depression Rating Scale

For depression, there are several commonly used rating scales to measure symptoms and severity of depression. The Hamilton Depression Rating Scale (HDRS) consists of 17 or 21 items (Hamilton, 1961). It is the most widely used continuous measure to determine severity of depressive symptoms in adults and adolescents because of its comprehensive coverage of depressive symptoms. The HDRS is the standard depression outcome measure used in clinical trials presented to the U.S. Food and Drug Administration by pharmaceutical companies seeking approval of new drug applications and is the standard by which all other depression scales are measured. Although other depressive scales exist, including some developed and used for adults, the Hamilton remains the most reliable and valid. The scale takes approximately 30 minutes to complete and score.

The scale contains items defined by anchor-point descriptions that increase in intensity. The rater is instructed to begin each query with the first recommended depression symptom question. Raters consider intensity and frequency of symptoms when assigning values. Total possible scores range from 0 to 63. Ten of the 21 items are rated on a scale from 0 to 4, nine items are rated from 0 to 2, and two are rated from 0 to 3. Each item score is summed to calculate total HDRS scores. Since the test's development in the 1950s, total HDRS scores have demonstrated reliability and a high degree of concurrent and discriminant validity (Carroll, Fielding, & Blashki, 1973).

Beck Depression Inventory

The Beck Depression Inventory (BDI, BDI-II; Beck & Steer, 1993; Beck, Steer, & Garbing, 1988) is a self-report depression severity scale, designed for individuals 13 and older, that consists of 21 multiple-choice questions. It is one of the most commonly used scales in both the clinical and the research arenas. Participants are asked to rate their depressive symptoms and behaviors during the past week. The BDI assesses common symptoms of depression such as hopelessness, irritability, guilt, and self-harm, as well as physical symptoms such as fatigue, weight loss, and lack of interest in sex, with four possible forced-choice answers that range in intensity, such as:

(0) I do not feel sad.
(1) I feel sad.
(2) I am sad all the time and I can't snap out of it.
(3) I am so sad or unhappy that I can't stand it.

Values are assigned to each question and then totaled, and the total score is compared to validated scores to determine the severity of depression. Total scores from 0 to 9 indicate few to no depressive symptoms; 10 to 18 indicate mild to moderate depression; 19 to 29 indicate moderate to severe depression; and 30 to 63 indicate severe depression (Beck & Steer, 1993; Beck et al., 1988). The BDI is a copyrighted scale. Therefore, the researcher needs to request permission and actually purchase the instrument for use.

Conners' Rating Scale–Revised

The Conners' Rating Scale–Revised (CRS–R) consists of several versions, with differing numbers of items, aimed specifically at parents, teachers, or adolescents, that allows them to rate childhood behaviors (Conners, Sitarenios, Parker, & Epstein, 1998). The CRS–R is a means of standardized evaluation in children and adolescents aged 3 to 17 for emotional, behavioral, and attentional symptoms, particularly attention deficit hyperactivity disorder. It takes several to 20 minutes to complete, depending on the version. A 10-item short version may be used to assess baseline severity of behavioral problems and to assess treatment response over time.

Short and long versions of the Conners' Parent Rating Scales (CPRS), Teacher Rating Scales (CTRS), and Adolescent Self-Report (CASS) exist; the longer versions are more comprehensive and provide a more thorough psychosocial evaluation. The parent version consists of either 80 or 27 items that focus on inattention, opposition, and hyperactive behaviors. The teacher versions, consisting of 87 or 27 items, cover similar domains. Age- and gender-based norms are available for comparison for each of the subscales and overall score.

Instruments for Measurement of Anxiety

For anxiety, there are several rating scales available. The most common tool is the Beck Anxiety Inventory (Beck, Epstein, Brown, & Steer, 1988); in which 21 items are rated by the clinician. For children aged 6 to 19, the revised Children's Manifest Anxiety Scale consists of 37 items completed by the child (Reynolds & Richmond, 1994). Obsession symptoms or those that reflect obsessive–compulsive disorder can be measured by the Yale Brown Obsessive Compulsive Scale (Y-BOCS; Goodman et al., 1989). The adult version contains about 20 items rated by the clinician, whereas the child version (CY-BOCS), targeted at children aged 6 to 14, contains approximately 40 items (Scahill et al., 1997).

SUMMARY

Much of what nurses do as part of daily practice can be based on systematic research. Once the research question(s) are identified and the design elucidated, APNs can focus on specific existing instruments that are valid and reliable to measure the concept of interest. Psychosocial data collection tools commonly address mood (e.g., depression and anxiety), behavior, general psychiatric or psychological symptoms, and measures of global impression. The APN or researcher may complete some instruments, and the participant may complete others. Using appropriate tools to elicit psychological or behavioral content helps quantify and answer the question under investigation. Data derived using these methods can provide documentation to answer relevant clinical questions or test an intervention. As a result, the APN can use evidence to direct and guide practice and contribute to knowledge development in a given domain.

SUGGESTED ACTIVITIES

1. Find a recent newspaper or Internet article of interest that reports the results of a study. Go to the original source (peer-reviewed article), and examine which instruments were used. For example, did the authors develop a survey, or did they use an existing measurement tool? What was the underlying concept that was being measured?
2. Next, read the description of the instrument in the journal article. What key characteristics are outlined about the instrument? What type of reliability and validity were used, and what is your interpretation of them?
3. Select a concept related to your practice as a nurse/APN. Using established procedures and references, find at least two relevant instruments that reflect the concept. If your search results in no appropriate tool, describe at least three steps to consider in instrument development.

REFERENCES

Achenbach, T. M. (1991). *Integrative guide for the 1991 CBCL/4–18, YSR, and TRF profiles*. Burlington, MA: University of Vermont, Department of Psychiatry.

Beck, A. T., Epstein, N., Brown, G., & Steer, R. A. (1988). An inventory for measuring clinical anxiety: Psychometric properties. *Journal of Consulting and Clinical Psychology, 56*(6), 893–897.

Beck, A. T., & Steer, R. A. (1993). *Manual for the Beck Depression Inventory*. San Antonio, TX: Psychological Corporation.

Beck, A. T., Steer, R. A., & Garbing, M. G. (1988). Psychometric properties of the Beck Depression Inventory: Twenty-five years of evaluation. *Clinical Psychology Review, 8,* 77–100.

Biggs, J. T., Wylie, L. T., & Ziegler, V. E. (1978). Validity of the Zung Self-rating Depression Scale. *British Journal of Psychiatry, 132,* 381–385.

Bobes, J. (1998). How is recovery from social anxiety disorder defined? *Journal of Clinical Psychiatry, 59*(Suppl. 17), 12–19.

Burns, N., & Grove, S. K. (2005). *The practice of nursing research: Conduct, critique and utilization.* Philadelphia, PA: Elsevier Health Sciences.

Carroll, B. J., Fielding, J. M., & Blashki, T. G. (1973). Depression rating scales. *Archives of General Psychiatry, 28,* 361–366.

Conners, C. K., Sitarenios, G., Parker, J. D., & Epstein, J. N. (1998). The revised Conners' Parent Rating Scale (CPRS-R): Factor structure, reliability and criterion validity. *Journal of Abnormal Child Psychology, 26*(4), 257–268.

Crum, R. M., Anthony, J. C., Bassett, S. S., & Folstein, M. F. (1993). Population-based norms for the Mini-Mental State Examination by age and education level. *Journal of the American Medical Association, 269,* 2386–2391.

Ewing, J. A. (1984). Detecting alcoholism: The CAGE questionnaire. *Journal of the American Medical Association, 252,* 1905–1907.

Folstein, M., Folstein, S. E., & McHugh, P. R. (1975). "Mini-Mental State." A practical method for grading the cognitive state of patients for the clinician. *Journal of Psychiatric Research, 12*(3), 189–198.

Frank-Stromborg, M., & Olsen, S. J. (2004). *Instruments for clinical health-care research* (3rd ed.). Sudbury, MA: Jones & Bartlett.

Goodman, W. K., Price, L. H., Rasmussen, S. A., Mazure, C., Delgado, P., Heninger, G. R., & Carney, D. S. (1989). The Yale-Brown Obsessive Compulsive Scale (Y-BOCS), Part I: Development, use, and reliability. *Archives of General Psychiatry, 46,* 1006–1011.

Guy, W. (1976). *Clinical global impression. ECDEU assessment manual for psychopharmacology, revised.* Rockville, MD: National Institute of Mental Health.

Hamilton, M. (1961). Development of a rating scale for primary depressive illness. *British Journal of Social and Clinical Psychology, 6*(4), 278–296.

Lachar, D., Bailley, S., Rhoades, H., Espadas, A., Aponte, M., & Cowan, K., et al. (2001). New subscales for an anchored version of the Brief Psychiatric Rating Scale: Construction, reliability, and validity in acute psychiatric admissions. *Psychological Assessment, 13*(3), 384–395.

Mateo, M. A., & Kirchhoff, K. T. (1999). Using and conducting nursing research in the clinical setting. Philadelphia, PA: W.B. Saunders.

Overall, J. L., & Gorham, D. R. (1962). The Brief Psychiatric Rating Scale. *Psychological Reports, 10,* 799–812.

Overall, J. L., & Gorham, D. R. (1976). Brief Psychiatric Rating Scale. In W. Guy (Ed.), *ECDEU assessment manual for psychopharmacology* (pp. 157–160). Rockville, MD: U.S. Department of Health, Education & Welfare.

Reynolds, C. R., & Richmond, B. O. (1994). *Revised Children's Manifest Anxiety Scale.* Los Angeles, CA: Western Psychological Services.

Scahill, L., Riddle, M. A., McSwiggin-Hardin, M., Ort, S. I., King, R. A., Goodman, W. K., Cicchetti, D., & Leckman, J. F. (1997). Children's Yale-Brown Obsessive Compulsive Scale: Reliability and validity. *Journal of American Academy of Child & Adolescent Psychiatry, 36*(6), 844–852.

Zung, W. W. (1965). A self-rating depression scale. *Archives of General Psychiatry, 12,* 63–70.

PART III

Using Available Evidence

Systematic Reviews

Kathleen R. Stevens

Once a number of studies on the same topic accumulate, the challenge becomes determining whether they have implications for clinical care. The systematic review (SR) is regarded as the most scientific way to summarize research evidence in evaluating health care interventions intended to prevent and treat illness. SRs can distinguish interventions that work from those that are ineffective, harmful, or wasteful. SRs give reliable estimates about how well various options work and identify gaps in knowledge requiring further research.

The SR is a type of research design within the larger field of the science of *research synthesis*. SRs have emerged as an integral part of the evolution of evidence-based practice (EBP), and are considered foundational not only to effective clinical practice but also to further research. When done well, SRs are considered the highest level of evidence for clinical decision making.

A primary value of SRs is that they generate new knowledge that is not otherwise apparent from examining the set of primary research studies. This summary is accomplished by the use of rigorous scientific methods. As in other research designs, application of research methods is central in constructing accurate and valid results.

The primary purpose of this chapter is to highlight the need for SRs in research; to introduce the methodology necessary to produce rigorous, credible conclusions; and to discuss who produces SRs and where SRs may be found.

DEFINITIONS OF SYSTEMATIC REVIEW

Early in the evolution of the design of scientific methods for conducting SRs, the Cochrane Collaboration advanced the following definition: "Systematic reviews are concise summaries of the best available evidence that address sharply defined clinical questions" (Cochrane Collaboration, 1999, n.p.). Systematic reviews are further described as a review of a clearly formulated question that uses systematic and explicit methods to identify, select, and critically appraise relevant research and to collect and analyze data from the studies that are included in the review; statistical methods (meta-analysis) may or may not be used to analyze and summarize the results of the included studies (Higgins & Green, 2011, n.p.).

In short, the SR is a type of evidence summary that uses a rigorous scientific approach to combine results from a body of original research studies into a clinically meaningful whole (Stevens, 2004).

As a scientific investigation, the SR focuses on a specific type of research question and uses explicit, transparent methods through each step of identifying, selecting, assessing, and summarizing individual research studies (Haynes, Sackett, Guyatt, & Tugwell, 2006; West et al., 2002). Essential aspects of each of these steps in the SR methodology are discussed later in this chapter. It is crucial that SR investigative methods be preplanned, transparent, and replicable, as is true in other research designs. The SRs may or may not include a quantitative analysis of the results of selected studies to develop inferences (conclusions) about the population of interest (Institute of Medicine [IOM], 2008, 2011).

HIGHLIGHTS OF THE EVOLUTION OF SYSTEMATIC REVIEWS

Because of the nascence of SRs as a research design, the broader scientific field uses multiple terms to refer to similar, sometimes overlapping, sometimes less rigorous approaches to summarizing the science on a given topic. These terms are *review* (used in the medical literature), *state-of-the-science review* (used in the nursing literature), and *review of literature* (commonly used in research methods textbooks). There are, however, important distinctions to be made. Today, all terms but the systematic review are considered to be flawed and to produce biased conclusions. Even the review of literature, performed to demonstrate a gap in knowledge, and therefore a need for a research study, has come under scrutiny for lack of rigor (Chalmers, 2005).

This new level of scientific rigor in research synthesis is not yet reflected in all published SRs. In seminal research, Mulrow (1987) created a strong case for moving from the then loosely performed "review" in medicine to the more scientifically performed systematic review. Mulrow's assessment of 50 "reviews" published in the medical literature showed that the rigor of the reviews was woefully lacking and that, therefore, the conclusions were not trustworthy.

The distinction between SRs and traditional literature reviews is the strict scientific design that is employed in SRs. As in other research designs, if strict methods are not employed, then the conclusion is called into question for bias and accuracy. Because clinicians rely on SRs to summarize what is known about a clinical intervention, it is crucial that we "get the evidence straight" (Glasziou & Haynes, 2005) before applying it in clinical decision making. It is equally important to understand what is known before investing additional resources to conduct primary research—perhaps over questions for which the answers are already known.

Since Mulrow (1987), several other studies have appraised the quality of reviews in the medical literature. Kelly, Travers, Dorgan, Slater, and Rowe (2001) conducted a study in which they assessed the quality of SRs in the emergency medicine literature. Likewise, Choi et al. (2001) conducted a critical appraisal of SRs in the anesthesia literature. Dixon, Hameed, Sutherland, Cook, and Doig (2005) completed a critical appraisal study in which they evaluated meta-analyses in the surgical literature. In each case, the rigor of the published SRs was found to be lacking.

Stevens (2006) demonstrated that SRs published in the nursing literature also reflected a lack of rigor. In a study similar to Mulrow's (1987), SRs were located in nursing journals. Randomly selected articles classified in the Cumulative Index of Nursing and Allied Health Literature (CINAHL) as of the publication type "systematic review" were evaluated using the Overview Quality Assessment Questionnaire (OQAQ; Oxman & Guyatt, 1991), a widely used critical appraisal instrument. This study showed that "systematic reviews" are overclassified in CINAHL, with classification as SR occurring when the article did not specify that the SR methods were used. In addition, 90% of the SRs fell short of the expected level of rigor.

The poignant chiding of an early EBP leader drives home the point for rigorous SRs:

> More than a decade has passed since it was first shown that patients have been harmed by failure to prepare scientifically defensible reviews of existing research evidence. There are now many examples of the dangers of this continuing scientific sloppiness. Organizations and individuals concerned about improving the effectiveness and safety of health care now look to systematic reviews of research—not individual studies—to inform their judgments. (Chalmers, 2005)

Recognizing the poor state of rigor of SRs and the significance of "getting the evidence straight," the Institute of Medicine (IOM, 2008) assessed what is needed to move the synthesis of science forward. Their report acknowledged the great strides made in the new science of SRs. However, it called for more methodological research to produce better SRs. The report suggested that investing in the science of research synthesis will increase the quality and value of evidence in SRs. The IOM committee recommended establishment of EBPs for SRs (IOM, 2008, 2011).

A primary mover in the field of SRs, the Cochrane Collaboration methodology workgroup continues to evolve methods for conducting SRs. Likewise, the IOM strongly urges continued development of methodological foundations and rigorous standards for SRs (2008).

THE NEED FOR SYSTEMATIC REVIEWS

Science is largely composed of two types of research: (1) primary research—original studies based on observation or experimentation on subjects; and (2) secondary research—reviews of published research that draws together the findings of two or more primary studies.

Systematic reviews offer a number of advantages to practice and in planning the next primary study. An SR distills a volume of data into a manageable form, clearly identifies cause-and-effect relationships, increases generalizability across settings and populations, reduces bias, resolves complexity and incongruence across single studies, increases rate of adoption of research into care, and offers basis for ease of update as new evidence emerges (Mulrow, 1994). With such advantages, the need for rigorous execution of SRs is clear.

Systematic reviews are a type of secondary research that follows highly rigorous and prescribed methods to produce an unbiased summary of what is known on a particular topic. In science, there is general agreement about a hierarchy of knowledge produced through various methods. In this hierarchy, the SR is considered the most robust, producing the most accurate view of objective truth. That is, SRs are deemed the most reliable form of research that provides conclusions about "what works" in health care to produce intended patient outcomes (IOM, 2008, 2011).

Moreover, given their value in determining state of the science and the rigorous scientific standards now supporting the conduct of SRs, these reviews are considered a research design worthy of specific funding and support. This point was demonstrated in a study of the relative citation impact of study designs in the health sciences (Patsopoulos, Apostolos, & Ioannidis, 2005). The investigators compared the frequency of citation across a variety of research designs (SR, true experiment, cohort, case control, case report, nonsystematic review, and decision analysis). Meta-analyses were cited significantly more often than all other designs after adjusting for year of publication, high journal impact factor, and country of origin. When limited to studies that addressed treatment effects, meta-analyses received more citations than randomized trials (Patsopoulos et al., 2005).

The purpose of an SR is twofold: (1) to indicate what we know about the clinical effectiveness of a particular health care process; and (2) to identify gaps in what is known, pointing to a need for further research. So valuable is the SR in setting the stage for further research that leaders have recommended denial of funding of proposals that are not preceded by an SR on the topic (Chalmers, 2005).

Three of the most important reasons for conducting SRs are (1) to reduce the volume of literature that must guide clinical decisions, (2) to reduce bias arising from several sources, and (3) to provide a resolution among single primary studies that draw conflicting conclusions about whether an intervention is effective.

Reducing Volume of Literature

An oft-cited benefit of an SR is that it reduces a number of single research studies into one, harmonious statement reflecting the state of the science on a given topic. Literally thousands of new health research studies are published weekly. Each year, MEDLINE indexes more than 560,000 new articles, and Cochrane Central adds about 20,000 new randomized trials to its database. This represents about 1,500 new articles and 55 new trials per day (Glasziou & Haynes, 2005). Individual readers are daunted by the challenge of reading and staying abreast of the published literature. The SR offers a solution in that it reduces the world's scientific literature to a readable summary of synthesized knowledge.

For example, a CINAHL search on "falls in the elderly" yields 1,500 articles. Even limiting the search to "research publications" reduces the list to 830 articles. Narrowing the search to "systematic reviews" yields 15 articles for review. The SRs range in rigor; however, one article on the subject (Gillespie et al., 2009) was published in the Cochrane Database of Systematic Reviews, ensuring that the synthesis was conducted in a highly systematic (scientific) way. This SR report notes that, after searching multiple bibliography databases and screening studies for relevance and quality, the authors included 62 trials involving 21,668 people in the SR (Gillespie et al., 2009). Upon synthesizing effects using meta-analysis, the researchers drew conclusions about interventions that are likely to be beneficial in reducing falls and interventions whose effectiveness is unknown. Results are expressed in terms of relative risk and confidence intervals. An example of a beneficial intervention is expressed as follows. A significant pooled relative risk (0.86 with a 95% confidence interval of 0.76–0.98) from five studies representing 1,176 participants suggests the clinical effectiveness of a multidisciplinary multifactorial risk screening and an intervention program for elders with a history of falling or those at high risk to reduce falls (Gillespie et al., 2009).

SRs consolidate research results from multiple studies on a given topic to increase the power of what we know about cause and effect, making an excellent foundation for clinical decision making.

Avoiding Bias

The term *bias* refers to a deviation in accuracy of the conclusion (Cochrane Collaboration, 2008). An SR reduces bias and provides a true representation of the science. Common sources of bias are (1) an incomplete literature search, (2) biased selection of literature, and (3) exclusion of nonpublished literature. Conducting SRs according to a structured scientific approach ensures that a true representation of knowledge is presented.

Resolving Conflicting Results

Rapid growth in the number of health care studies has sharpened the need for SRs to assist clinicians, patients, and policymakers in sorting through the confusing and sometimes conflicting array of available evidence. Although one study may conclude that an intervention is effective, a second study may conclude that the intervention offers no advantage over the comparison. The simplistic approach of comparing the number of studies that favor an intervention and the number that do not yields an erroneous conclusion. Some studies have larger sample sizes or higher-quality methodologies and therefore carry more weight. Some studies of poor quality may be excluded by using preset criteria.

The growth and maturation of methods and expertise for conducting and using SRs have increased the reliability of evidence for use in making health care decisions. It is crucial that nurses engage in conducting rigorous SRs and critically appraise those that are presented in the literature.

FUNDAMENTALS OF SYSTEMATIC REVIEWS

Whether they are serving as the lead investigator or as a member of an interprofessional team, nurses should have knowledge and skills related to SRs. Essential competencies for nurses include locating, critically appraising, and conducting SRs (Stevens, 2009).

Two primary organizations, the Agency for Healthcare Research and Quality (AHRQ) and the Cochrane Collaboration, have established guidelines for conducting SRs. The process has been adapted and renamed by others; however, there are commonly accepted principles for conducting an SR.

An SR should consist of a detailed description of the approach and parameters used to ensure completeness in identifying the available data, the rationale for study selection, the method of critical appraisal of the primary studies (evidence), and the method of analysis and interpretation. Documentation of each step is requisite and provides the necessary transparency so that the SR may be replicated. It is strongly suggested that persons well versed in SR methods be part of the research team for all SR studies.

The five basic steps listed here should be followed, and the key decisions that constitute each step of the review should be clearly documented (IOM, 2011).

Step 1: Formulate the research question
Step 2: Construct an analytic (or logic) framework
Step 3: Conduct a comprehensive search for evidence
Step 4: Critically appraise the evidence
Step 5: Synthesize the body of evidence

Step 1: Formulate the Research Question

Like other research designs, SRs use specific methods of inquiry to yield new and valid knowledge. The aim of an SR is to create a summary of scientific evidence related to the effects (outcome) produced by a specific action (intervention). Therefore, the research question used in an SR is designed in a very specific way. A well-formulated, clearly defined question lays the foundation for a rigorous SR. The question guides the analytic framework; the overall research design, including the search for evidence; decisions about types of evidence to be included; and critical appraisal of the relevant evidence from single research studies.

The SR research question must define a precise, unambiguous, answerable research question. The mnemonic PICO was devised (Richardson, Wilson, Nishikawa, & Hayward, 1995) to reflect the four key elements of the SR question:

1. Patient population
2. Intervention
3. Comparison
4. Outcome(s) of interest

An example of a well-stated SR question is as follows:

> What is the evidence that physical activity interventions, alone (I) or combined with diet modification or smoking cessation (C), are effective in helping cancer survivors (P) improve their psychosocial or physiological outcomes (O)? (Holtzman et al., 2004)

A second question, in which the comparison condition is implied, is as follows:

> What are the effects of smoking cessation programs (I) implemented during pregnancy on the health (O) of the fetus, infant, mother, and family (P)? (Lumley, Oliver, Chamberlain, & Oakley, 2004)

Note that, in this example, the implied comparison is the absence of smoking-cessation programs.

The population characteristics, such as age, gender, and comorbidities, usually vary across studies and are likely to be factors in the effect of an intervention. In addition, a given intervention may produce a number of outcomes of interest. The SR question is formulated so that it includes beneficial and adverse outcomes. For example, although prostate cancer treatment reduces mortality, the SR should also examine harmful effects of treatment such as urinary incontinence (IOM, 2008, 2011).

Depending on the specific SR question, different types of original studies will be of interest. For example, questions about effectiveness of prescription drugs will generate searches for randomized, controlled trials. On the other hand, a question about the effects of illicit drug use will find no trials that assign one group to such drug use; in this case, the question will generate a search for observational studies that compare the health of otherwise similar groups of users and nonusers.

The SR question is typically formulated during initial literature searches and evolves as the SR team examines background literature. In addition, a broader group of stakeholders is often involved in question formulation. These may include policymakers, managers, health professionals, and consumers (Agency for Healthcare Research and Quality [AHRQ], 2005).

Step 2: Construct an Analytic (or Logic) Framework

After stating the SR question, the researcher then constructs a framework. This framework maps the relations between the intervention and the outcomes of interest. In the case of the relations between screening and various outcomes as depicted in Figure 14.1, the analytic framework was developed by the U.S. Preventive Services Task Force to depict causal pathways (Harris et al., 2001).

The analytic framework demonstrates which factors are intermediate to the outcomes of interest and guides the construction of the search.

Step 3: Conduct a Comprehensive Search for Evidence

The comprehensive search for evidence is the most important—and time-consuming—step in conducting a reliable and valid SR (Higgins & Green, 2011). The search is crucial to identifying *all* relevant studies; in addition, search details must be documented so that the search can be replicated. The comprehensiveness of the search is what distinguishes an SR from a traditional narrative review (Moynihan, 2004). The question asked generates the specific search for evidence from original studies.

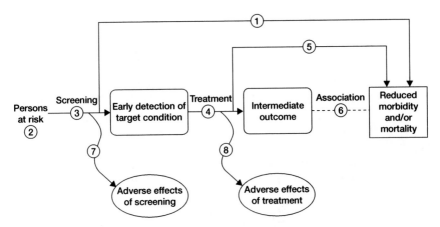

Figure 14.1   Generic analytic framework used by the U.S. Preventive Services Task Force for topics about health screening.
From "Translating Evidence into Recommendations," Agency for Healthcare Research and Quality, Rockville, MD. Retrieved from http://www.ahrq.gov/clinic/ajpmsuppl/harris3 .htm#source

Constructing an adequate search strategy requires the skills of a librarian knowledgeable about EBP. The expert search strategy may consist of more than three pages of search terms, limited, for example, to human research, randomized control trials, the specific intervention, outcomes of interest, and multiple bibliographic databases. The world's literature is searched across databases such as CINAHL, MEDLINE, Embase, and others. Often, the initial search may yield 2,000 to 3,000 articles. In addition to these databases, other sources are searched, including review group registers (e.g., Cochrane Central Register of Controlled Trials Database), and hand searches of textbook bibliographies, citation indexes, and website resources are also conducted.

The inclusion of unpublished studies reduces publication bias. Because studies that find no effect are less likely to be published (Dickersin, 2005), reliance on published studies produces an overestimate of the effects of interventions. To minimize publication bias, it is important to find "fugitive" or "grey" literature—for example, conference proceedings and unpublished studies. Researchers often contact experts directly to locate articles that were not found in the literature.

Step 4: Critically Appraise the Evidence

Once found, studies are screened to select the highest-quality studies available and to guard against selection bias. Studies are judged according to explicit criteria for design quality, strength of findings, and consistency with other studies in the set. Each study is examined to determine its applicability to the population and outcomes of interest and internal and external validity (AHRQ, 2005; Cochrane Collaboration, 2008; Glasziou & Haynes, 2005).

Using specifically designed forms, the researcher extracts data from the studies that meet the quality criteria for inclusion. This abstraction process treats each study as a "subject" of the SR. The data extracted primarily include the effect size of the intervention on the outcome. Typically, at least two investigators independently extract data; if opinions about either quality or data extraction diverge, consensus is gained through discussion and/or third-party adjudication (Higgins & Green, 2011).

Step 5: Synthesize the Body of Evidence

Summarizing Across Studies

SRs originally were developed to summarize quantitative research using statistical techniques. Summary approaches in synthesizing nonexperimental and qualitative research are also used. To synthesize a body of quantitative evidence, many SRs use meta-analyses. This is an approach that statistically combines results of separate original studies into a single result, originated by Glass (1976) and advanced by the Cochrane Collaboration and AHRQ as useful in SRs. The meta-analytic method provides a more precise estimate of the effect of the intervention than other methods such as vote counting, in which the number of positive studies is compared to the number of negative studies. Meta-analysis takes into account the weight of the effect of each individual study.

The results of a meta-analysis are often displayed in a forest plot (Figure 14.2). The plot provides a simple visual representation of the information from the individual studies that went into the meta-analysis. The graphical display conveys the strength of evidence in quantitative studies.

Forest plots are usually presented in two columns. The left column lists studies, and the right column is a plot of the measure of effect for each study. Effect estimates and confidence intervals for both individual studies and meta-analyses are displayed (Lewis & Clarke, 2001). Single-study estimates are represented by a square, the size of which reflects its weight in the meta-analysis. The confidence interval for that study is represented by a horizontal line extending on either side of the block. The length of the line is an indication of the width of the confidence interval around the result; the longer the line, the wider the confidence interval and the less precise the estimate of effect size. The meta-analyzed measure of effect (pooled result across all

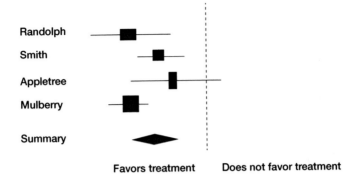

Figure 14.2   **Example of a forest plot.**

the included studies) is plotted as a diamond, with the lateral points reflecting the synthesized confidence interval (Higgins & Green, 2011).

A vertical line is also plotted, representing "no effect." If the confidence interval line crosses the vertical line, it cannot be said that the result was different from no effect—that is, there was no statistically significant difference between intervention and comparison conditions. The same applies for the meta-analyzed measure of effect (the diamond) (Higgins & Green, 2011).

Analyzing Bias

Two primary types of bias can occur: bias in the individual studies that are incorporated into the SR and biases resulting from the selection of studies into the SR. To examine bias of individual studies, researchers use traditional design critique. Bias in study selection is examined using approaches that detect publication bias (studies that show an effect are more likely to be published), citation bias (studies that show an intervention effect are more often cited), language bias (large studies are typically published in English-language journals), and multiple publication bias (the same study results are sometimes published multiple times). All of these biases are in the same direction, indicating that the intervention was effective.

The funnel plot is the primary analytic technique employed to assess bias. The funnel plot detects publication bias by examining the range of effect sizes represented in the set of studies. If small studies are represented, then the funnel plot is asymmetric (AHRQ, 2005; Higgins & Green, 2011). In the absence of bias, the funnel plot is symmetric, as represented in Figure 14.3. Note that the points in the figure form an upside down funnel. Figure 14.4 depicts a funnel plot reflecting bias, probably arising from publication bias.

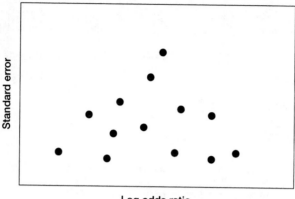

Figure 14.3   Funnel plot representing no bias.

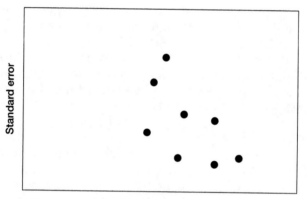

Figure 14.4   Funnel plot representing bias.

BEYOND THE SYSTEMATIC REVIEW

The variety of knowledge generated from primary research is valuable to clinical decision making. Although SRs remain the "gold standard" for summarizing randomized controlled trials (RCTs) about intervention studies, other forms of evidence summaries have emerged to service other purposes. Approaches to non-RCT bodies of evidence include scoping review, narrative review, integrative review, and qualitative review (IOM, 2008). The underlying rationale for using one approach over the other largely depends on the nature of the body of literature.

Nursing is rich with qualitative evidence; in tandem, approaches to synthesizing this type of evidence have emerged (e.g., Barnett-Pate & Thomas, 2009). Although not a cause-and-effect conclusion, evidence summaries of qualitative research offer insights into the meaning of health care and patient preferences that are valuable in guiding clinical decisions. On a specific topic, a number of qualitative studies may provide a valuable array of evidence that could be summarized to inform practice (Sandelowski, Barroso, & Voils, 2007). Another evidence summary approach is the scoping study. The scoping review is deemed most appropriate when there is a need to determine the gaps in science with regard to setting a research agenda (Arksey & O'Malley, 2005).

SUMMARY

All systematically derived evidence has value for advancing the scientific foundations of nursing care. Evidence summaries transform the multitude of studies on a topic into a usable form for clinical decision making. SRs put the "science" into reviews of literature. The rigorous approach used in producing SRs ensures that the synthesis of studies is valid, representing accuracy and truth. The IOM notes, "Systematic reviews of evidence on the effectiveness of health care services provide a central link between the generation of research and clinical decision making. SR is itself a science and, in fact, is a new and dynamic science with evolving methods" (IOM, 2008, p. 108).

If nursing care is to be effective in producing intended outcomes, it must be based on rigorously conducted SRs. Nurse scientists make significant contributions to the evolution of methodologies that match the science of nursing. High priority should be given to conducting quantitative and qualitative SRs and carefully employing the methodologies that guide these processes (Higgins & Green, 2011; IOM, 2008, 2011) to transform research evidence into a useable form of knowledge. Nurse scientists and clinical experts are called on to engage in the conduct of SRs to guide clinical decision making in nursing and health care.

SUGGESTED ACTIVITIES

1. Visit the Cochrane Collaboration website at http://www.cochrane.org/. Read the introduction. Search for "logo" in the website search box, and read the explanation of the Cochrane Collaboration logo.
2. Visit the website for the Agency for Healthcare Research and Quality at http://www.ahrq.gov
   Go to http://www.ahrq.gov/research/findings/evidence-based-reports/gaphaistp.html and read about Prevention of Healthcare Associated Infections. Read the structured abstract.

a. What four infections were studied? (Answer: central line-associated bloodstream infections [CLABSI], ventilator-associated pneumonia [VAP], surgical site infections [SSI], and catheter-associated urinary tract infections [CAUTI]).
b. What was shown to be effective and to what strength of evidence? There is moderate strength of evidence across all four infections that both adherence and infection rates improve when either audit and feedback plus provider reminder systems or audit and feedback alone are added to the base strategies of organizational change and provider education.

References for Suggested Activities

Balk, E., Chung, M., Chew, P., Ip, S., Raman, G., Kupelnick, B., ... Lau, J. (2005, August). *Effects of soy on health outcomes.* Evidence Report/Technology Assessment No. 126. (Prepared by Tufts-New England Medical Center Evidence-Based Practice Center under Contract No. 290-02-0022.) AHRQ Publication No. 05-E024-2. Rockville, MD: Agency for Healthcare Research and Quality.

Kane, R. L., Shamliyan, T., Mueller, C., Duval, S., & Wilt, T. J. (2007, March). *Nurse staffing and quality of patient care.* Evidence Report/Technology Assessment No.151 (Prepared by the Minnesota Evidence-Based Practice Center under Contract No. 290-02-0009.) AHRQ Publication No. 07-E005. Rockville, MD: Agency for Healthcare Research and Quality.

Definitive Resources on Conducting Systematic Reviews

The Agency for Healthcare Research and Quality's *EPC Partner's Guide* details information on the Evidence-Based Practice Center program for current and potential partner organizations. It also presents background on the program and the roles and responsibilities of key participants, including the Agency for Healthcare Research and Quality (AHRQ), the partners, the EPCs, and the EPC Coordinating Center. Additional information is available at http://www.ahrq.gov/legacy/clinic/epc/#Devt

Cochrane Handbook for Systematic Reviews of Interventions provides guidance on how to prepare and maintain Cochrane Intervention reviews. The handbook may be found at http://www.cochrane.org/training/cochrane -handbook

REFERENCES

Agency for Healthcare Research and Quality (AHRQ). (2005). *Evidence-based Practice Centers partner's guide.* Washington, DC: Agency for Healthcare Research and Quality.

Arksey, H., & O'Malley, L. (2005). Scoping studies: Towards a methodological framework. *International Journal of Social Research Methodology: Theory and Practice, 8*(1), 19–32.

Barnett-Page, E., & Thomas, J. (2009). Methods for the synthesis of qualitative research: A critical review. *BMC Medical Research Methodology, 9*(59). doi:10.1186/1471-2288-9-59

Chalmers, I. (2005). Academia's failure to support systematic reviews. *Lancet, 365*(9458), 469.

Choi, P. T.-L., Halpern, S. H., Malik, N., Jadad, A. R., Tramer, M. R., & Walder, B. (2001). Examining the evidence in anesthesia literature: A critical appraisal of systematic reviews. *Anesthesia and Analgesia, 92*(3), 700–709.

Cochrane Collaboration. (1999). *Cochrane handbook for systematic reviews of interventions.* The Cochrane Collaboration (out of print). Available from: http://www.cochrane.org/training/cochrane-handbook

Cochrane Collaboration. (2008). *Glossary of Cochrane Collaboration and research terms.* Retrieved March 7, 2013, from http://www.cochrane.org/glossary

Dickersin, K. (2005). Publication bias: Recognizing the problem, understanding its origins and scope, and preventing harm. In H. Rothstein, A. Sutton, & M. Borenstein (Eds.), *Publication bias in meta-analysis: Prevention, assessment, and adjustments.* London, UK: John Wiley.

Dixon, E., Hameed, M., Sutherland, F., Cook, D. J., & Doig, C. (2005). Evaluating meta-analyses in the general surgical literature: A critical appraisal. *Annals of Surgery, 241*(3), 450–459.

Gillespie, L. D., Gillespie, W. J., Robertson, M. C., Lamb, S. E., Cumming, R. G., & Rowe, B. H. (2009). Interventions for preventing falls in elderly people. *Cochrane Database of Systematic Reviews 4,* CD000340.

Glass, G. V. (1976). Primary, secondary and meta-analysis. *Educational Researcher, 5*(10), 3–8.

Glasziou, P., & Haynes, B. (2005). The paths from research to improved health outcomes. *ACP Journal Club, 142*(2, Suppl.), A-8–A-10.

Harris, R. P., Helfand, M., Woolf, S. H., Lohr, K. N., Mulrow, C. D., Teutsch, S. M., ... Third US Preventive Services Task Force. (2001). Current methods of the U.S. Preventive Services Task Force: A review of the process. *American Journal of Preventive Medicine, 20*(3, Suppl.), 21–35.

Haynes, R. B., Sackett, D. L., Guyatt, G. H., & Tugwell, P. (2006). *Clinical epidemiology: How to do clinical practice research* (3rd ed.). Philadelphia, PA: Lippincott, Williams & Wilkins.

Higgins, J. P. T., & Green, S. (Eds.). (2011). *Cochrane handbook for systematic reviews of interventions* (Version 5.1.0). The Cochrane Collaboration. Available from www.cochrane-handbook.org. Accessed March 7, 2013.

Holtzman, J., Schmitz, K., Babes, G., Kane, R. L., Duval, S., Wilt, T. J., ... Rutks, I. (2004). *Effectiveness of behavioral interventions to modify physical activity behaviors in general populations and cancer patients and survivors.* Evidence Report/Technology Assessment No. 102. AHRQ Publication No. 04-E027-2. Rockville, MD: Agency for Healthcare Research and Quality.

Institute of Medicine (IOM). (2008). *Knowing what works in health care.* In J. Eden, B. M. Wheatley, & H. Sox (Eds.). Washington, DC: National Academies of Science.

Institute of Medicine (IOM). (2011). *Finding what works in health care: Standards for systematic reviews.* Washington, DC: National Academies Press (Committee on Standards for Systematic Reviews of Comparative Effective Research; Board on Health Care Services).

Kelly, K. D., Travers, A., Dorgan, M., Slater, L., & Rowe, B. H. (2001). Evaluating the quality of systematic reviews in the emergency medicine literature. *Annals of Emergency Medicine, 38*(5), 518–526.

Lewis, S., & Clarke, M. (2001). Forest plots: Trying to see the wood and the trees. *British Medical Journal, 322,* 1479–1480.

Lumley, J., Oliver, S. S., Chamberlain, C., & Oakley, L. (2004). Interventions for promoting smoking cessation during pregnancy. *Cochrane Database of Systematic Reviews,* 4(Article No. CD001055). doi: 10.1002/14651858 .CD001055.pub2

Moynihan, R. (2004). *Evaluating health services: A reporter covers the science of research synthesis.* New York, NY: Milbank Memorial Fund.

Mulrow, C. (1987). The medical review article: State of the science. *Annals of Internal Medicine, 106*(3), 485–488.

Mulrow, C. (1994). Rationale for systematic reviews. *British Medical Journal, 309,* 597–599.

Oxman, A. D., & Guyatt, G. H. (1991). Validation of an index of the quality of review articles. *Journal of Clinical Epidemiology, 4*(411), 1271–1278.

Patsopoulos, N. A., Apostolos, A. A., & Ioannidis, J. P. A. (2005). Relative citation impact of various study designs in the health sciences. *Journal of the American Medical Association, 293,* 2362–2366.

Richardson, W. S., Wilson, M. C., Nishikawa, J., & Hayward, R. S. A. (1995). The well-built clinical question: A key to evidence-based decisions. *ACP Journal Club, 123,* A12–A13.

Sandelowski, M., Barroso, J., & Voils, C. I. (2007). Using qualitative meta-summary to synthesize qualitative and quantitative descriptive findings. *Research in Nursing and Health, 30*(1), 99–111.

Stevens, K. R. (2004). *The ACE star model of knowledge transformation.* San Antonio, TX: The University of Texas Health Science at San Antonio. Retrieved November 20, 2008, from www.acestar.uthscsa.edu

Stevens, K. R. (2006). Evaluation of systematic reviews in nursing literature. Proceedings of the Summer Institute on Evidence-Based Practice. San Antonio, TX: University of Texas Health Science Center.

Stevens, K. R. (2009). *Essential competencies for evidence-based practice in nursing* (2nd ed.). San Antonio, TX: University of Texas Health Science Center.

West, S., King, V., Carey, T., Lohr, K., McCoy, N., Sutton, S., & Lux, L. (2002). *Systems to rate the strength of scientific evidence.* Evidence Report/ Technology Assessment No. 47. (Prepared by the Research Triangle Institute, University of North Carolina Evidence-Based Practice Center under Contract No. 290-97-0011.) AHRQ Publication No. 02-E016. Rockville, MD: Agency for Healthcare Research and Quality.

15

Program Evaluation

Karen J. Saewert

The use of program evaluation has grown rapidly to meet the obligation to provide effective services, make subsequent decisions about continuing specific programs, and improve future programming (Posavac & Carey, 2010; Shadish, Cook, & Leviton, 1991). Program evaluation has its roots in sociology, education, public health, and other related fields (Shadish et al., 1991; Stufflebeam & Shinkfield, 2007). As a type of research, program evaluation helps society and those responsible for various social and service programs to understand the context of the program (e.g., schools and primary care) and whether the program meets goals and objectives. At first glance, program evaluation appears simple. However, entire books, collegiate courses, and doctoral programs focus on program evaluation theories, methods, and models (Stufflebeam & Shinkfield, 2007). Although it is beyond the scope of this chapter to provide a comprehensive understanding of program evaluation, the reader can gain basic knowledge about the process and stimulate his or her interest in learning more, especially about the principles and steps of program evaluation and their application to health care. Application of program evaluation to health care is essential as economic resources for new clinical programs shrink and the viability and impact of existing programs are questioned. Examples of areas in health care subject to program evaluation include case management, health education, faculty practice, hospital-based nursing orientation, school-based health centers, tobacco-cessation programs, pregnancy prevention, hospital-based pain management programs, and hospital-based fall-prevention programs (Barkauskas et al., 2004; Becker et al., 2007; Chan, Mackenzie, Tin-Fu, & Leung, 2000; Cramer, Mueller, & Harrop, 2003; Dykeman, MacIntosh, Seaman, & Davidson, 2003; Hackbarth & Gall, 2005; Hulton, 2007; Jacobson Vann, 2006; Logan, Boutotte, Wilce, & Etkind, 2003; Menix, 2007; Meyer & Meyer,

2000). These studies have used various frameworks and methods, but common across them were three goals: to analyze new or existing programs within a specific social context (e.g., school setting, hospital, and community); to produce information for evaluating the programs' effectiveness; and, to use this information to make decisions about program refinement, revisions, and/or continuation.

OVERVIEW AND PRINCIPLES OF PROGRAM EVALUATION

Program evaluation is defined as the systematic collection, analysis, and reporting of descriptive and judgmental information about the merit and worth of a program's goals, design, process, and outcomes to address improvement and accountability and to increase understanding of the phenomenon (Posavac & Carey, 2010; Stufflebeam & Shinkfield, 2007). A distinguishing feature of program evaluation is that it examines programs—a set of specific activities designed for an intended purpose that has quantifiable goals and objectives. Because programs come in a variety of shapes and sizes, the models and methods for evaluating them are also varied (Stufflebeam & Shinkfield, 2007).

A number of different models of program evaluation are available and are briefly summarized in Table 15.1 (Posavac & Carey, 2010; Stufflebeam & Shinkfield, 2007).

There is no clear consensus or agreement about use of any one model in program evaluation. An overriding principle in selecting a model is to understand completely the program that is being evaluated; the context and history of the program; the intended purpose of undertaking a program evaluation; and the time, expertise, and resources required for conducting a program evaluation (Billings, 2000; Hackbarth & Gall, 2005; Posavac & Carey, 2010; Shadish et al., 1991; Spaulding, 2008; Stufflebeam & Shinkfield, 2007). Selection of an evaluation model should consider the needs of stakeholders who will use the evaluation results; evaluators should look for a program that will help organize the evaluation and yield the most useful information for various stakeholders (Hackbarth & Gall, 2005).

Of particular interest in health care is the Centers for Disease Control and Prevention (CDC) framework for program evaluation that was set forth to ensure that amid the complex transitions in health care, program directors, funders, and leaders remain accountable and committed to achieving measurable health outcomes (Billings, 2000; Centers for Disease Control and Prevention, 2012; Logan et al., 2003). This framework, illustrated in Figure 15.1, is a practical, nonprescriptive tool, designed to summarize and organize the essential elements of program evaluation; it includes recommended steps in evaluation and standards for effective evaluation; and is a starting point for tailoring a program evaluation.

TABLE 15.1 Overview of Selected Models for Program Evaluation

MODEL	DESCRIPTION	CONSIDERATIONS
Objective based	Uses objectives written by the creators of the program and the evaluator. The objectives depict the overarching purpose of the evaluation and guide the type of information to be used in the evaluation. This approach includes an emphasis on and an evaluation based on the stated program goals and objectives. Evaluation data collection activities stem from the objectives.	Most prevalent model used for program evaluation. Some evaluators become so focused on the objectives that that they neglect to examine why programs succeed or fail, to consider any additional positive effects or undesired side effects of the program, or to ask whether the program objectives were the best ones for the people served.
Goal-free evaluation	Assumption is that evaluators work more effectively if they do not know the goals of a program. Considerable effort is spent studying the program as administered, the staff, the clients, the setting, and records to identify all positive and negative impacts of the program. The program staff and funders decide whether evaluation findings demonstrate that the program meets the needs of the clients.	This approach is expensive, and the rather open-ended nature may be threatening to staff. Projects that receive funding are required to show specific outcomes based on objectives, and, if the outcomes are not included in the evaluation, the appropriate data may not be collected.
Expert-oriented model	The focus is on the evaluator as a content expert who carefully examines a program to render a judgment about its quality. The evaluators judge a program or service on the basis of an established set of criteria as well as their own expertise in the area. Some decisions are based on objective quantified information as well as on qualitative impressions. This approach is often used when the entity being evaluated is large, complex, and unique.	Agencies that grant accreditation to institutions, programs, or services send program evaluators to the sites to conduct an expert-oriented evaluation. Examples include health care accrediting bodies and accrediting agencies for specific health care programs such as organ transplant programs. Issues include specificity of criteria, interpretation of criteria by various experts, and level of content expertise of the evaluator.

(continued)

285

TABLE 15.1 **Overview of Selected Models for Program Evaluation (continued)**

MODEL	DESCRIPTION	CONSIDERATIONS
Naturalistic model	A naturalist evaluation is used to develop a deep and thorough understanding of a program. The evaluator becomes the data gather, using a variety of observation and qualitative techniques. By personally observing all phases of the program and holding detailed conversations with stakeholders, the evaluator attempts to gain a rich understanding of the program, its clients, and the social environment and setting.	Because of the detail included, reports often become quite lengthy. The advantage is that personal observations are often necessary to understand the meaning of numerical information about the program.
Participative-oriented model	Evaluators seek to involve program participants in the evaluation of the program. Evaluators invite stakeholders to participate actively in the evaluation and gain skills from the experience. Participants may develop instruments, analyze data, and report findings.	This requires close contact with community stakeholders. Some argue that this approach can compromise the validity of the evaluation. The potential benefits are that the stakeholders may be more likely to enact recommendations and that the process for improvement may take less time.
Improvement-focused model	Evaluators adopt an explicit assumption that program improvement is the focus of the evaluation. Evaluators help program staff discover discrepancies between program objectives and the needs of the target population, between program implementation and program plans, and between expectations of the target population and the services actually delivered. Objective information is needed, but this information should be interpreted using qualitative information, as well. Evaluators look for strengths of the program (merit and worth) and ways that the program may fall short of its goals and thus require improvement.	This approach tends to lead to an integrated understanding of the program and its effects. Some experts believe that an improvement-focused approach best meets the criteria necessary for effective evaluation. To carry out this evaluation without threatening the staff is challenging.

Success case model	Detailed information is sought from those who benefit most from the program.	Applied naively, this approach could lead to program managers tailoring programs to those most likely to succeed, rather than those most in need of the program.
Theory-driven model	Evaluations are based on a careful description of the service to be offered in the program (individuals in need), and the way the program is expected to change the participants and the outcomes to be achieved are specified. Analysis consists of discovering the relationships among (1) the services and characteristics of the participants, (2) the services and immediate changes, and (3) immediate changes and outcome variables.	Complex correlation techniques are used to analyze data and relationships. Qualitative understanding of the program may be ignored in place of quantitative approaches. This may require resources and expertise that are not available or funded.

287

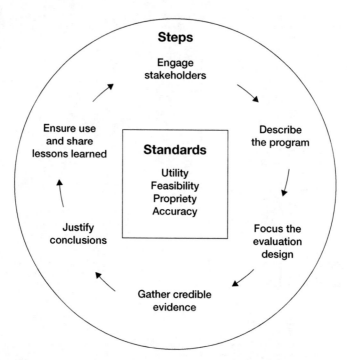

FIGURE 15.1   Recommended framework for program evaluation.
From Centers for Disease Control and Prevention (2012).

Standards of Program Evaluation

Program evaluations are expected to meet specific standards based
on four fundamental concepts: *utility, feasibility, propriety*, and *accuracy*. These concepts and related standards are central to the CDC
framework and represent the four fundamental categories of evaluation quality recommended by the Joint Committee on Standards for
Educational Evaluation (Stufflebeam & Shinkfield, 2007).

In brief, *utility* refers to the usefulness of an evaluation for those
persons or groups involved with or responsible for implementing the
program. Evaluators should ascertain the users' information needs and
report the findings in a clear, concise, and timely manner. The general
underlying principle of utility is that program evaluations should effectively address the information needs of clients and other audiences
with a right to know and inform program improvement processes. If
there is no prospect that the findings of a contemplated evaluation will
be used, the evaluation should not be done.

Program evaluation should employ procedures that are *feasible,* parsimonious, and operable in the program's environment without disrupting or impairing the program. Feasibility also addresses the control of political forces that may impede or corrupt the evaluation. Feasibility standards require evaluations to be realistic, prudent, diplomatic, politically viable, frugal, and cost-effective.

Evaluations should meet conditions of *propriety.* They should be grounded in clear, written agreements that define the obligations of the evaluator and program client with regard to supporting and executing the evaluation and protecting the rights and dignity of all involved. In general, the propriety standards require that evaluations be conducted legally, ethically, and with due regard for the welfare of those involved in the evaluation and those affected by the results.

Accuracy includes standards that require evaluators to describe the program as it was planned and executed, present the program background and setting, and report valid and reliable findings. This fundamental concept and related standards require that evaluators obtain sound information, analyze it correctly, report justifiable conclusions, and note any pertinent caveats (Stufflebeam & Shinkfield, 2007).

Guiding Principles

In addition to these fundamental concepts and related standards of evaluation, the American Evaluation Association has set forth guiding principles for evaluators intended to guide the professional practice of evaluators and to inform evaluation clients and the general public about the principles they can expect to be upheld by professional evaluators (American Evaluation Association, n.d.). These principles focus on the following areas and are fully detailed at the association's website:

1. *Systematic inquiry*: Evaluators conduct systematic, data-based inquiries about whatever is being evaluated.
2. *Competence*: Evaluators provide competent performance to stakeholders.
3. *Integrity and honesty*: Evaluators ensure the honesty and integrity of the entire evaluation process.
4. *Respect for people*: Evaluators respect the security, dignity, and self-worth of the respondents, program participants, clients, and other stakeholders with whom they interact.
5. *Responsibilities for general and public welfare*: Evaluators articulate and take into account the diversity of interests and values that may be related to the general and public welfare.

FORMATIVE AND SUMMATIVE EVALUATION

Formative and *summative* evaluations are common components of program evaluation. Experts have noted that the role of formative evaluation is to assist in developing and implementing programs, whereas summative evaluation is used to judge the value of the program. It is not the nature of the collected data that determines whether an evaluation is formative or summative but the purpose for which the data are used (Stufflebeam & Shinkfield, 2007). Data for summative and formative evaluation can be *qualitative* and/or *quantitative* in nature; the former is a nonnumerical (e.g., narrative and observation) approach (quality), whereas the latter is a numerical or statistical approach (quantity).

Formative Evaluation

Formative evaluations are used to assess, monitor, and report on the development and progress of implementing a program (Stetler et al., 2006; Stufflebeam & Shinkfield, 2007; Wyatt, Krauskopf, & Davidson, 2008). This type of evaluation is directed at continuously improving operations and offers guidance to those who are responsible for ensuring the program's quality. A well-planned and executed formative evaluation helps ensure that the purpose of the program is well defined, its goals are realistic, and its variables of interest are measurable. In addition, formative evaluation may focus on the proper training of staff who will be involved in the program implementation. During this evaluation phase, data are collected that serve to monitor the project's activities. The evaluator should interact closely with program staff, and the evaluation plan needs to be flexible and responsive to the development and implementation of the program.

As an example of formative evaluation, we will perform such an evaluation of a hypothetical pulmonary rehabilitation program. As part of the initial implementation of a pulmonary rehabilitation program, it is important that a final decision be made during the program's planning phase about the overall purpose of the program and its component parts (see Table 15.2).

The knowledge and skills of the personnel regarding the components and purpose of the program need to be assessed. For example, a pulmonary clinical nurse specialist can provide oversight for program development and implementation This would include working with physical therapists, respiratory therapists, and physicians in making decisions regarding program personnel qualifications, program location, the referral base for program clients, the time frame for program implementation, and the projected outcomes that are to be used to assess the program's effectiveness.

TABLE 15.2 Example of Formative Evaluation in a Pulmonary Rehabilitation Program

Planning phase	▪ *Purpose of the Program:* To improve activity level, to reduce symptomatology, and to decrease health care resource use among patients with chronic obstructive pulmonary disease (COPD).
	▪ *Components of the Clinical Program:* To implement a pulmonary rehabilitation program in which physicians, clinical nurses, physical therapists, and occupational therapists collaborate to facilitate increasing activity tolerance among COPD patients through an outpatient rehabilitation program. The patients are required to learn and perform program exercises on an outpatient basis; perform these activities at home on their own or with the assistance of a friend or spouse; receive patient education about oxygen use, medication use, and management of symptoms; monitor their oxygen use; rate their ability to perform self-care behaviors; monitor their medication use; and rate their functional status on a continuing basis.
	▪ *Program Protocol:* Delineate the requirements of patients and the duties of staff to implement successfully the pulmonary rehabilitation program. This protocol should also include the plan for staff training and data collection and quality improvement methods. This protocol must also be clear to the staff involved in implementing the program. The patients must be clear on what is required for their participation in the rehabilitation program.
Implementation phase	▪ *Evaluate Staff Training Program:* Examine how staff are trained to follow the program protocol, how to answer patient questions, and ways to ensure patient adherence to the program. Staff need to be trained in the correct methods of increasing activity tolerance among COPD patients, in educating patients on how to monitor their medication use and oxygen use, and in rating levels of functional status and ability to manage self-care behaviors.
	▪ *Process Variables:* Assess how well the program protocol is being implemented. Measure timeline and frequencies for patient recruitment into the program, determine whether number of staff involved in the program is sufficient, run focus groups or use interviews or diary data with patients and staff to determine any problems with the program implementation, and determine the barriers to efficient running of the program. Most important, determine the level of adherence of patients to their exercise requirements, their self-monitoring requirements, and their self-rating requirements, and determine the level of adherence among staff to guidelines presented to them in the program protocol. By using direct-observation techniques, the evaluator can determine how well staff and patients are interacting during the outpatient phase of the program, how well the staff are collaborating to increase activity tolerance among the participating patients, and track other process variables of interest.

Key Aspects of Formative Evaluations

Delineate program phases and time frames.

Assess key stakeholder perceptions related to program implementation.

Examine program participant referrals and enrollments.

Obtain feedback from program participants.

Provide feedback to key program stakeholders, to promote continuous program improvement.

Summative Evaluation

In contrast, a summative evaluation focuses on measuring the general effectiveness or success of the program by examining its outcomes. A summative evaluation addresses whether the program reached its intended goals, upheld its purpose, and produced unanticipated outcomes; it may also compare the effectiveness of the program with that of other, similar interventions (Posavac & Carey, 2010). This type of evaluation is meant to assess a program at its completion. Summative evaluations might be used to compare the effectiveness of the different treatment programs, if more than one is implemented, or to make comparisons among the "treatment" group (e.g., those enrolled in a pulmonary rehabilitation program) and a natural comparison group (e.g., those not enrolled in a pulmonary rehabilitation program). Longitudinal comparisons may also be examined to determine the relative influence of the program at different stages. In other words, the summative evaluation also seeks to determine the long-term and lasting effects on clients of having participated in the program (Posavac & Carey, 2010; Stufflebeam & Shinkfield, 2007).

USE OF PROCESS AND OUTCOME DATA

Formative and summative evaluations can be further understood in terms of *process* (program implementation and progress) and *outcome* (program success). Process refers to *how* the program is run or *how* the program reaches its desired results. A formative evaluation is process focused and requires a detailed description of the operating structure required for a successful program. Outcome refers to the success of a program and the effects, including, but not limited to, cost and quality. Outcomes can be individualized to show the effects and determine the impact of the program on each program participant. Outcomes can also be program based to examine the success and determine the impact of the program on an organizational level. Program-based outcomes are often analyzed in terms of their fiscal impact or success through a comparison with similar programs.

USE OF QUALITATIVE AND QUANTITATIVE DATA

Qualitative and *quantitative* data are both useful for program evaluations. Qualitative data, with their rich and narrative quality, provide an understanding of the impact of the program on individuals enrolled in the program. The descriptive nature of qualitative data allows one to understand the operating structure of a program and the individualized outcomes of a program. On the other hand, quantitative data, with their strictly numerical nature, allow a mathematical understanding of the factors involved in a program (e.g., statistical significance and power analysis). In addition, quantitative data provide descriptive analysis (e.g., frequency counts, and means or averages) of the variables of interest. The statistical nature of quantitative data facilitates understanding of overall programmatic outcomes and makes possible direct comparisons among program participants and, if applicable, between program groups. Frequently, only one of these approaches is used, neglecting the often beneficial and complementary provisions of the other. For qualitative data, direct observation and description are emphasized, as these lead to a form of discovery or an understanding of individual level impact of program factors. Qualitative methods may also provide insight into the context in which the program is delivered. Quantitative data tend to rely on standardized instrumentation and variable control and provide numerical figures that depict level of program success.

Triangulation is one way that both qualitative and quantitative data can be incorporated into a program evaluation to enhance the validity of program evaluation findings. Denzin (1978) described four forms of triangulation: data, investigator, theory, and methodology focused on a technological solution for ensuring validity (Mathison, 1988). These forms, applied in the context of program evaluation are outlined below:

1. *Data triangulation:* Use of multiple data sources to conduct program evaluation that may include time and setting variations
2. *Investigator triangulation:* Involvement of more than one evaluator in the program evaluation process
3. *Theory triangulation:* Use of various perspectives to interpret evaluation results
4. *Methodological triangulation:* Application of different methods to different understandings related to program evaluation

Mathison (1988) proposed an alternative conceptualization of triangulation strategies useful to consider: convergence, inconsistency, and contradiction. This alternative perspective takes into account that triangulation results in convergent, inconsistent, and contradictory evidence that must be rendered sensible by the evaluator. This belief shifts the responsibility for constructing and making sense of program evaluation findings to the program evaluator and suggests that triangulation as a strategy provides evidence for the evaluator to consider, but the triangulation strategy does not, in and of itself, do this. This viewpoint, applied to program evaluation is extrapolated as follows:

1. *Convergence:* Occurs when program evaluation data collected from different sources, investigators, perspectives, and/or methods *agree*
2. *Inconsistency:* Occurs when program evaluation data collected from different sources, investigators, perspectives, and/or methods are *inconsistent but not confirmatory or contradictory*
3. *Contradiction:* Occurs when program evaluation data collected from different sources, investigators, perspectives, and/or methods are *not simply inconsistent, but contradictory*

Triangulation strategies explicate existing, often unarticulated problems realistically—rarely in agreement and frequently inconsistent and/or contradictory—challenging evaluators to make sense of evaluation finds within a holistic context and understanding (Mathison, 1988).

STEPS IN PROGRAM EVALUATION

Overview

Program evaluation should not focus solely on *proving* whether a program or initiative works, rather on *improving* the program. Historically, emphasis on the positivist scientific approach and on proving that programs work has created an imbalance in human service evaluation work—with a heavy emphasis on proving that programs work through the use of quantitative, impact designs and not enough attention to more naturalistic, qualitative designs aimed at improving programs (W. K. Kellogg Foundation, 2004). Program evaluation should consider a more pluralistic approach that includes a variety of perspectives. Questions to consider include:

- Does the program work? Why does it work or not work?
- What factors impact the implementation and effectiveness of the program?
- What are program strengths?
- What opportunities exist for program improvement?

Internal and External Evaluators

Evaluators can relate to an organization seeking program evaluation in two primary ways: internally or externally. Internal evaluators work for the organization seeking program evaluation and may do a variety of evaluations in that setting on an episodic or ongoing basis. External evaluators may be independent consultants or work for a research firm, university, or a government agency contracted to conduct a specific program evaluation. An evaluator's affiliation has implications for program evaluations and should be considered along with competence, personal qualities, and the purpose of the evaluation (Posavac & Carey, 2010).

Competence factors include methodological and knowledge expertise needed to conduct the program evaluation. Internal evaluators often have knowledge and access advantages consistent with an internal alliance with the program, its participants, and staff. The methodological expertise of an evaluator must also be considered; this includes the extent to which an evaluator has access to resources and individuals to bridge any knowledge and/or methodological disparities. Although not absolute, external evaluators frequently have access to a wider range of resources and methodological experts than are often available to an internal evaluator. Selecting an evaluator with the program content expertise and experience may enhance the evaluator's insight into crucial issues; conversely, an evaluator with limited expertise and experience may contribute avoidable interpretive errors.

A program evaluator's trustworthiness, objectivity, sensitivity, and commitment to program improvement are critical to a program evaluation effort. The perception of these attributes by others may vary depending on whether the evaluator is internal or external to the organization. For example, an internal evaluator might be expected to have a higher degree of commitment to improving the program and may be readily trusted by program participants, staff, and administrators. The internal evaluator's institutional credibility should be anticipated to influence his or her ability to conduct the evaluation. In contrast, an external evaluator may be perceived as more objective and may find it easier to elicit sensitive information. Developing a reputation for tackling sensitive issues is often made easier when evaluators consistently emphasize that the majority of program improvement opportunities are associated with system issues versus the performance of individuals. Regardless of internal or external organizational affiliation, individual qualities remain an important consideration in selecting a program evaluator.

Finally, the purpose of the evaluation can provide additional guidance to those charged with making an evaluator selection decision. The internal evaluator may have the advantage in performing formative evaluations and leveraging existing relationships with program participants, staff, and administrators and maximize the effectiveness of communication and adoption of program improvement recommendations. In contrast, if the primary purpose of the evaluation is summative in nature and is intended to decide whether a program is continued, expanded, or discontinued, an external evaluator may be a preferable choice (Posavac & Carey, 2010).

Initial Communication

When an evaluation is being conducted it is imperative that communication between the evaluator and program representatives be clear and agreements and expectations made explicit. Evaluators must acknowledge, be flexible, and willing to accommodate the competing demands of program administrators. Agreements, if written, advisably serve as both a reminder and record of decision making. Seeing evolving evaluation plans described in writing can draw attention to implications that neither evaluators nor administrators have previously considered.

PLANNING AND CONDUCTING THE EVALUATION: ESSENTIAL STEPS

Ideally, program evaluation should begin when programs are planned and implemented. Formative evaluation, described earlier in this chapter, is a technique often used during program planning and implementation. However, some programs may already be under way, and they may never have undergone a formal evaluation process. Evaluation of such programs requires that the evaluator understand the program and how it is being implemented as part of the evaluation process. For purposes of presenting the steps of program evaluation, the author is assuming that the program being discussed is currently under way. The CDC framework for evaluation (see Figure 15.1) will be used as the guide in describing the program evaluation steps (Centers for Disease Control and Prevention, 2012).

Step 1: Engaging Stakeholders

The evaluation cycle begins by engaging stakeholders—the persons or organizations that have an investment in what will be learned from an evaluation and what will be done with the knowledge. Stakeholders include program staff, those who derive some of their revenue or income from the program (e.g., program administrators), sponsors of the program (e.g., CEO of an organization, foundations, and government agencies), and clients or potential participants in the program. Understanding the needs of intended program recipients is necessary because it is for their welfare that the program has been developed. This may require undertaking a needs assessment and gathering information on the demographics and health status indicators of the target populations. These data may reside in existing data sources (e.g., health statistics from local or state health departments) or may be collected from key informants through surveys, focus groups, or observations (Hackbarth & Gall, 2005; Laryea, Sen, Gien, Kozma, & Palacio, 1999). Stakeholders must be engaged in the inquiry to ensure that their perspectives are understood. When stakeholders are not engaged, an evaluation may fail to address important elements of a program's objectives, operations, and outcomes (Hackbarth & Gall, 2005; Posavac & Carey, 2010).

Step 2: Describing the Program

Program descriptions convey the mission and objectives of the program being evaluated. Descriptions should be sufficiently detailed to ensure understanding of (a) program goals and strategies, (b) the program's capacity to effect change, (c) its stage of development, and (d) how it fits into the larger organization and community. Program descriptions set the frame of reference for all subsequent decisions in an evaluation. The description enables the evaluator to compare the program with similar programs and facilitates attempts to connect program components to their effects. Moreover, different stakeholders may have different ideas regarding the program's goals and purposes. Working with stakeholders to formulate a clear and logical program description will bring benefits even before data are available to evaluate the program's effectiveness. Aspects to include in a program description are need (nature and magnitude of the problem or opportunity addressed by the program, target populations, and changing needs), expected effects (what the program must accomplish to be considered successful, immediate and long-term effects, and potential unintended consequences), activities (what activities the program undertakes to effect change, how these activities are related, and who does them), resources (time, talent, technology, equipment, information, money, and other assets available to conduct program activities; congruence between desired activities and resources), stage of development (newly implemented or mature), and context (setting and environmental influences within which the program operates). An understanding of environmental influences such as the program's history, the politics involved, and the social and economic conditions within which the program operates is required to design a context-sensitive evaluation and to aid in interpreting findings accurately (Barkauskas et al., 2004; Jacobson Vann, 2006; Menix, 2007).

Questions to facilitate program descriptions include: (a) Who wants the evaluation? (b) What is the focus of the evaluation? (c) Why is the evaluation wanted? (d) When is the evaluation needed? and (e) What resources are available to support the evaluation? Addressing these questions will assist in helping individuals understand the goals of the program evaluation, arrive at an overall consensus on the purpose of evaluations, and determine the time and resources available to carry out the evaluation. These questions also assist in uncovering the assumptions and conceptual basis of the program. For example, diabetes care programs may be based on the chronic-care model, a disease-management model, or a health-belief model, and it is important that the evaluator understand the program's conceptual basis to understand essential information to include in the program evaluation (Berg & Wadhwa, 2007).

Development of a logic model is part of the work of describing the program. A logic model sequences the events for bringing about change by synthesizing the main program elements into a picture of how the program is supposed to work. Often, this model is displayed in a flow chart, map, or table to portray the sequence of steps that will lead to the desired results. One of the virtues of a logic model is its ability to summarize the program's overall mechanism of change by linking processes (e.g., exercise) to eventual effects (e.g., improved quality of life and decreased coronary risk). The logic model can also display the infrastructure needed to support program operations. Elements that are connected within a logic model generally include inputs (e.g., trained staff, exercise equipment, and space); activities (e.g., supervised exercise three times per week and education about exercise at home); outputs (e.g., increased distance walked); and results, whether immediate (e.g., decreased dyspnea with activities of daily living), intermediate (e.g., ability to participate in desired activities of life and improved social interactions), or long term (e.g., improved quality of life). Creating a logic model allows stakeholders to clarify the program's strategies and reveals assumptions about the conditions necessary for the program to be effective. The accuracy of a program description can be confirmed by consulting with diverse stakeholders and comparing reported program descriptions with direct observation of the program activities (CDC Evaluation Working Group, 2008; Dykeman et al., 2003; Ganley & Ward, 2001; Hulton, 2007).

Step 3: Focusing the Evaluation Plan

On the basis of the information gained in steps one and two, the evaluator needs to set forth a focused evaluation plan (see Table 15.3). A systematic and comprehensive plan anticipates the program's intended uses and creates an evaluation strategy with the greatest chance of being useful, feasible, ethical, and accurate. Although the components of the plan may differ somewhat depending on the information and understanding of the program gained in steps 1 and 2, essential elements of the evaluation plan are discussed here.

TABLE 15.3 Examples of Steps 3, 4, and 5 for Formative and Summative Evaluations

COMPONENTS	FORMATIVE EVALUATION	SUMMATIVE EVALUATION
Selecting and defining variables of interest	Focus on process variables that determine how well the program is running. Are patients being recruited? ▪ Has staff been properly trained in the program protocol? ▪ Are staff members following program protocol? ▪ Are patients adhering to program requirements?	Focus on outcome variables that determine the effectiveness of the program. ▪ Were patients and staff satisfied with the program? ▪ Did patient health improve significantly? ▪ Were medical resources reduced as a result of the program? ▪ Are patients continuing the program on their own once the program is completed?
Measuring variables of interest	Focus on ways to measure how well the program is being run. Use: ▪ Focus groups to discuss problem areas and ways to improve the program. ▪ Direct observation to measure how the staff are following the protocol. ▪ Staff diary data to measure problems that occur on a daily basis. ▪ Interviews of patients to determine how well they are adhering to the program requirements.	Focus on ways to measure the impact the program has had. Use: ▪ Self-reports of patients and staff to report on the progress of the patient in terms of health status, functioning, symptomatology. ▪ Collateral reports from spouses of patients to get a second rating on the patient's improvements. ▪ Biomedical data to determine changes in biological parameters of functioning. ▪ Chart abstractions to measure health care resource use.
Selecting a program evaluation design	Use descriptive designs or narrative accounts. ▪ Allow for a narrative account of how well the program is being run. ▪ Provide feedback from patients and staff on areas in need of improvement. ▪ Document patient adherence levels to the program requirements. ▪ Track process variables over the implementation of the program.	Use experimental, quasi-experimental, or sequential designs (when possible). ▪ Allow for a comparison among groups of patients that were assigned to groups that received the program or did not receive the program. ▪ Use random assignment to program groups whenever possible. ▪ Use over-time examinations, if resources permit. ▪ Allow for determination of impact that the program has had on patients' lives.

(continued)

299

TABLE 15.3 Examples of Steps 3, 4, and 5 for Formative and Summative Evaluations (*continued*)

COMPONENTS	FORMATIVE EVALUATION	SUMMATIVE EVALUATION
Collecting data	Use uniform collection procedures that do not disrupt the program implementation.	Use systematic procedures for collecting data across groups (if more than one) and across time.
	▓ Collected data must be coded according to a uniform system that translates narrative data into meaningful groupings. For example, focus group comments can be grouped into comments about staff-related problems, patient-related problems, recruitment difficulties, adherence difficulties, and so on.	▓ Collected data must be coded with a uniform system that translates the data into numerical values so that data analysis can be conducted. For example, responses to a question about health status that includes responses such as *poor, fair, good,* and *excellent* need to be coded as 0, 1, 2, or 3. Across-time data collection must follow the same
	▓ Program evaluators should not bias data collection strategies by holding preconceptions about how well the program is being run.	procedures. For example, all patients receive self-reports either in the mail or from the program site. The procedures must not vary.
Evaluating data analysis	Use both qualitative and quantitative approaches.	Use both qualitative and quantitative approaches.
	▓ Qualitative approaches provide a narrative description of the process variables and allow for descriptive understanding of how well the program is running.	▓ Qualitative approaches provide a narrative description of the impact that the program has had on individual patients. Quotes from patients to exemplify the personal impact can be used.
	▓ Quantitative approaches provide frequency counts and means or averages for some of the variables of interest. For example, frequencies for patient recruitment can be computed for time periods in order to determine when lags in recruitment occurred and give insights into possible reasons for the lag.	▓ Quantitative approaches provide a statistical comparison between groups (if more than one) or across time. Can determine whether the program was effective in increasing patient health status, increasing staff and patient satisfaction, and reducing health care resources utilized.
	▓ Allows evaluators to make recommendations based on data.	▓ Quantitative approaches can also be used to make comparisons with other similar clinical programs.
		▓ Enables evaluators to make recommendations based on data.

From Centers for Disease Control (1999).

Purpose

Articulating an evaluation's purpose (i.e., intent) prevents premature decision making regarding how the evaluation should be conducted. Characteristics of the program, particularly its stage of development and context, influence the evaluation's purpose. The purpose may include gaining insight into program operations that affect program outcomes so that knowledge can be put to use in designing future program modifications; describing program processes and outcomes for the purpose of improving the quality, effectiveness, or efficiency of the program; and assessing the program's effects by examining the relationships between program activities and observed consequences. It is essential that an evaluation purpose be set forth and agreed on, as this will guide the types and sources of information to be collected and analyzed.

Selecting and Defining Variables of Interest

Defining the *independent* (process and context) and *dependent* (outcome) variables to be measured carefully and accurately is an essential part of focusing the evaluation plan. This step is likely to be the most daunting, as well as the most important. Selection and definition of the variables must be precise enough so as not to generate unwieldy data management and analysis, yet retain variables that are both meaningful and measurable. During formative evaluations, *process* variables are of primary interest, whereas during summative evaluations both *process* and *outcome* variables are of interest. Returning to the previously discussed pulmonary rehabilitation example, a *process* variable of importance might address whether or not program clients were learning how to exercise on their own while at home. A related *outcome* variable in this example might be defined as the level at which program clients were still exercising 6 months to 1 year following the completion of the formal program.

Independent or Process Variables

An example of an important independent or process variable is the level of adherence to any treatments or self-care regimens prescribed by a program. More than 25 years of research indicates that, on average, 40% of patients fail to adhere to the recommendations prescribed to them to treat their acute or chronic conditions (DiMatteo & DiNicola, 1982). How well participants adhere to program requirements, a focus of formative evaluation, is intimately linked to a program's overall effectiveness. Nonadherence has been found to be a causal factor in the time and money wasted in health care visits (Haynes, Taylor, & Sackett, 1979) and must not be overlooked in determining how well a program is being implemented. As an illustration, if a program introduces barriers to adherence (e.g., by requiring time-intensive self-care routines, by introducing complex treatments with numerous factors to remember, by making it difficult to get questions answered, or by having uninformed or untrained staff), program client adherence will likely be diminished. An accompaniment to adherence is the issue of how well the program staff maintains or adheres to the program's protocol. The integrity of an intervention or program is not upheld unless the staff members assigned to carry it out are diligent in following procedures and protocol (Kirchhoff & Dille, 1994). In addition to assessing adherence, program evaluators need to ascertain the level at which staff members are adhering to the program protocols.

Process variables include how well participants are recruited into the program, how well trained and informed the staff members are about the program's purpose and importance, identified barriers (if any) to the implementation of the program, the level at which the program site is conducive to conducting a well-run program, and the perceptions held by program staff and participants related to the usefulness of the program. These factors generally are easier to realign than are issues of participant and staff adherence. For this reason, evaluators need to spend a considerable amount of time formatively assessing and adjusting program procedures and protocols to maximize participant and staff adherence.

All programs are situated within a community or organization. This context exerts some degree of influence on how the program works and on its effectiveness. The need to examine which contextual factors have the greatest impact on program success and which context factors may help or hinder the optimization of the program's goals and objectives is likely to arise in program evaluations. Variables such as leadership style, cultural competence, organizational culture, and collaboration are all examples of contextual factors that the evaluator should consider. Gathering this type of information through either quantitative or qualitative techniques will help the evaluator understand why some component of the program worked or did not work (Greenhalgh, Robert, Bate, Macfarlane, & Kyriakidou, 2005; Stetler, McQueen, Demakis, & Mittman, 2008). Other areas worthy of examination include the federal and state climates, the impact of these climates on program processes and effectiveness, and how these climates have changed over time (Randell & Delekto, 1999). As an example, if payment for a pulmonary rehabilitation program is not available through third-party payors, including Medicare, the impact of this contextual factor should be considered in the evaluation of the program.

Dependent or Outcome Variables

Examples of dependent or outcome variables (Fitzgerald & Illback, 1993) that are measured by social scientists and health care services evaluators in determining the effectiveness of health care programs include:

- Participant health status and daily functioning
- Client satisfaction with program providers and care received
- Program provider satisfaction
- Cost containment

Evaluators and nurses alike should consider each of these variables as outcomes of a clinical program. The evaluator who conducts a program evaluation and who attempts to determine the effectiveness or success of a program should pay particular attention to these four outcomes.

The first important outcome variable defines and measures whether the program has facilitated the client's ability to improve his or her health and/or functional status. The outcome of importance is whether the program has improved quality of life and whether health goals have been achieved. If the program does not increase these outcome variables and the protocol or intervention has been followed (i.e., client and staff have adhered to the program), then the program's effectiveness is questionable. Although expectations for health improvements may not be a focus of the program, client health status is an important outcome variable that needs to be examined. For this reason, health status measurements taken multiple times and in multiple ways using triangulation techniques over the course of the program and even after the program is completed must be considered.

An important outcome of the health care delivery and program evaluation is client satisfaction. Research suggests that an intervention that decreases satisfaction with health care may lead to poorer health (Kaplan, Greenfield, & Ware, 1989), poorer adherence to treatments (Ong, de Haes, Hoos, & Lammes, 1995), poorer attendance at follow-up appointments (DiMatteo, Hays, & Prince, 1986), and greater interest in obtaining health care elsewhere (Ross & Duff, 1982) than is the case among those whose satisfaction has increased. Evaluators need to take into account changes in client satisfaction with the program, in particular, and with their health care in general, because any decrease in satisfaction can point to problems in the program's purpose, scope, and execution.

Another outcome that is often overlooked is that of nursing staff satisfaction. Slevin, Somerville, and McKenna (1996) measured staff satisfaction during the evaluation of a quality improvement initiative and found that satisfaction among the nurses was related to better interpersonal care of patients. Level of satisfaction can pertain directly to the process and implementation of the intervention or can be more generally defined and include professional satisfaction. Any program that introduces frustrations for its staff may risk contributing to it being conducted in the manner other than intended, serve to diminish the quality of care delivered, and perhaps negatively influence client satisfaction and health status. The satisfaction of program staff who implements the intervention on a daily basis and interacts and negotiates with clients must be addressed. Evaluation of programs must attend to the impact that the program has on the staff involved, and not simply the impact that it has on the patients (Slevin et al., 1996).

Finally, of considerable importance to program evaluation is the outcome variable of cost containment and/or reduction. An effective program is one that improves the quality and delivery of care, while maintaining and perhaps even reducing costs to both the organization and the client. This evaluation outcome, however, is generally long term in nature and requires multiple follow-ups; this can pose a considerable burden for programs with limited resources. Data that may be available to assist in this aspect of outcome evaluation include, information about any program client hospitalizations and related lengths of stay, emergency room visits, regular doctor office visits, supplies and equipment costs, and personnel time. It is beneficial for program evaluators to work collaboratively with financial management personnel to obtain this important information.

Measuring Variables

The next step is to select the way in which each variable of interest will be measured. In making this decision, it is important to consider, first, the many ways in which variables can be assessed and measured (e.g., self-reports, biomedical instrumentation, direct observation, or chart abstraction) and, second, the source from which the data will be collected (e.g., program client, program staff, health care records, or other written documents). Measurement is an important element of program evaluation, for without rigorous, reliable, and valid information, the data obtained and subsequent recommendations are questionable.

Program evaluators need to consider, if possible, the use of valid and reliable research instruments, rather than develop new instruments to measure the variables of interest. Many forms of instrumentation exist that have been used for purposes of program evaluations.

Potential Benefits of Using Published Instruments to Gather Self-Report Information

- Gathered information has a greater chance of being reliable and valid. That is, the instrument measures what it intends to measure and has internal consistency.
- The program evaluator has a normative group by which to compare ranges, means, and standard deviations on the instrument to the sample being evaluated.
- The instrument is composed of items or questions that are understandable by the majority of respondents.
- The instrument has a response format that both fits with the stem of the question and is responded to with relative ease.

Several reference books are available that have compiled a multitude of research instruments and normative data for measures (Frank-Stromberg & Olsen, 2004; Robinson, Shaver, & Wrightsman, 1991; Stewart & Shamdasani, 1990).

Fitzgerald and Illback (1993) delineate the various methods of obtaining information and corresponding data sources to consider in program evaluation. *Self-reports* from program clients and staff are likely the most widely used technique for acquiring information about the process and effects of an intervention. These measures, completed by program participants and staff, can often be completed at the individual's leisure. These measures can either be user friendly, allowing the individual to complete the questionnaire by circling his or her response to the various items, or research friendly, requiring the individual to transfer his or her responses onto a computer-scannable form. The main advantages of self-reports include ease of use, cost-efficiency, limited coding, and data-entry requirements, and reduced need for highly trained staff to implement their use. The main disadvantage is the prevalent belief that self-report instruments elicit self-presentation tendencies (i.e., the tendency of individuals to present themselves in a socially desirable manner or in a positive light). This view is often unfounded, as many measurement experts now hold the view that most of the people, most of the time, are accurate in their self-reported responses (Stewart & Ware, 1992; Ware, Davies-Avery, & Donald, 1978).

In addition to self-report inventories completed by the program participant, *collateral reports* can also be obtained. These reports rely on the same instruments as those used for self-reports, with slight modifications in wording. These measures can provide additional information about the program client. Collateral reports are completed by an individual closely related to the study participant. These types of reports have not been used to a great extent in nursing research, though they have been used extensively in psychological research. These collateral measures have been found to be highly correlated with the self-report data and can serve as either a validity check on the self-report data or an additional source of variant information to be used in the program evaluation.

Use of *structured* and *unstructured interviews* is another method for acquiring information. The practice of interviewing program participants either in face-to-face interactions or over the telephone provides benefits beyond those of self-report questionnaires but also introduces a few drawbacks. The benefits of interviews include the ability to clarify any confusing questions or items, increase response rates, obtain more complete information (individuals are often more likely to leave questions blank on questionnaires), and obtain narrative accounts unrestricted by standardized questions and response formats. The main drawback to interviews, however, is the need for interviewers trained to avoid leading and introducing bias. Another drawback includes the reduced ability to acquire vast amounts of information, which self-report questionnaires more easily achieve.

Direct observation is an alternative method of measurement that does not rely on the reports of the program participants in the project. Observations, like interviews, require highly trained observers. To effectively obtain data, observers must record very specific and narrow pieces of information often limiting the amount of time a particular action is observed. For instance, a program client may be observed through the use of time-sampling techniques in which only the first 5 minutes or last 5 minutes of every hour are observed and recorded. In addition, direct observations can provide information only about observable behaviors and does not allow insight into the perceptions or attitudes of the program participants.

A variation on interviews and direct observations is the use of *focus groups* (Becker et al., 2007; Laryea et al., 1999; Packer, Race, & Hotch, 1994; Wyatt et al., 2008). The qualitative information obtained from focus groups helps evaluators performing formative and summative evaluations to assess areas that need to be further refined, changed altogether, or even eliminated. Focus groups were first used by market researchers and have been a favored method by which to obtain information about consumer preferences (Stewart & Shamdasani, 1990). The use of focus groups, however, is becoming more widespread among program evaluators seeking to understand program client preferences and expectations. For example, a focus group can be used to gather pertinent information about a group of clients participating in a program or to obtain process feedback about how the program is proceeding. Focus groups can also be used to learn about how clients talk about a program or its directive and to ascertain perceptions about program effectiveness and utility (Morgan, 1988; Stewart & Shamdasani, 1990).

Stewart and Shamdasani (1990) discuss the role of focus groups in program evaluation and define the focus group technique as the collective interview of usually 8 to 12 individuals who are brought together to discuss a particular topic for an hour or two. The group is generally directed by a trained moderator who keeps the discussion focused on the topic of interest, enhances group interaction, and probes for necessary details. Morgan (1988) points out that information acquired from group discussions is often more readily accessible than it would be for individual interviews, as individual members are cued or primed to give information that they might not give in an interview. The topic of interest can vary depending on whether this technique is used for the purpose of formative or summative program evaluation.

Biomedical data include laboratory tests, blood pressure, heart and respiratory rates, and other types of data that require the use of a bioinstrument for collection (e.g., use of blood pressure monitor, heart rate monitor, or stress tests). Because of the expense of medical tests, their use as the sole means of data collection in program evaluation may not be practical. If the program requires use of biomedical data collection as part of its protocol, however, the evaluator might be able to acquire this information. The type of biomedical information collected for program evaluations must provide information relevant to the program and its evaluation and must hold meaning outside basic medical parameters. In other words, biomedical information is useless unless it can be translated into information that is directly meaningful in the determination of a program's effectiveness (e.g., if the program's goal is to reduce hypertension, then the bioinstrumentation must demonstrate that blood pressure has been lowered among the program's participants).

Health care record reviews or *written document abstractions* are another source of data to consider when conducting a program evaluation. Use of health care records as a data source requires development of a standardized evaluation form and coding scheme to use in abstracting data. These types of reviews need trained abstractors who are clear about the information to be gathered and the need to be systematic in the review process. These types of reviews often allow for the gathering of information that cannot be found in any other manner. The main drawback to this data collection method is associated with document completeness, readability, and accuracy. The primary advantage of this method is the evaluator's ability to rely on existing data.

Diary data (self-report) are another source of data that can be used to measure variables of interest. Diary data can be completed by either the health care provider or the client and provide information that is immediate and time relevant. Data can be collected once a day (a nightly count of food consumed for that day), several times a day (when every prescription medication is taken), or even randomly (prompted by some form of an alert). The main disadvantage of using diary data is that individuals may not always take the necessary time to complete the forms completely or accurately. Diary data, however,

Ways to Measure Variables

Self-reports obtained from program clients or staff

Collateral reports obtained from family members

Structured or unstructured interviews conducted by a trained interviewer

Direct observation of the program implementation mechanisms

Focus groups on program benefits and problems

Biomedical information to substantiate program client progress

Health care record or other written document abstractions

Diary data obtained from program clients or staff

represent an advance in data collection methods when used in combination with other forms of data previously discussed.

Selecting the Design

The next step is to select the method that will provide the information necessary to determine a program's effectiveness. Numerous evaluation methods are available that serve as both practical and efficient means to determine the effectiveness of clinical programs. For program evaluations to determine whether or not the outcomes of interest have improved, the program evaluation must be conducted with precision and rigor. A brief review of evaluation methods or designs that an evaluator can consider in selecting a technique for program evaluation is provided in terms outlined by Rossi, Lipsey, and Freeman (2004) that include the amount of the time and financial expense required to implement it, the type of analysis plan necessary, the level of control it offers the evaluator over the variables of interest, and the level of associated statistical power.

True *randomized controlled trials* (RCTs) involve a comparison between one or more experimental groups that have an intervention group and a control group that does not receive the intervention. Participants in the experimental group(s) participate in the program that is intended to affect a measurable outcome, whereas those in the control group serve as a comparison (Chan et al., 2000). The key component to true experiments is the random assignment of subjects to either the experimental or the control group. This assignment theoretically eliminates any individual differences among the groups prior to the implementation of the program. For this reason, in experimental designs the outcomes can be attributed to the program and not to differences among the participants of the program. Observed group differences in the selected program outcomes determine the level of program success or failure. In other words, for the program to be deemed a success, it must have a significant, beneficial effect on the experimental group in comparison to its effect on individuals in the comparison (control) group. If the program is conducted in an experimental manner, program evaluators can decide to incorporate this design into the evaluation by either assigning all of the participants to be evaluated or by randomly selecting an equal number of participants from each group (experimental and control) for the evaluation.

According to program evaluation experts, this type of design is difficult to implement in the dynamic, real-world setting where programs reside. Furthermore, this design requires withholding ongoing feedback regarding information related to program improvement during the experiment (Stufflebeam & Shinkfield, 2007). Opportunities to meet the requirements of randomized experiments in program evaluation, particularly in service fields such as health care and social service, are quite limited. This type of design is costly and may not be feasible, and the information it provides may not be useful in addressing the purpose of the program evaluation. The expectation of federal agencies and government mandates—that program evaluations employ RCTs—has had a crippling and wasteful influence on the practice of program evaluations (Stufflebeam & Shinkfield, 2007).

Both quantitative and qualitative approaches to data collection are appropriate in experimental designs. Before comparing group data, however, the evaluator should perform a formative evaluation that focuses on how well the experiment is being conducted and whether random assignment to the groups is being upheld. The summative evaluation will allow for comparisons between the groups in an attempt to illustrate the program's causal effect on outcomes. Qualitative data are useful in experimental designs because they can make it clear whether the program is being carried out as intended and can clarify differences in perceptions among members of the experimental and the control groups. By providing a narrative description of the impact of the program on the individuals, qualitative data provide further support for the evaluator's conclusions about the program's effectiveness. By offering a narrative of the way in which the program or intervention is being carried out, qualitative data give the evaluator information that elucidates the quantitative findings.

Quasi-experiments involve the same intervention and comparison component as true experiments, except that quasi-experiments differ in one critical way: random assignment of subjects or participants to a "treatment" group is not feasible. For instance, a program may have the goal of understanding the effect of gender differences on some health-related area. Since we cannot randomly assign individuals to be in a gender-specific group this design inherently involves a quasi-experimental approach. The evaluation process for quasi-experiments is similar to that for true experiments. The main difference, however, occurs during the summative evaluation. Since random assignment to treatment groups is not feasible, it is not possible to be certain that changes in outcome variables are the result of the intervention or program. Differences among the individuals in the assigned groups or other factors cannot be ruled out as the cause for observed changes in the outcome variable(s) of interest.

One drawback to both experiments and quasi-experiments is the need for a control or natural comparison group. This need for an additional group can pose a limitation for sites where client participation is limited, recruitment takes a great deal of time, or there is no natural comparison group readily available. In addition, some have argued the ethical implications of providing some clients with care or experimental care and not providing equivalent care to others. For these reasons, a *cross-sequential design* might be the most practical. In the cross-sequential design, the program evaluator observes or assesses several different groups of patients over several time periods, but each group is observed initially in the same period, for example, 6 weeks after admission to the program (Rosenthal & Rosnow, 1991). This type of design allows the time of measurement and the client group to serve as the basis for comparison, eliminating the need for a control group. In essence, a cross-sequential design simultaneously compares several different groups of clients on a set of variables observed during a single designated time period. The evaluator is able to assess for possible variations in how the program is conducted. If clients observed during the beginning of the program have different outcomes from those recruited later in the program, the evaluator can attempt to determine whether these differences are due to individual differences among the clients or to differences in program implementation.

Finally, *descriptive designs* are also useful to employ in program evaluations. These designs serve to track and describe key outcome variables over time and examine data for patterns and trends. Descriptive designs can be employed that use a cross-sectional examination of the reports of program clients and staff or a longitudinal examination of trends in relationships among variables of interest and provide narrative descriptions of the component parts of the program as viewed by clients and staff. These designs are particularly relevant for formative evaluations, because this phase of evaluation is focused on the process of planning and implementing the program as well as on *how* the program is being executed. Descriptions of the program can help to illuminate problems in program execution, especially in program client and staff adherence. For example, by examining the changes in functional status in a group of pulmonary rehabilitation program participants over a 1-year period (by including measurements before the program, during the program, and after the program), the evaluator can determine to some degree the level of success of the program in increasing functional status. If all program participants are observed to have functional status improvements corroborated by biomedical tests, staff reports, and diary data, then the program will likely be deemed effective.

Sample Size in Program Evaluations

When selecting a design for program evaluation, the evaluator must consider effective sampling and representation as an important aspect of meaningful evaluation. Sample size depends on several factors. Among these are the expected effect size of the intervention (i.e., whether the intervention will produce a small amount or a large amount of change), type of design used, plan for data analysis, and budgetary constraints. For a further explanation of sample size and its related statistical power to detect significant effects, please refer to Chapter 10 on sampling.

Step 4: Gathering Credible Evidence: Data Collection

The collection of valid, reliable, and systematic information provides the foundation of an effective program evaluation and requires establishing the conditions and systematic procedures for data collection. Establishing clear procedures for data collection and training staff to collect high-quality data must occur. Consistent procedures must be used to collect data for the results of the evaluation to enhance the evaluation's utility, accuracy, and trustworthiness.

Data Collection Quality

Once the evaluator has identified the sources of information and data collection strategies, quality control mechanisms must be established to protect data integrity. These quality control mechanisms should include periodic monitoring of the quality of information obtained and taking practical steps to improve the quality of data and/or data collection procedures if indicated. Similar problems may become evident with all forms of data. Data collection procedures and data analysis are highly sensitive to variations. Goals of the evaluator include ensuring uniformity across the program, maintaining systematic procedures, and eliminating sources of potential bias.

Data Coding

One of the most tedious components of the evaluation process is the coding and entering of all relevant data (Coffey & Atkinson, 1996; Keppel & Zedeck, 1989; Lipsey, 1994). The protocol for coding data needs to be well developed early in program planning and, whenever possible, to follow a standardized and published method. Because data collected during an evaluation may be narrative, the coding scheme for analyzing the accounts must be succinct, time efficient, and meaningful. The accounts are usually sorted through and divided into a manageable number of conceptual or programmatic categories. Often, not all of these categories will be used in the evaluation of the program, but, nonetheless, a systematic coding scheme needs to be followed. Additionally, all self-report data, biomedical data, and document-based data need to be coded into numerical values that can be used in the computations for the final evaluations. Again, these coding procedures need to be uniform across all participants (participant and staff reports) and across all forms of data. For instance, item anchors should be consistent and not vary throughout the coding scheme (if the first response is "poor," the code should be "0"; if the first response is "none of the time," the code should be "0"; if the first response is "never," the code should be "0," and so forth).

The evaluator must also remember to keep track of the manner in which items are phrased or data from written documents and bioinstruments are abstracted so that these can be accurately recoded. Items may be phrased in an alternate manner to reduce acquiescent and response biases that may require recoding. Multiple items that measure the same variable should be analyzed only when they are all directionally coded for consistency.

Step 5: Justifying Conclusions: Data Analysis, Interpretation, and Recommendations

Techniques for analyzing, synthesizing, and interpreting findings should be agreed on before data collection begins and guide this phase of program evaluation. Once all data are accurately coded and entered into a database, the evaluator can move forward with data analysis. The reader is referred to Chapter 13 for a thorough discussion of how to conduct a proper analysis. Analysis and synthesis of an evaluation's findings may detect patterns in the evidence, either by isolating important findings (analysis) or by combining sources of information to reach a broader understanding (synthesis). Mixed-method evaluations require the separate analysis of each evidence element and a synthesis of all sources to allow for an examination of patterns of agreement, convergence, or complexity.

The program evaluator must be cautious in interpreting the results of an evaluation once it has been completed. Interpretation is the process of determining the significance of results before determining what the findings mean and is part of the overall effort to understand the evidence gathered in an evaluation. The uncovering of facts regarding a program's performance is not a sufficient basis on which to draw evaluative conclusions. Evaluation evidence must be interpreted to determine the practical significance of what has been learned. Interpretations draw on information and perspectives that stakeholders bring to the evaluation inquiry.

The results of data analysis can sometimes be confusing but are often unassuming. Effect size refers to the magnitude of the relationship between two variables; the smaller the related coefficient, the smaller the effect. The evaluator must keep in mind that the effect size coefficient is meaningful only in a statistical sense and does not mean that the effect it has on the lives of individuals is small (Cohen, 1988; Rosenthal & Rosnow, 1991). The determination, based on quantitative data analysis, that a program has a small effect may be predominant; however, a small effect does not mean that the effect is unimportant. To interpret qualitative data, the evaluator should employ standard qualitative analysis techniques, using quotations and stories to illustrate themes and concepts. Qualitative information is important to include; it illustrates the basis for recommendations derived from the data, particularly for components that address program implementation.

Judgments about the program are made on the basis of data analysis and interpretation. Statements about the program are set forth, and they focus on the merit, worth, or significance of the program and are based on the agreed-upon values or standards set by the stakeholders in the planning stages of program evaluation. They are formed by comparing the findings and interpretations regarding the program against one or more of the selected standards. Because multiple standards can be applied to a given program, some evaluative statements may be incongruent. However, one of the unique features of program evaluation is that the evaluator makes judgment statements based on standards that are set a priori and reflect the perspectives of various stakeholder groups. For example, a 10% increase in pulmonary rehabilitation program annual enrollment may be viewed as positive by the program manager, whereas potential participants in the program may view this figure differently and argue that a critical threshold for access to this service has not been reached. Conflicting statements regarding a program's quality, value, or importance may suggest that stakeholders are using different standards on which to base their judgment. In the context of an evaluation, such disagreement can be a catalyst for clarifying relevant values and the worth of the program (Centers for Disease Control and Prevention, 2012).

Recommendations

Recommendations are proposed actions for consideration that grow out of the evaluation. Forming recommendations is a distinct element of program evaluation that requires information beyond what is necessary to form judgments regarding program performance (Centers for Disease Control and Prevention, 2012). Knowing that a program is able to reduce the risk of disease does not necessarily translate into a recommendation to continue the effort, particularly when competing priorities or other effective alternatives exist. Thus, summative evaluation recommendations related to continuing, expanding, redesigning, or terminating a program are separate from judgments regarding a program's effectiveness. Making recommendations requires information concerning the context, particularly the organizational context, in which programmatic decisions will be made. Recommendations that lack sufficient evidence or those that are not aligned with stakeholders' values can undermine an evaluation's credibility. By contrast, an evaluation can be strengthened by recommendations that anticipate the political sensitivities of intended users and that highlight areas that users can control or influence. Sharing draft recommendations, soliciting feedback from multiple stakeholders, and presenting alternative options instead of directive advice increase the likelihood that recommendations will be relevant and well received.

Conclusions and recommendations are strengthened by (a) summarizing the plausible mechanisms of change, (b) delineating the temporal sequence between activities and effects, (c) searching for alternative explanations and showing why they are unsupported by the evidence, and (d) showing that the effects can be repeated (Centers for Disease Control and Prevention, 2012). When different but equally well-supported conclusions exist, each can be presented with a summary of its strengths and weaknesses.

Step 6: Ensure Use and Share Lessons Learned: The Written Report and Follow-Up

Lessons learned in the course of an evaluation do not automatically translate into informed decision making and appropriate action. Deliberate effort is needed to ensure that the evaluation processes and findings are used and disseminated appropriately (Centers for Disease Control and Prevention, 2012).

Writing an Evaluation Plan and Report

Writing an *evaluation report* and disseminating the report to key stakeholders are essential final steps in program evaluation (see also Chapter 21, on reporting results through publication).

Checklist for Ensuring Effective Evaluation Reports

- Provide interim and final reports to intended users in time for use.
- Tailor the report content, format, and style for the audience(s) by involving audience members.
- Include an executive summary.
- Summarize the description of the stakeholders and how they were engaged.
- Describe essential features of the program (e.g., in appendices).
- Explain the focus of the evaluation and its limitations.
- Include an adequate summary of the evaluation plan and procedures.
- Provide all necessary technical information (e.g., in appendices).
- Specify the standards and criteria for evaluative judgments.
- Explain the evaluative judgments and how they are supported by the evidence.
- List both strengths and weaknesses of the evaluation.
- Discuss recommendations for action with their advantages, disadvantages, and resource implications.
- Ensure protection for program clients and other stakeholders.
- Anticipate how people or organizations might be affected by the findings.
- Present minority opinions or rejoinders where necessary.
- Verify that the report is accurate and unbiased.
- Organize the report logically and include appropriate details.
- Remove technical jargon.
- Use examples, illustrations, graphics, and stories.

Adapted from Worthen, Sanders, and Fitzpatrick (1997).

A full report addressing these elements and supported by evidence contributes to the usefulness, the primary purpose, of the program evaluation. An *executive summary* is useful for administrators and those individuals with program decision-making responsibilities. It is also critical that the executive summary clearly document the association between the program and the outcomes of interest, demonstrate program benefits, cost savings, and the number of program participants served. The executive summary is usually written after the evaluator has completed the final summative report designed to be a more comprehensive report of the program evaluation. The executive summary needs to succinctly address the outcomes of the program evaluation linked to the evidence gathered and be consistent with the agreed-upon standards of the stakeholders. Writing the final report and the subsequent executive summary for a new or continuing program may seem like a daunting task, but it can serve as a useful template for subsequent program reviews.

Follow-Up

Follow-up refers to the support provided to users to enable them to disseminate and enact the program evaluation findings as appropriate (Centers for Disease Control and Prevention, 2012). Active follow-up might be necessary to remind intended users of the planned use of the report. Follow-up might also be required to ensure that lessons learned are not lost or ignored in the process of making complex or politically sensitive decisions. To guard against such oversight, someone involved in the evaluation process should serve as an advocate for the evaluation's findings during the decision-making phase. This type of advocacy increases appreciation of what was discovered and what actions are consistent with the findings.

Facilitating use of evaluation findings also carries with it the responsibility for preventing misuse. Evaluation results are always bound by the context in which the evaluation was conducted. However, some results may be interpreted or taken out of context and used for purposes other than those agreed on. For example, individuals who seek to undermine a program might misuse results by overemphasizing negative findings without giving regard to the program's positive attributes. Active follow-up can help prevent these and other forms of misuse by ensuring that evidence is not misinterpreted and is not applied to situations, time periods, persons, contexts, and purposes other than those for which the finds are applicable and that were the central focus of the evaluation (Centers for Disease Control and Prevention, 2012).

SUMMARY

The process of planning, conducting, and analyzing a well-devised and comprehensive program evaluation is time-consuming, creative, and challenging. The effort put forth in an evaluation can be rewarded with fiscal reinforcement, community recognition, and a sound future for the program. Programs that are found to be effective in terms of increasing participant and staff satisfaction, increasing health status, and cost savings are likely the ones that will receive continued or increased funding. Ultimately, the program evaluator needs to examine and protect the program's integrity at all levels, for, if integrity is not maintained, the outcomes of the program are questionable.

SUGGESTED ACTIVITIES

1. You have been asked by the chief nursing officer to evaluate the cardiovascular case management program at your community hospital. Describe how you will proceed in developing an evaluation plan for this program. Include a purpose statement for the evaluation, a list of the key stakeholders you will need to communicate with, and the program evaluation methods you will use to gather information to include in the evaluation.
2. Compare and contrast the use of an internal evaluator and an external evaluator for program evaluation. For example, what are the advantages and disadvantages of having an individual employed by the institution conduct the evaluation and of contracting with an external program evaluator?

ACKNOWLEDGMENTS

The author acknowledges the important foundational work for this chapter developed by Marita G. Titler, PhD, RN, FAAN, in the previous edition of this book.

REFERENCES

American Evaluation Association. (n.d.). *Guiding principles for evaluators.* Retrieved April 9, 2013, from www.eval.org/p/cm/id/fid=51

Barkauskas, V. H., Pohl, J., Breer, L., Tanner, C., Bostrom, A. C., Benkert, R., & Vonderheid, S. (2004). Academic nurse-managed centers: Approaches to evaluation. *Outcomes Management, 8*(1), 57–66.

Becker, K. L., Dang, D., Jordan, E., Kub, J., Welch, A., Smith, C. A., & White, K. M. (2007). An evaluation framework for faculty practice. *Nursing Outlook, 55*(1), 44–54.

Berg, G. D., & Wadhwa, S. (2007). Health services outcomes for a diabetes disease management program for the elderly. *Disease Management, 10*(4), 226–234.

Billings, J. R. (2000). Community development: A critical review of approaches to evaluation. *Journal of Advanced Nursing, 31*(2), 472–480.

Centers for Disease Control. (1999). Framework for program evaluation. *Morbidity and Mortality Weekly Report, 48* (RR 11). Retrieved from http://www.cdc.gov/eval/framework.htm#graphic

Centers for Disease Control and Prevention. (2012). *A framework for program evaluation.* Retrieved April 9, 2013, from http://www.cdc.gov/eval/framework/index.htm

Chan, S., Mackenzie, A., Tin-Fu, D., & Leung, J. K. (2000). An evaluation of the implementation of case management in the community psychiatric nursing service. *Journal of Advanced Nursing, 31*(1), 144–156.

Coffey, A., & Atkinson, P. (1996). *Making sense of qualitative data: Complementing research strategies.* Thousand Oaks, CA: Sage.

Cohen, J. (1988). *Statistical power analysis for the behavioral sciences* (2nd ed.). Hillsdale, NJ: Erlbaum.

Cramer, M. E., Mueller, K. J., & Harrop, D. (2003). Comprehensive evaluation of a community coalition: A case study of environmental tobacco smoke reduction. *Public Health Nursing, 20*(6), 464–477.

Denzin, N. K. (1978). *The research act.* New York, NY: McGraw-Hill.

DiMatteo, M. R., & DiNicola, D. D. (1982). *Achieving patient compliance: The psychology of the medical practitioner's role.* New York, NY: Pergamon Press.

DiMatteo, M. R., Hays, R. D., & Prince, L. M. (1986). Relationship of physicians' nonverbal communication skill to patient satisfaction, appointment noncompliance, and physician workload. *Health Psychology, 5*(6), 581–594.

Dykeman, M., MacIntosh, J., Seaman, P., & Davidson, P. (2003). Development of a program logic model to measure the processes and outcomes of a nurse-managed community health clinic. *Journal of Professional Nursing, 19*(4), 197–203.

Fitzgerald, E., & Illback, R. J. (1993). Program planning and evaluation: Principles and procedures for nurse managers. *Orthopaedic Nursing, 12*(5), 39–44, 70.

Frank-Stromberg, M., & Olsen, S. J. (2004). *Instruments for clinical health care research.* Boston, MA: Jones & Bartlett.

Ganley, H. E., & Ward, M. (2001). Program logic: A planning and evaluation method. *Journal of Nursing Administration, 31*(1), 4, 39.

Greenhalgh, T., Robert, G., Bate, P., Macfarlane, F., & Kyriakidou, O. (2005). *Diffusion of innovations in health service organisations: A systematic literature review.* Malden, MA: Blackwell.

Hackbarth, D., & Gall, G. B. (2005). Evaluation of school-based health center programs and services: The whys and hows of demonstrating program effectiveness. *Nursing Clinics of North America, 40*(4), 711–724.

Haynes, R. B., Taylor, D. W., & Sackett, D. L. (1979). *Compliance in health care.* Baltimore, MD: Johns Hopkins University Press.

Hulton, L. J. (2007). An evaluation of a school-based teenage pregnancy prevention program using a logic model framework. *Journal of School Nursing, 23*(2), 104–110.

Jacobson Vann, J. C. (2006). Measuring community-based case management performance: Strategies for evaluation. *Lippincott's Case Management, 11*(3), 147–159.

Kaplan, S. H., Greenfield, S., & Ware, Jr., J. E. (1989). Assessing the effects of physician-patient interactions on the outcomes of chronic disease. *Medical Care, 27*(3), S110–S127.

Keppel, G., & Zedeck, S. (1989). *Data analysis for research designs: Analysis of variance and multiple regression correlation approaches.* New York, NY: W. H. Freeman.

Kirchhoff, K. T., & Dille, C. A. (1994). Issues in intervention research: Maintaining integrity. *Applied Nursing Research, 7*(1), 32–38.

Laryea, M., Sen, P., Gien, L., Kozma, A., & Palacio, T. (1999). Using focus groups to evaluate an education program. *International Journal of Psychiatric Nursing Research, 4*(3), 482–488.

Lipsey, M. W. (1994). Identifying potentially interesting variables and analysis opportunities. In H. Cooper & L. V. Hedges (Eds.), *The handbook of research synthesis* (pp. 111–123). New York, NY: Russell Sage Foundation.

Logan, S., Boutotte, J., Wilce, M., & Etkind, S. (2003). Using the CDC framework for program evaluation in public health to assess tuberculosis contact investigation programs. *International Journal of Tuberculosis and Lung Disease, 7*(12), S375–S383, S389.

Mathison, S. (1988). Why triangulate. *Educational Researcher, 17*(2), 13–17.

Menix, K. D. (2007). Evaluation of learning and program effectiveness. *Journal of Continuing Education in Nursing, 38*(5), 201–208.

Meyer, R. M., & Meyer, M. C. (2000). Utilization-focused evaluation: Evaluating the effectiveness of a hospital nursing orientation program. *Journal for Nurses in Staff Development, 16*(5), 202–208.

Morgan, D. L. (1988). *Focus groups as qualitative research.* Sage University paper series on qualitative research methods (Vol. 16). Beverly Hills, CA: Sage.

Ong, L. M. L., de Haes, J. C. J. M., Hoos, A. M., & Lammes, F. B. (1995). Doctor-patient communication: A review of the literature. *Social Science & Medicine, 40*(7), 903–918.

Packer, T., Race, K. E. H., & Hotch, D. F. (1994). Focus groups: A tool for consumer-based program evaluation in rehabilitation agency settings. *Journal of Rehabilitation, 60*(3), 30–33.

Posavac, E. J., & Carey, R. G. (2010). *Program evaluation: Methods and case studies* (8th ed.). Upper Saddle River, NJ: Pearson Education.

Randell, C. L., & Delekto, M. (1999). Telehealth technology evaluations process. *Journal of Healthcare Information Management, 13*(4), 101–110.

Robinson, J. P., Shaver, P. R., & Wrightsman, L. S. (Eds.). (1991). *Measures of personality and social psychological attitudes* (Vol. 1). San Diego, CA: Academic Press.

Rosenthal, R., & Rosnow, R. L. (1991). *Essentials of behavioral research: Methods and data analysis.* New York, NY: McGraw-Hill.

Ross, C. E., & Duff, R. S. (1982). Returning to the doctor: The effects of client characteristics, type of practice, and experience with care. *Journal of Health and Social Behavior, 23*(2), 119–131.

Rossi, P., Lipsey, M. W., & Freeman, H. E. (2004). *Evaluation: A systematic approach* (7th ed.). Newbury Park, CA: Sage.

Shadish, W. R., Jr., Cook, T. D., & Leviton, L. C. (1991). *Foundations of program evaluation: Theories of practice.* Thousand Oaks, CA: Sage.

Slevin, E., Somerville, H., & McKenna, H. (1996). The implementation and evaluation of a quality improvement initiative at Oaklands. *Journal of Nursing Management, 4*(1), 27–34.

Spaulding, D. T. (2008). *Program evaluation in practice: Core concepts and examples for discussion and analysis.* San Francisco, CA: Jossey-Bass.

Stetler, C. B., Legro, M. W., Wallace, C. M., Bowman, C., Guihan, M., Hagedorn, H., kimmel, B., Sharp, N. D., & Smith, J. L. (2006). The role of formative evaluation in implementation research and the QUERI experience. *Journal of General Internal Medicine, 21*(2), S1–S8.

Stetler, C. B., McQueen, L., Demakis, J., & Mittman, B. S. (2008). An organizational framework and strategic implementation for system-level change to enhance research-based practice: QUERI services. *Implementation Science, 3*(30), 1–11.

Stewart, A. L., & Ware, J. E., Jr. (Eds.). (1992). *Measuring functioning and well-being: The medical outcomes study approach.* Durham, NC: Duke University Press.

Stewart, D. W., & Shamdasani, P. M. (1990). *Focus groups: Theory and practice.* Applied social research methods series (Vol. 20). Newbury Park, CA: Sage.

Stufflebeam, D. L., & Shinkfield, A. J. (2007). *Evaluation theory, models and applications.* San Francisco, CA: Jossey Bass.

Ware, J. E., Jr., Davies-Avery, A., & Donald, C. A. (1978). *Conceptualization and measurement of health for adults in the health insurance study: Vol. V, General health perceptions.* Santa Monica, CA: RAND Corporation.

W. K. Kellogg Foundation. (2004). *Evaluation handbook.* Retrieved April 9, 2013, from http://www.wkkf.org/knowledge-center/resources/2010/w-k -kellogg-foundation-evaluation-handbook.aspx

Worthen B. R., Sanders, J. R., & Fitzpatrick, J. L. (1997). *Program evaluation: Alternative approaches and practical guidelines* (2nd ed.). New York, NY: Addison, Wesley Longman.

Wyatt, T. H., Krauskopf, P. B., & Davidson, R. (2008). Using focus groups for program planning and evaluation. *Journal of School Nursing, 24*(2), 71–77.

ADDITIONAL RESOURCES

American Evaluation Association. (n.d.). Retrieved April 9, 2013, from http://www.eval.org

Holden, D. J., & Zimmerman, M. A. (Eds.) (2009). *A practical guide to program evaluation planning: Theory and case examples.* Thousand Oaks, CA: Sage.

Western Michigan University. (n.d.). *The evaluation center.* Retrieved April 9, 2013, from http://www.wmich.edu/evalctr

Yarbrough, D. B., Shulha, L. M., Hopson, R. K., & Caruthers, F. A. (2011). *The program evaluation standards: A guide for evaluations and evaluation users* (3rd ed.). Thousand Oaks, CA: Sage.

16

Implementing Evidence-Based Practice

Susan Adams and Marita G. Titler

The use of evidence-based practice (EBP) has become the expected standard in health care; yet in spite of decades of high-quality health care research and a growing evidence base, its impact at the point of care remains inconsistent. It has long been recognized that the availability of high-quality research does not ensure that findings will be used to improve patient outcomes (Clancy, Slutsky, & Patton, 2004; Institute of Medicine, 2001; McGlynn et al., 2003). In fact, recent findings in both the United States and the Netherlands indicate that 30% to 40% of patients do not receive evidence-based care, and 20% to 25% of patients receive unneeded or potentially harmful care (Graham et al., 2006).

In an effort to improve patient care, government bodies and individual organizations have focused time, attention, and resources on compiling and evaluating research findings, as shown by the increase in published systematic reviews (Institute of Medicine, 2008). The findings from these reviews on topics relevant to preventive, acute, and chronic health care have been used to develop behavioral interventions, evidence-based health care programs, and evidence-based guidelines and protocols. However, despite these efforts, use of EBPs at the point of care remains inconsistent (Clancy et al., 2004; Grimshaw et al., 2004; Institute of Medicine, 2007b; Srinivasan & Fisher, 2000; Taylor, Auble, Calhoun, & Mosesso, 1999; Wang, Berglund, & Kessler, 2000).

There is a need for focused research to identify effective strategies to increase the use of evidence-based programs, guidelines, and protocols (Institute of Medicine, 2007a; Leape, 2005; Rubenstein & Pugh, 2006; Sung et al., 2003) and to answer questions such as these: What strategies are effective in increasing the use of EBP? Are these strategies effective in all settings (e.g., acute care, long-term care, school health, and primary care)? Are they effective with all end users (e.g., nurses, physicians, pharmacists, and housekeeping staff)? And are they effective with different evidence-based health care practices (prescribing drugs, hand washing, and fall prevention)? In summary, we need to know what strategies to use in what setting and with whom for varying topics when implementing EBPs in an organization.

This chapter describes the field of implementation science, a relatively new area of study that is addressing these questions through research. Included are emerging definitions, an overview of promising models, the current state of the science, and information on developing a program of research. The chapter concludes with suggestions for future research needed to move the field forward.

DEFINITION OF TERMS

Implementation, simply stated, is putting into effect the decision to adopt a change in practice (e.g., a research finding or an evidence-based health care practice). *Implementation research* is the investigation of strategies to increase the rate and extent of adoption and sustainability of EBP by individuals and organizations to improve clinical and operational decision making (Eccles & Mittman, 2006; Titler, Everett, & Adams, 2007). It includes research to (a) understand context variables that influence adoption of EBPs, and (b) test the effectiveness of interventions to promote and sustain use of evidence-based health care practices. *Implementation science* denotes both the systematic investigation of methods, interventions, and variables that influence adoption of evidence-based health care practices and the organized body of knowledge gained through such research (Eccles & Mittman, 2006; Rubenstein & Pugh, 2006; Sussman, Valente, Rohrbach, Skara, & Pentz, 2006; Titler & Everett, 2001; Titler et al., 2007).

Because implementation research is a young science, there are no standardized definitions of commonly used terms (Graham et al., 2006). This is evidenced by differing definitions and the interchanging of terms that, in fact, may represent different concepts to different people. Adding to the confusion, terminology may vary depending on the country in which the research was conducted. A recent study done by Graham et al. (2006) reported identifying 29 terms in nine countries that refer to some aspect of translating research findings into practice. For example, researchers in Canada may use the terms *research utilization, knowledge-to-action, knowledge transfer,* or *knowledge translation* interchangeably, whereas researchers in the United States, the United Kingdom, and Europe may be more likely to use the terms *implementation* or *research translation* to express similar concepts (Graham & Logan, 2004; Graham et al., 2006; Titler & Everett, 2001). Table 16.1 provides examples of currently used definitions of common terms describing concepts related to implementation science. Although

TABLE 16.1 Definitions Associated With Evidence-Based Practice

	DEFINITION	SOURCE
Diffusion	"The process by which an innovation is communicated through certain channels over time among members of a social system."	Rogers, E. (2003). *Diffusion of innovations* (5th ed., p. 5). New York, NY: Simon & Schuster.
Dissemination	"The targeted distribution of information and intervention materials to a specific public health or clinical practice audience. The intent is to spread knowledge and the associated evidence-based intervention."	NIH. Retrieved September 22, 2007, from http://grants .nih.gov/grants/guide/pa-files/PAR-07-086.html
Dissemination research	"The study of the processes and variables that determine and/or influence the adoption of knowledge, interventions or practice by various stakeholders."	Dobbins, M., Ciliska, D., Cockerill, R., Barnsley, J., & DiCenso, A. (2002). A framework for the dissemination and utilization of research for health-care policy and practice. *Online Journal of Knowledge Synthesis for Nursing, 9*(7), 2.
	Research about "how, when, by whom, and under what circumstances research evidence spreads throughout the agencies, organizations, and front line workers providing public health and clinical services."	NIH. Retrieved April 6, 2009, from http://grants.nih.gov /grants/guide/pa-files/PAR-07-086.html
Evidence	"Knowledge that has been derived from a variety of sources and that has been tested and found to be credible."	Jones, M., & Higgs, J. (2000). Will evidence-based practice take the reasoning out of practice? In J. Higgs, & M. Jones (Eds.), *Clinical reasoning in the health professions* (p. 311). Boston, MA: Butterworth Heinemann.
Implementation	"The use of strategies to adopt and integrate evidence-based health interventions and change practice patterns within specific settings."	NIH. Retrieved April 26, 2009, from http://grants.nih .gov/grants/guide/pa-files/PAR-07-086.html

(continued)

323

TABLE 16.1 Definitions Associated With Evidence-Based Practice (*continued*)

	DEFINITION	SOURCE
Implementation research	"The scientific study of methods to promote the systematic uptake of clinical research findings and other evidence-based practices into routine practice" in order to improve the quality and effectiveness of health care.	Graham, I. D., Logan, J., Harrison, M. B., Straus, S. E., Tetroe, J., Caswell, W., et al. (2006). Lost in knowledge translation: Time for a map? *Journal of Continuing Education in the Health Professions, 26*(1), 13–24.
Implementation science	"The investigation of methods, interventions, and variables that influence adoption of evidence-based healthcare practices by individuals and organizations to improve clinical and operational decision making and includes testing the effectiveness of interventions to promote and sustain use of evidence-based healthcare practices."	Titler, M. G., Everett, L. Q., & Adams, S. (2007). Implications for implementation science. *Nursing Research, 56*(4 Suppl.), S53–S59, S53.
	"All aspects of research relevant to the scientific study of methods to promote the uptake of research findings into routine health care in both clinical and policy contexts."	Graham, I. D., Logan, J., Harrison, M. B., Straus, S. E., Tetroe, J., Caswell, W., & Robinson, N. (2006). Lost in knowledge translation: Time for a map? *Journal of Continuing Education in the Health Professions, 26*(1), 13–24.
Knowledge to action	A broad concept that encompasses both the transfer of knowledge and the *use* of knowledge by practitioners, policymakers, patients, and the public, including use of knowledge in practice and/or the decision-making process. The term is often used interchangeably with knowledge transfer or knowledge translation.	Graham, I. D., Logan, J., Harrison, M. B., Straus, S. E., Tetroe, J., Caswell, W., & Robinson, N. (2006). Lost in knowledge translation: Time for a map? *Journal of Continuing Education in the Health Professions, 26*(1), 13–24.
Knowledge transfer	"Knowledge transfer is used to mean the process of getting knowledge used by stakeholders."	Graham, I. D., Logan, J., Harrison, M. B., Straus, S. E., Tetroe, J., Caswell, W., & Robinson, N. (2006). Lost in knowledge translation: Time for a map? *Journal of Continuing Education in the Health Professions, 26*(1), 13–24.

	"The traditional view of 'knowledge transfer' is a unidirectional flow of knowledge from researchers to users."	Canadian Institutes of Health Research. Retrieved April 26, 2009, from http://www.cihr-irsc.gc.ca/e/26574.html
Knowledge translation	"Knowledge translation is the exchange, synthesis and ethically-sound application of knowledge within a complex system of interactions among researchers and users."	Canadian Institutes of Health Research. Retrieved April 26, 2009, from http://www.cihr-irsc.gc.ca/e/26574.html
Research utilization	A process directed toward transfer of specific research into practice through the systematic use of a series of activities.	Horsley, J., Crane, A., Crabtree, M., & Wood, D. (1983). *Using research to improve nursing practice: A guide.* Philadelphia, PA: W. B. Saunders.
Translation research	Testing the effectiveness of interventions on the rate and extent of adoption of evidence-based practices by nurses, physicians, and other health care providers.	Titler, M., & Everett, L. (2001). Translating research into practice. *Critical Care Nursing Clinics of North America, 12*(4), 587–604.
	Translation research broadly studies and examines factors that facilitate efficacious and effective translation of research into everyday health policies and programs; evaluates the effectiveness of the administrative, management, policy, healthcare and health practice decisions and/or use of research knowledge; and describes the experience and roles of the stakeholders, practitioners, and participants.	National Institutes of Health, retrieved September 22, 2007, from http://grants.nih.gov/grants/guide/rfa-files/RFA-CD-07-005.html

From Adams (2007). Reprinted with permission.

these definitions provide an explanation of terms used in articles about implementation science, terms such as *implementation, dissemination, research translation,* and *knowledge transfer* may be used interchangeably, and the reader must determine the exact meaning from the content of the article.

The interchange of terms leads to confusion about how implementation research fits into the broader picture of conduct and use of research. One way to understand this relationship is to compare implementation research and the commonly used scientific terms for the steps of scientific discovery: basic research, methods development, efficacy trials, effectiveness trials, and dissemination trials (Sussman et al., 2006). For example, the term *translation* denotes the idea of moving something from one form to another. The National Institutes of Health (NIH) uses this term to describe the process of moving basic research knowledge that may be directly or indirectly relevant to health behavior changes into a form that eventually has impact on patient outcomes (Sussman et al., 2006). The NIH has increased emphasis on translation research and has divided the concept into Type I and Type II. Type I translation research focuses on the first three steps of research, that is, basic, or "bench" research, and the movement of that research forward through methods development and efficacy trials. Type II describes the movement through the last two steps of the research process: effectiveness trials and dissemination trials. Implementation research is a subset of Type II translation research as denoted by NIH and focuses on the last step of the research process: actual use of the information to change practice. Building a common taxonomy of terms in implementation science is of primary importance to this field and must involve input from a variety of stakeholders and researchers from various disciplines (e.g., health care, organizational science, psychology, and health services research) (Institute of Medicine, 2007b).

IMPLEMENTATION MODELS

Several models are available to guide the overall process of EBP (Rosswurm & Larrabee, 1999; Stetler, 2001; Titler et al., 2001). Most of these models include implementation as a concept, but the focus of EBP models is primarily on identifying clinical problems, collecting and analyzing evidence, making the decision to use the evidence to change practice, and evaluating the change after implementation. Little detail and little guidance are provided regarding the actual process of implementation. Users of these models are told to "implement," a directive that fails to take into account the complexity of the process of implementation. Implementing and sustaining change is a complex and multifaceted process, requiring attention to both individual and organizational factors (Titler, 2008).

Many experts believe that using a model specifically focused on implementation provides a framework for identifying factors that may be pertinent in different settings or circumstances, and allows for testing and comparing tailored strategies for individual settings. The hope is this will allow for some generalization of results (Grimshaw, Eccles, Walker, & Thomas, 2002; Improved Clinical Effectiveness through Behavioural Research Group [ICEBeRG], 2006). Although no single model may apply to all situations, a model must be sufficiently specific to guide both implementation research and implementation at the point of care but general enough to cross various populations.

Several attempts have been made to search for and organize the multitude of theories, models, and frameworks that are used to promote changes in practice or behavior. Just as the terms for implementation science are often used interchangeably, although technically they are not the same, the terms *conceptual frameworks/models* and *theoretical framework/models* are often used interchangeably, although they differ in their level of abstraction (ICEBeRG, 2006; Kitson et al., 2008; Meleis, 2005). In this discussion, the term *model* will be used as a general term, unless the model is specifically identified as a theory or conceptual framework by its creator. A model, then, for our purposes, is a set of general concepts and propositions that are integrated into a meaningful configuration to represent how a particular theorist views the phenomena of interest, in this case the transfer of evidence into practice (Fawcett, 2005).

Although an extensive review of all models suggested for possible use in implementation science is beyond the scope of this chapter, several promising models are discussed in some detail. For a summary of additional models, the review by Grol, Bosch, Hulscher, Eccles, and Wensing (2007) is recommended. Included in their recent review of models relevant to quality improvement and implementation of change in health care are cognitive, educational, motivational, social interactive, social learning, social network, social influence theories, as well as models related to team effectiveness, professional development, and leadership. Additional work by ICEBeRG has resulted in the development of an implementation database consisting of planned action models, frameworks and theories that explicitly describe both the concepts and the action steps to be considered or taken. This database was developed from a search of social science, education, and health literature that focused on practitioner or organizational change (http://www .iceberg-grebeci.ohri.ca/research/kt_theories_db.html).

Diffusion of Innovations

Probably the most well known and frequently used theory for guiding change in practice is the Diffusion of Innovations Theory by Everett Rogers. Rogers (2003) proposed that the rate of adoption of an innovation is influenced by the nature of the innovation, the manner in which the innovation is communicated, and the characteristics of the users and the social system into which the innovation is introduced. Rogers's theory has undergone empirical testing in a variety of different disciplines (Barta, 1995; Charles, 2000; Feldman & McDonald, 2004; Greenhalgh, Robert, Macfarlane, Bate, & Kyriakidou, 2004; Lia-Hoagberg, Schaffer, & Strohschein, 1999; Michel & Sneed, 1995; Rogers, 2003; Rutledge, Greene, Mooney, Nail, & Ropka, 1996; Wiecha et al., 2004).

According to Rogers, an innovation can be used to describe any idea or practice that is perceived as new by an individual or organization; evidence-based health care practices are considered an innovation according to this theory. Rogers acknowledges the complex, nonlinear interrelationships among organizational and individual factors as people move through five stages when adopting an innovation: knowledge/awareness, persuasion, decision, implementation, and evaluation (2003).

Translation Research Model

The Translation Research Model by Titler and Everett (2001), which is built on Rogers's Diffusion of Innovation Theory, provides a way to develop and test strategies to implement EBPs in health care (see Figure 16.1). According to Titler, the rate and extent of adoption can be influenced by using empirically tested strategies to affect each area identified by Rogers: the characteristics of the innovation (e.g., the use of EBP guidelines and practice prompts), the communication channels (e.g., use of opinion leaders, change champions, and outreach), the social system (e.g., modifying policies and procedures, and obtaining leadership support), and individual users (e.g., performance gap assessment and focus groups).

The Translation Research Model has been used as the framework in a series of multisite experimental studies funded by the Agency for Healthcare Research and Quality (AHRQ) (PI Titler, RO1 HS10482, and PI Titler AHRQ RO2) and the National Cancer Institute (PI Herr R01-CA115363–01). Strong points of this model are its simplicity and its focus on specific implementation strategies that have been tested for effectiveness, that is, the "how" of implementation which is often overlooked in other models.

The PARiHS Framework

The PARiHS framework (Promoting Action on Research Implementation in Health Services) is another promising model proposed to help practitioners understand and guide the implementation process. Developed

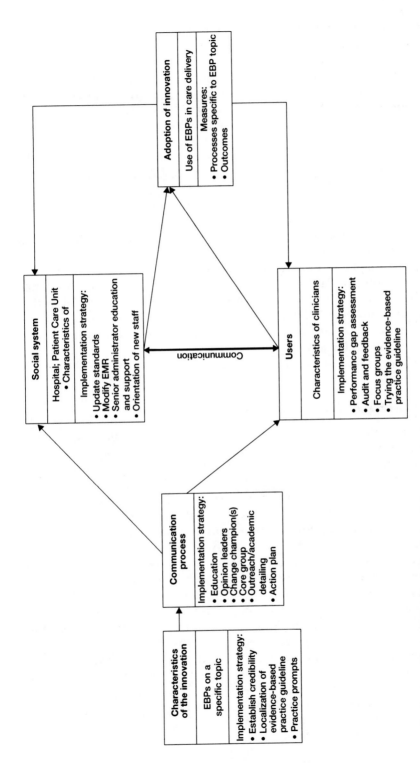

FIGURE 16.1   Translation research model.
From Titler and Everett (2001).

in 1998 as a result of work with clinicians to improve practice, the framework has undergone concept analysis and has been used as a guide for structuring research and implementation projects at the point of care (Ellis, Howard, Larson, & Robertson, 2005; Wallin, Ewald, Wikblad, Scott-Findlay, & Arnetz, 2006; Wallin, Rudberg, & Gunningberg, 2005). This framework proposes that implementation is a function of the relationship among the nature and strength of the evidence, the contextual factors of the setting, and the method of facilitation used to introduce the change. Kitson and colleagues suggested that the model may be best used as part of a two-stage process: first, the practitioner uses the model to perform a preliminary evaluation measure of the elements of the evidence and the context and, second, the practitioner uses the data from the analysis to determine the best method to facilitate change. A strong point of this model is its ability to adapt the facilitation process to the level of evidence and the level of context support available, making it adaptable to various situations. For example, if one or two of the components are weak (e.g., poor organizational support), this may be overcome by increased or targeted facilitation. Although the model is promising, it offers few specifics to guide the actual facilitation process. According to Kitson, the PARiHS framework is still under development and has not been tested as a conceptual framework, and its usefulness has not been quantified (Kitson et al., 2008).

The Knowledge Transfer Framework

The Knowledge Transfer Framework (KTF) (see Figure 16.2) was developed by the Agency for Healthcare Research and Quality (AHRQ) to speed up the transfer of results from AHRQ's safety research portfolio into health care practice (Nieva et al., 2005). This framework uses the term *knowledge transfer* to denote a three-stage process that includes (1) knowledge creation and distillation; (2) diffusion and dissemination; and (3) end-user adoption, implementation, and institutionalization.

Although originally designed for the translation of safety research into health care practice, the creators of the framework suggest that it may be relevant to other research initiatives whose focus is the uptake of evidence into practice settings. The framework is broad in scope, but the final stage is pertinent to our discussion of implementation. The suggested strategies are similar to those proposed by both Rogers and Titler; however, there are a few key differences, most notably the use of partnerships and the inclusion of the end users throughout the entire research process. Because implementation of evidence-based health care practices in actual practice settings involves complex and unpredictable interactions, external partnerships may be useful in providing the network of support needed to assess and evaluate these complex relationships and to facilitate the transfer of evidence into practice.

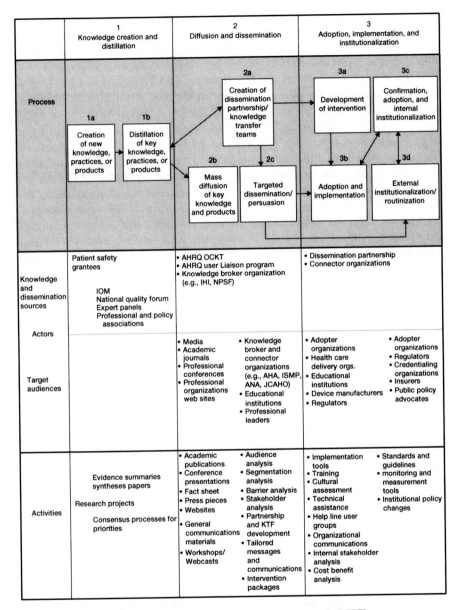

	1 Knowledge creation and distillation		2 Diffusion and dissemination		3 Adoption, implementation, and institutionalization	
Process	**1a** Creation of new knowledge, practices, or products	**1b** Distillation of key knowledge, practices, or products	**2a** Creation of dissemination partnership/ knowledge transfer teams **2b** Mass diffusion of key knowledge and products	**2c** Targeted dissemination/ persuasion	**3a** Development of intervention **3b** Adoption and implementation	**3c** Confirmation, adoption, and internal institutionalization **3d** External institutionalization/ routinization
Actors — Knowledge and dissemination sources	Patient safety grantees IOM National quality forum Expert panels Professional and policy associations		• AHRQ OCKT • AHRQ user Liaison program • Knowledge broker organization (e.g., IHI, NPSF)		• Dissemination partnership • Connector organizations	
Actors — Target audiences			• Media • Academic journals • Professional conferences • Professional organizations web sites	• Knowledge broker and connector organizations (e.g., AHA, ISMP, ANA, JCAHO) • Educational institutions • Professional leaders	• Adopter organizations • Health care delivery orgs. • Educational institutions • Device manufacturers • Regulators	• Adopter organizations • Regulators • Credentialing organizations • Insurers • Public policy advocates
Activities	Evidence summaries syntheses papers Research projects Consensus processes for priorities		• Academic publications • Conference presentations • Fact sheet • Press pieces • Websites • General communications materials • Workshops/ Webcasts	• Audience analysis • Segmentation analysis • Barrier analysis • Stakeholder analysis • Partnership and KTF development • Tailored messages and communications • Intervention packages	• Implementation tools • Training • Cultural assessment • Technical assistance • Help line user groups • Organizational communications • Internal stakeholder analysis • Cost benefit analysis	• Standards and guidelines • monitoring and measurement tools • Institutional policy changes

FIGURE 16.2   AHRQ Knowledge Transfer Framework (KTF).
AHA, American Heart Association; ANA, American Nurses Association; IHI, Institute for Healthcare Innovation; IOM, Institute of Medicine; ISMP, Institute for Safe Medication Practices; JCAHO, Joint Commission on Accreditation of Healthcare Organizations; NPSF, National Patient Safety Foundation.

From Nieva, Murphy, Ridley, Donaldson, Combes, Mitchell, et al. (2005).

Conceptual Model of Diffusion in Service Organizations

Although it does not provide specific strategies for the implementation process, the *conceptual model of diffusion in service organizations* by Greenhalgh, Robert, Bate, Macfarlane, and Kyriakidou (2005) provides a framework for identifying variables that should be considered when implementing change in organizations. Based on a systematic review of literature on diffusion and sustainability of innovations in organizations, the model is intended primarily as a memory aid for those considering different aspects of a complex situation and their interaction. As such, it does not provide specific strategies to achieve implementation but rather provides general points to remember. For example, the model suggests that when looking at the characteristics of the adopter the practitioner should consider the adopter's needs, motivation, values and goals, skills, learning styles, and social networks (Greenhalgh et al., 2005). The conceptual model of diffusion in service organizations provides an understanding of the variables that should be considered when conducting implementation research or implementing a change in practice.

STATE OF THE SCIENCE

When implementing EBP, as previously stated, it is helpful to use a model to provide structure and guidance in targeting interventions to increase the rate of adoption. For this discussion, we will use the Translation Model (see Figure 16.1) as a guide for providing an overview of implementation strategies. To be effective, it is recommended that the practitioner use multifaceted strategies to affect the various areas identified in the model, that is, the characteristics of the innovation (in this case, an evidence-based health care practice), the communication channels, the social system, and the individual users (Feldman, Murtaugh, Pezzin, McDonald, & Peng, 2005; Greenhalgh et al., 2004; Nieva et al., 2005; Rogers, 2003; Rubenstein & Pugh, 2006).

Innovation

The nature or characteristics of the EBP influence the rate of adoption; however, the attributes of an evidence-based health care practice as perceived by the users and stakeholders are not stable but change depending on the interaction between the users and the context of practice (Dopson, FitzGerald, Ferlie, Gabbay, & Locock, 2002; Greenhalgh et al., 2005). For example, an identical guideline for improving pain management may be viewed as pertinent and not complex by users in one setting (e.g., labor and delivery) but as less of a priority and as difficult to implement by staff in another unit (e.g., geropsychiatry).

Although a positive perception of the EBP alone is not sufficient to ensure adoption, it is important that the information be perceived as pertinent and presented in a way that is credible and easy to understand (Greenhalgh et al., 2004, 2005; Kitson, Harvey, & McCormack, 1998; Rogers, 2003; Rycroft-Malone et al., 2004; Titler, 2008). Some characteristics of the innovation known to influence the rate of adoption are the complexity or simplicity of the evidence-based health care practice, the credibility and pertinence of the evidence-based health care practice to the user, and the ease or difficulty of assimilating the change into existing behavior (Rogers, 2003; Titler & Everett, 2001). However, although these characteristics are important, the decision to use and sustain an EBP is complex. This is evident in the continued failure to achieve a consistent high rate of adherence to hand-washing recommendations in spite of the relative simplicity of the process and the knowledge of its pertinence to optimal patient outcomes.

EBP guidelines are one tested method of presenting information (Grimshaw et al., 2004; Guihan, Bosshart, & Nelson, 2004). EBP guidelines are designed to assimilate large, complex amounts of research information into a usable format (Grimshaw et al., 2004; Lia-Hoagberg et al., 1999). Appropriately designed guidelines are adaptable and easy to assimilate into the local setting. Empirically tested methods of adapting guidelines and protocols to the local practice setting include practice prompts, quick reference guides, decision-making algorithms, and computer-based decision support systems (Eccles & Grimshaw, 2004; Feldman et al., 2005; Grimshaw, Eccles, Thomas, et al., 2006; Wensing, Wollersheim, & Grol, 2006).

Communication

The method and the channels used to communicate with potential users about an innovation influence the speed and extent of adoption of the innovation (Rogers, 2003; Titler & Everett, 2001). Communication channels include both formal methods of communication that are established in the hierarchical system and informal communication networks that occur spontaneously throughout the system. Communication networks are interconnected individuals who are linked by patterned flows of information (Rogers, 2003).

Mass-media communication methods are effective in raising awareness at the population or community level, for example, of public health issues such as the need for immunizations and screenings and include the use of television, radio, newspapers, pamphlets, posters, and leaflets (Grilli, Ramsay, & Minozzi, 2002; Lam et al., 2003; Randolph & Viswanath, 2004; Rogers, 2003; Silver, Rubini, Black, & Hodgson, 2003). Many acute-care EBP implementation projects also use awareness campaigns in the early stages that may include similar strategies (e.g., bulletin boards, flyers, posters, and newsletters). Although research has been done on the effectiveness of mass-media campaigns at the population level to guide message content and delivery to the general public (Grilli et al., 2002; Randolph & Viswanath, 2004), less evidence is available to guide the message content or delivery methods needed to affect the rate of adoption of EBP among health care workers (Titler, 2008).

Interpersonal communication is more effective than mass-media communication in persuading people to change practice (Rogers, 2003). Communication strategies tested in health care systems that use interpersonal communication channels include education (Davis, Thomson, Oxman, & Haynes, 1995; Forsetlund et al., 2009; Grimshaw et al., 2001), opinion leaders (Doumit, Gattellari, Grimshaw, & O'Brien, 2007; Locock, Dopson, Chambers, & Gabbay, 2001), change champions (Guihan et al., 2004), facilitators (Kitson et al., 1998; Stetler et al., 2006), audit and feedback (Grimshaw et al., 2004; Hysong, Best, & Pugh, 2006; Jamtvedt, Young, Kristoffersen, O'Brien, & Oxman, 2006), and outreach consultation and education by experts (Bero et al., 1998; Davis et al., 1995; Feldman & McDonald, 2004; Hysong et al., 2006; Titler, 2008).

The literature indicates that education using didactic teaching strategies such as the traditional dispersion of educational material and formal conference presentations may increase awareness but has little impact on changing practice. Interactive teaching methods, especially when combined with other methods, have proven more effective (Bero et al., 1998; Forsetlund et al., 2009; Grimshaw et al., 2001). Educational strategies that lead to improvement in EBP adherence include educational meetings with an interactive component, small-group educational meetings (which are more effective than large-group meetings), and educational meetings that include an opportunity to practice skills (Forsetlund et al., 2009).

Opinion leaders are informal leaders from the local peer group who are viewed as respected sources of information and judgment regarding the appropriateness of the innovation (Rogers, 2003). They are trusted to evaluate new information and to determine the appropriateness of the innovation for the setting. Opinion leaders have been effective in promoting the adoption of EBP (Doumit et al., 2007), especially in combination with other strategies such as outreach and performance feedback (Dopson et al., 2002; Doumit et al., 2007; Forsetlund et al., 2009; Locock et al., 2001; Soumerai et al., 1998). Although the effects of opinion leaders on natural settings have been well documented, selecting and engaging opinion leaders for specific projects is complex (Greenhalgh et al., 2004; Grimshaw, Eccles, Greener et al., 2006; Titler, 2008). For changes in practice that involve multiple disciplines, opinion leaders should be selected from each of the various disciplines involved. These opinion leaders must be respected members of their group, competent, knowledgeable, and enthusiastic about the innovation, and able to understand how the new practice fits with the group norms (Collins, Hawks, & Davis, 2000). Opinion leaders can be self-selected (e.g., volunteer to be a leader for a particular EBP), identified by program implementers as known leaders, selected as a result of their position (e.g., local advanced practice nurse), or nominated by staff members to lead the project (Titler, 2002).

Change champions are expert practitioners from the local peer group who promote the use of the innovation (Rogers, 2003). Change champions are nurses who provide information and encouragement, are persistent, and have positive working relationships with their colleagues (Titler, 2008). The use of change champions has proven effective in many settings (Estabrooks, O'Leary, Ricker, & Humphrey, 2003; Rycroft-Malone et al., 2004; Titler, 2002). Research suggests that nurses prefer interpersonal communication with peers rather than other sources of information, so the presence of a change champion is crucial in facilitating the adoption of the innovation (Adams & Barron, 2009; Estabrooks, Chong, Brigidear, & Profetto-McGrath, 2005; Estabrooks, O'Leary, et al., 2003).

Using a core group or team that has the same goal of promoting EBP, along with the change champion, increases the likelihood of obtaining the critical mass of users necessary to promote and sustain the adoption of the practice change (Dopson et al., 2002; Nelson et al., 2002; Rogers, 2003; Titler, 2006, 2008). Members of the core group should represent the various shifts and days of the weeks and should assume responsibility for providing information, daily reinforcement of the change, and positive feedback to several of their peers. Conferencing with the core group, opinion leaders, and change champions during implementation of the innovation is recommended to provide additional support and guidance (Horbar et al., 2004; Titler, 2008; Titler & Everett, 2001).

Educational outreach, also called academic detailing, is one-on-one communication between an external topic expert and health care practitioners in their practice setting to provide information on the practice change. The expert should be knowledgeable about the research base for the EBP change and able to respond to questions and concerns that arise during implementation. Feedback on performance and/or education may be provided at that time. When used alone or in combination with other strategies, outreach has proven effective in the adoption of EBP (Feldman & McDonald, 2004; Hendryx et al., 1998; Horbar et al., 2004; O'Brien et al., 2007).

A related concept is the facilitator role identified as an essential component in the PARiHS model of translation of EBP (Harvey et al., 2002). The facilitator role may range from task-focused activities (e.g., outreach and academic detailing) to holistic interactions designed to enable individuals, teams, and organizations to change practice (Harvey et al., 2002; Kitson et al., 1998; Stetler et al., 2006). The facilitator may be internal to the organization or external to the organization, and facilitation may encompass more than one individual (both internal and external), in contrast to outreach, which is typically external to the organization (Greenhalgh et al., 2005; Stetler et al., 2006; Titler, 2008).

Users of the Innovation

Several studies have analyzed attitudes and characteristics that influence adoption of EBP by individual users (Estabrooks, Floyd, Scott-Findlay, O'Leary, & Gushta, 2003; Milner, Estabrooks, & Myrick, 2006; Rogers, 2003). Characteristics such as favorable attitude toward research and previous involvement in research studies are consistently associated with use of research findings in practice (Estabrooks, Floyd, et al., 2003). Additional characteristics such as educational level, professional role (e.g., management versus staff nurse), autonomy, conference attendance, cooperativeness and self-efficacy, job satisfaction, professional association membership, and time spent reading professional journals may influence one's readiness to adopt EBP, but the findings are not consistent across various studies (Estabrooks, 1999; Hutchinson & Johnston, 2004; McKenna, Ashton, & Keeney, 2004; Milner et al., 2006).

Implementation strategies targeted at the individual user include audit and feedback and performance gap assessment (PGA). Performance gap assessment and audit and feedback have consistently shown positive effects on changing practice behavior of providers (Berwick, 2003; Bradley, Holmboe et al., 2004; Horbar et al., 2004; Hysong et al., 2006; Jamtvedt et al., 2006; McCartney, Macdowall, & Thorogood, 1997). Performance gap assessment provides *baseline* performance data specific to the EBPs being implemented (e.g., pain assessment and fall rates) prior to the implementation process (Jamtvedt et al., 2006), accompanied by a discussion about the gap between current practices and the desired EBPs. For example, investigators who were testing the effectiveness of a translating-research-into-practice intervention for acute pain management in older adults met with physicians and nurses at each experimental site at the beginning of the implementation process to review indicators of acute pain management (e.g., avoid meperidine prescription) specific to their setting and to discuss gaps between current practices and recommended EBPs in areas such as frequency of pain assessment, dosing of opioids, and around-the-clock administration of analgesics (Titler et al., 2009). Audit and feedback follows PGA and consists of ongoing audit of performance indicators specific to the EBP being implemented (e.g., pain assessment and fall rates), followed by presentation and discussion of the data with staff members. For example, investigators testing the translating research into practice (TRIP) intervention followed the PGA strategy, with ongoing audit and feedback of pain data collected by concurrent medical record abstraction of older adult patients admitted during the implementation phase and presentation of data in graph form to nurses and physicians every 6 weeks for 10 months (six reports). Although these strategies show a consistently positive effect on adoption of EBPs, the effect size varies among studies. Greater effectiveness is associated with additional factors such as low baseline compliance and increased intensity of the feedback (Bero et al., 1998; Davis et al., 1995; Grimshaw et al., 2001, 2004; Hysong et al., 2006; Jamtvedt et al., 2006). Organizations with a successful record of EBP guideline adherence provide nonpunitive, individualized feedback in a timely manner throughout the implementation process (Hysong et al., 2006). Timely feedback is feedback that is provided monthly or more frequently; those organizations that provide feedback at longer intervals or inconsistently have lower adherence to guidelines (Hysong et al., 2006). Providing individual feedback, as opposed to unit or facility-level feedback, is also associated with better adherence to EBP guidelines. Offering positive feedback, in addition to pointing out areas where the practitioner can improve performance, provides better results than providing feedback only when staff members fall short of optimal performance (Hysong et al., 2006).

Social System

The social system or context of care delivery influences adoption of an innovation (Fraser, 2004a, 2004b; Institute of Medicine, 2001; Rogers, 2003; Vaughn et al., 2002). To date, much of implementation research has focused on acute and primary care. However, health care is delivered in a wide variety of health care delivery systems, including occupational settings, school settings, long-term care and assisted-living facilities, and homes and community settings through public health and home health care agencies. These settings have obvious differences because of their unique natures, but, even within similar settings, each organization has its own character and feel. This is a result of the interaction of individuals through communication channels and social networks within the organizational structure and hierarchy, as well as interaction with the larger community as a whole. It is important to remember that the resulting social system is unique to each setting and is complex and dynamic (Garside, 1998; Greenhalgh et al., 2005; Scott, Mannion, Davies, & Marshall, 2003a, 2003b).

When choosing strategies to increase adoption of EBP, it is necessary to focus on both the organizational structures and the individual adopters within the social system. For example, requiring a change in pain-assessment frequency by individual caregivers but not providing the accompanying organizational changes (appropriate forms, changes in the electronic charting system, and inclusion of the new standards in performance evaluations) is shortsighted and reduces the likelihood that the change will be sustained in practice. Organizational procedures and policies should support the use of EBPs and should contain language explicitly requiring their use in all policies and protocols instituted in the organization (Titler & Everett, 2001). The expectation that practice will be based on evidence and participation in research activities should be a written part of job evaluations, as well.

There are several structural characteristics that are consistently associated with increased use of EBP, such as size, slack resources, and urbanicity. Organizations that are larger in size and divided into differentiated and specialized semiautonomous units are associated with innovativeness. Slack resources (i.e., uncommitted resources) are associated with larger organizations and may be partially responsible for the impact of organization size on adoption rates. Larger organizations may have more resources available, both financial and human, to support EBP in practice. Urbanicity provides organizations with access to more interpersonal and mass-media channels, access to resources and education opportunities, exposure to new ideas, and contact with other innovative organizations (Greenhalgh et al., 2005; Rogers, 2003; Titler, 2008).

There is no question that leadership at all levels in the organization is critical to adoption of EBP. The leader defines and communicates the organization's goals and vision (Bradley, Holmboe, et al., 2004; Bradley, Schlesinger, Webster, Baker, & Inouye, 2004; Institute of Medicine, 2001). Most early studies focused on measurable characteristics such as educational background and tenure of individuals holding key leadership positions (Greenhalgh et al., 2005). The wider contribution of leadership is harder to explicitly measure but includes efforts in areas such as promoting a climate that facilitates adoption, which can include communication style, providing a nonpunitive environment for risk taking, providing resources for EBP projects, providing time for research activities, and promoting a learning environment (Greenhalgh et al., 2005; Stetler, 2003; Titler, 2002, 2008). Other influences of leadership include setting role expectations that include the use of research in practice, providing role clarity, and supporting democratic and inclusive decision-making processes (Bradley, Webster, et al., 2004; Institute of Medicine, 2001; McCormack et al., 2002; Meijers et al., 2006; Rutledge & Donaldson, 1995). However, little research has been done on specific leadership strategies at the unit manager level that may impact the adoption of EBP.

Additional strategies are (a) the use of multidisciplinary teams, especially in the care of chronic illnesses, and (b) the revising of professional roles (Wensing et al., 2006). Both strategies have been effective in improving patient outcomes through better adherence to recommended EBP guidelines and also have resulted in reduced health care costs (Wensing et al., 2006). The use of multidisciplinary teams seeks to improve communication and cooperation between professional groups (e.g., physicians and nurses) and also to streamline services (Zwarenstein & Reeves, 2006). However, all teams are not created equal, and measuring characteristics of teams that improve patient outcomes is difficult. Some characteristics of high-functioning teams that show positive impact on patient care include team composition; stability; collaboration; time allotted for the various tasks; explicit, appropriate task and role definitions; and having a team leader (Schouten et al., 2008). A related strategy, revision of professional roles (e.g., reassigning prevention interventions to nonphysician staff, such as nurses), has also resulted in improved patient outcomes through better adherence to EBP guidelines (Zwarenstein & Reeves, 2006).

Documentation systems for effective data recording aid in the implementation and sustainability of guidelines and protocols by providing appropriate forms for outcome measurement and information for quality-improvement programs (Garside, 1998; Greenhalgh et al., 2004; Titler, 2008; Wensing et al., 2006). In addition, access to computer technology can improve professional performance and client outcomes in two ways. First, use of data recording, patient record keeping, computer prompts, and reminders increase adherence to EBP (Rappolt, Pearce, McEwen, & Polatajko, 2005; Wensing & Grol, 1994; Wensing et al., 2006). Second, information systems, including computer technology, allow for better knowledge acquisition and management (Bradley, Holmboe, et al., 2004; Titler, 2008; Wensing et al., 2006). The Institute of Medicine's 2001 report, *Crossing the Quality Chasm: A New Health System for the 21st Century,* stresses the importance of computerized information technology systems, but in order to take advantage of these systems, health care workers need not only access to the systems but the skills to use them (Institute of Medicine, 2001). Organizations that provide needed resources and access to support for EBP, such as technology and sufficient training to allow staff to become proficient, libraries, research findings, computer databases, journals, time and financial support for continuing education, and time for research participation and implementation, are more likely to implement and sustain EBP in practice (Bryar et al., 2003; Dopson, Locock, Chambers, & Gabbay, 2001; Estabrooks, 2003; Estabrooks, O'Leary, et al., 2003; Meijers et al., 2006; Pravikoff, Tanner, & Pierce, 2005; Titler, 2008).

DESIGNING IMPLEMENTATION STUDIES

The Institute of Medicine Forum on the Science of Quality Improvement and Implementation Research has sponsored several workshops on implementation science in which researchers have addressed various perspectives in conducting studies in this field (http://www.nap.edu). Methods used in implementation studies range from qualitative, phenomenological studies to randomized controlled trials (RCTs). Links between generalizable scientific evidence for a given health care topic and specific contexts create opportunities for experiential learning in implementation science (Institute of Medicine, 2007a). Given this perspective, qualitative methods may be used to better understand why specific implementation strategies work in some settings and not in others. For example, an investigator might ask why Centers for Medicare & Medicaid Services (CMS)-regulated EBPs for heart failure patients are adhered to in some hospitals and not others. A study designed to understand these differences might use qualitative approaches such as interviews with front-line staff, observation of clinical care delivery, and practitioner focus groups (Tripp-Reimer & Doebbeling, 2004). This qualitative study would generate hypotheses for future investigations. Such studies provide a sound basis for empirical studies on the effectiveness of implementation interventions.

Rigorous evaluations of implementation interventions provide a solid base of research that can be built upon. Much can be learned from empirical evaluation of naturally occurring adoption efforts such as the implementation of rapid-response teams in acute-care settings. Implementation studies that investigate natural experiments provide several benefits, including testing the relationships among various individual and system factors and the level of practice adoption. Understanding these factors and their relationships is important as one designs studies to test the effectiveness of implementation interventions.

At the IOM workshops, Grimshaw discussed the disagreement in the field of implementation science regarding the use of RCTs to evaluate the effectiveness of implementation interventions (Institute of Medicine, 2007a, 2007b). There is some antipathy to the use of RCTs in complex social contexts such as the process of implementation of EBPs, although others believe RCTs to be an extremely valuable method of evaluating these interventions. Randomized trials of implementation interventions tend to be pragmatic and focus on effectiveness in order to elucidate whether an intervention will be effective in a real-world setting. Such RCTs, unlike RCTs that focus on efficacy (e.g., drug trials), have broad inclusion criteria and are designed to improve our understanding of both the influence of context on the effectiveness of the intervention and why changes occurred. One method of achieving this understanding is to use observational approaches in conjunction with data from the RCT to test multilevel hypotheses about which interventions work and which do not. RCTs build on the knowledge generated by observational studies and case studies (Institute of Medicine, 2007a). The best method to evaluate a given intervention depends on the research question(s), hypotheses, and the specifics of the implementation intervention. One should always attempt to choose a mixture of the best possible methods, given the individual circumstances.

Building this body of research knowledge will require development in many areas. Theoretical developments are needed to provide frameworks and predictive theories that will lead to generalizable research such as studies on how to change individual and organizational behavior. Methodological developments are also required, as are exploratory studies aimed at improving our understanding of the experiential and organizational learning that accompanies implementation. Rigorous evaluations are needed to evaluate the effectiveness and efficiency of implementation interventions, and partnerships are needed to encourage communication among researchers, theorists, and implementers and to help researchers understand what types of knowledge are needed and how that knowledge can best be developed (Dawson, 2004; Titler, 2004a, 2004b; Tripp-Reimer & Doebbeling, 2004).

FUTURE DIRECTIONS

Although the evidence base for implementation strategies is growing, there is much work to be done. In 2003, the U.S. Invitational Conference "Advancing Quality Care Through Translation Research" convened, funded in part by the Agency for Healthcare Research and Quality (1 R13 HS014141–01). The objective was to set forth a future research agenda for translation (or implementation) science. Seventy-seven participants representing 25 states and all geographic regions of the United States were selected to attend on the basis of their knowledge and skills in research, education, practice, and public policy; the goal was to advance a translation science agenda.

Conference participants recommended giving high priority to testing multifaceted, interdisciplinary implementation interventions in a variety of settings, and to designing multisite studies that increase understanding about what interventions work in similar types of settings (e.g., acute care) with different contextual factors. Priority was also given to comparing the effectiveness of implementation interventions in different types of clinical settings (e.g., acute versus home health) to foster understanding of the components of the intervention that need modification depending on the type of setting. These implementation priorities are congruent with recommendations of others (Dopson et al., 2002; Greenhalgh et al., 2004; Grimshaw et al., 2004; Kirchhoff, 2004).

A unique finding of the U.S. Invitational Conference was the call to prioritize research on (1) methods for engaging stakeholders to increase their support and (2) implementation of clinical topics for nursing practice based on existing guidelines and synthesis reports.

The conference attendees identified these recommended research priorities for implementation science:

- Test implementation strategies across different types and contexts of care delivery to determine which strategies are most effective for which type of health care setting and context.
- Test interdisciplinary approaches (e.g., physicians, nurses, and physical therapists) to implementation.
- Test combined or multiple implementation strategies such as education plus use of opinion leaders plus audit and feedback.
- Test various dissemination methods and implementation strategies such as electronic information technology, communication strategies, and facilitator roles.
- Determine best methods for engaging stakeholders to promote the use of evidence in practice.
- Focus on measurement and methodological issues encountered in translation science regarding process measures, outcome measures, intervention/TRIP dose, core dependent measures (e.g., process versus outcome measures), organizational context, nested designs, and qualitative methods.
- Investigate leadership and organizational context variables and measures that promote EBPs.
- Develop and test measures of organizational readiness for EBP.
- Determine ways to create practice cultures that facilitate change.
- Test organizational-level interventions that promote EBPs.

SUMMARY

The use of EBP remains sporadic in spite of a growing evidence base and the increasing availability of systematic reviews and predeveloped EBP guidelines. Implementation science provides a research focus for identifying effective strategies to increase the use of evidence-based programs, guidelines, and protocols in different settings and among different end users. Because this is a young science, standardized definitions have not been established. Commonly used terms were identified in this chapter, along with promising models to guide implementation at the point of care. The current evidence base for implementation strategies is growing, and, although additional research is needed, there is sufficient evidence to warrant use of evidence-based strategies when implementing a change in practice.

SUGGESTED ACTIVITIES

1. You are the nurse manager of an adult surgical inpatient unit (30 beds) at a 500-bed community hospital. Staff members are changing practice for assessment of bowel mobility following abdominal

surgery. The practice change includes "giving up" listening for bowel sounds. Describe an implementation plan with specific implementation strategies for making this change in practice.

2. You are the school nurse supervising other school nurses in a rural consolidated school district. This school district includes three high schools, five elementary schools, and four middle schools. There are nine school nurses: two covering the high schools, two covering the middle schools, and five covering the elementary schools.

   a. Select a topic of interest to school nurses to promote the health of the population of students with a rationale for why this topic was selected.

   b. Identify evidence sources for each topic.

   c. Describe implementation strategies for the selected topics.

REFERENCES

Adams, S. (2007). *Understanding the context for translation of evidence-based practice into school nursing.* Unpublished dissertation. University of Iowa College of Nursing, Iowa City.

Adams, S., & Barron, S. (2009). Use of evidence-based practice in school nursing: Prevalence, associated variables and perceived needs. *Worldviews on Evidence-Based Nursing, 5*(4), 1–11.

Barta, K. M. (1995). Information-seeking, research utilization, and barriers to research utilization of pediatric nurse educators. *Journal of Professional Nursing: Official Journal of the American Association of Colleges of Nursing, 11*(1), 49–57.

Bero, L. A., Grilli, R., Grimshaw, J. M., Harvey, E., Oxman, A. D., & Thomson, M. A. (1998). Closing the gap between research and practice: An overview of systematic reviews of interventions to promote the implementation of research findings. The Cochrane effective practice and organization of care review group. *British Medical Journal (Clinical Research Edition), 317*(7156), 465–468.

Berwick, D. M. (2003). Disseminating innovations in health care. *Journal of the American Medical Association, 289*(15), 1969–1975.

Bradley, E. H., Holmboe, E. S., Mattera, J. A., Roumanis, S. A., Radford, M. J., & Krumholz, H. M. (2004). Data feedback efforts in quality improvement: Lessons learned from U.S. hospitals. *Quality & Safety in Health Care, 13*(1), 26–31.

Bradley, E. H., Schlesinger, M., Webster, T. R., Baker, D., & Inouye, S. K. (2004). Translating research into clinical practice: Making change happen. *Journal of the American Geriatrics Society, 52*(11), 1875–1882.

Bradley, E. H., Webster, T. R., Baker, D., Schlesinger, M., Inouye, S. K., Barth, M. C., Palane, K. L., Lipson, D., Stone, R., & Koren, M. J. (2004). Translating research into practice: Speeding the adoption of innovative health care programs. *Issue Brief (Commonwealth Fund), 724*, 1–12.

Bryar, R. M., Closs, S. J., Baum, G., Cooke, J., Griffiths, J., & Hostick, T., Kelly, S., Knight, S., Marshall, K., & Thompson, D. R. (2003). The Yorkshire BARRIERS project: Diagnostic analysis of barriers to research utilisation. *International Journal of Nursing Studies, 40*(1), 73–84.

Charles, R. (2000). The challenge of disseminating innovations to direct care providers in health care organizations. *Nursing Clinics of North America, 35*(2), 461–470.

Clancy, C. M., Slutsky, J. R., & Patton, L. T. (2004). Evidence-based health care 2004: AHRQ moves research to translation and implementation. *Health Services Research, 39*(5), xv–xxiii.

Collins, B. A., Hawks, J. W., & Davis, R. (2000). From theory to practice: Identifying authentic opinion leaders to improve care. *Managed Care, 9*(7), 56–62.

Davis, D. A., Thomson, M. A., Oxman, A.D., & Haynes, R. B. (1995). Changing physician performance. A systematic review of the effect of continuing medical education strategies. *Journal of the American Medical Association, 274*(9), 700–705.

Dawson, J. D. (2004). Quantitative analytical methods in translation research. *Worldviews on Evidence-Based Nursing, 1*(Suppl. 1), S60–S64.

Dopson, S., FitzGerald, L., Ferlie, E., Gabbay, J., & Locock, L. (2002). No magic targets! Changing clinical practice to become more evidence based. *Health Care Management Review, 27*(3), 35–47.

Dopson, S., Locock, L., Chambers, D., & Gabbay, J. (2001). Implementation of evidence-based medicine: Evaluation of the promoting action on clinical effectiveness programme. *Journal of Health Services Research & Policy, 6*(1), 23–31.

Doumit, G., Gattellari, M., Grimshaw, J., & O'Brien, M. A. (2007). Local opinion leaders: Effects on professional practice and health care outcomes. *Cochrane Database of Systematic Reviews, 1,* CD000125.

Eccles, M. P., & Grimshaw, J. M. (2004). Selecting, presenting and delivering clinical guidelines: Are there any "magic bullets"? *Medical Journal of Australia, 180* (6 Suppl.), S52–S54.

Eccles, M. P., & Mittman, B. S. (2006). Welcome to implementation science. *Implementation Science, 1*(1). Retrieved April 22, 2009, from http://www.implementationscience.com

Ellis, I., Howard, P., Larson, A., & Robertson, J. (2005). From workshop to work practice: An exploration of context and facilitation in the development of evidence-based practice. *Worldviews on Evidence-Based Nursing, 2*(2), 84–93.

Estabrooks, C. A. (1999). Modeling the individual determinants of research utilization. *Western Journal of Nursing Research, 21*(6), 758–772.

Estabrooks, C. A. (2003). Translating research into practice: Implications for organizations and administrators. *The Canadian Journal of Nursing Research = Revue Canadienne De Recherche En Sciences Infirmières, 35*(3), 53–68.

Estabrooks, C. A., Chong, H., Brigidear, K., & Profetto-McGrath, J. (2005). Profiling Canadian nurses' preferred knowledge sources for clinical practice. *Canadian Journal of Nursing Research = Revue Canadienne de Recherche en Sciences Infirmières, 37*(2), 118–140.

Estabrooks, C. A., Floyd, J. A., Scott-Findlay, S., O'Leary, K. A., & Gushta, M. (2003). Individual determinants of research utilization: A systematic review. *Journal of Advanced Nursing, 43*(5), 506–520.

Estabrooks, C. A., O'Leary, K. A., Ricker, K. L., & Humphrey, C. K. (2003). The Internet and access to evidence: How are nurses positioned? *Journal of Advanced Nursing, 42*(1), 73–81.

Fawcett, J. (2005). *Contemporary nursing knowledge: Analysis and evaluation of nursing models and theories* (2nd ed.). Philadelphia, PA: F. A. Davis.

Feldman, P. H., & McDonald, M. V. (2004). Conducting translation research in the home care setting: Lessons from a just-in-time reminder study. *Worldviews on Evidence-Based Nursing, 1*(1), 49–59.

Feldman, P. H., Murtaugh, C. M., Pezzin, L. E., McDonald, M. V., & Peng, T. R. (2005). Just-in-time evidence-based e-mail "reminders" in home health care: Impact on patient outcomes. *Health Services Research, 40*(3), 865–885.

Forsetlund, L., Bjørndal, A., Rashidian, A., Jamtvedt, G., O'Brien, M. A, Wolf, F., Davis, D., Odgaard-Jensen, J., & Oxman, A. D. (2009). Continuing education meetings and workshops: Effects on professional practice and health care outcomes. *Cochrane Database of Systematic Reviews, 2*, CD003030.

Fraser, I. (2004a). Organizational research with impact: Working backwards. *Worldviews on Evidence-Based Nursing, 1*(Suppl. 1), S52–S59.

Fraser, I. (2004b). Translation research: Where do we go from here? *Worldviews on Evidence-Based Nursing, 1*(Suppl. 1), S78–S83.

Garside, P. (1998). Organisational context for quality: Lessons from the fields of organisational development and change management. *Quality in Health Care, 7*(Suppl.), S8–S15.

Graham, I. D., & Logan, J. (2004). Innovations in knowledge transfer and continuity of care. *Canadian Journal of Nursing Research = Revue Canadienne de Recherche en Sciences Infirmières, 36*(2), 89–103.

Graham, I. D., Logan, J., Harrison, M. B., Straus, S. E., Tetroe, J., Caswell, W., & Robinson, N. (2006). Lost in knowledge translation: Time for a map? *Journal of Continuing Education in the Health Professions, 26*(1), 13–24.

Greenhalgh, T., Robert, G., Bate, P., Macfarlane, F., & Kyriakidou, O. (2005). *Diffusion of innovations in health service organisations: A systematic literature review.* Malden, MA: Blackwell.

Greenhalgh, T., Robert, G., Macfarlane, F., Bate, P., & Kyriakidou, O. (2004). Diffusion of innovations in service organizations: Systematic review and recommendations. *Milbank Quarterly, 82*(4), 581–629.

Grilli, R., Ramsay, C., & Minozzi, S. (2002). Mass media interventions: Effects on health services utilisation. *Cochrane Database of Systematic Reviews, 1*, CD000389.

Grimshaw, J. M., Eccles, M. P., Greener, J., Maclennan, G., Ibbotson, T., Kahan, J. P., & Sullivan, F. (2006). Is the involvement of opinion leaders in the implementation of research findings a feasible strategy? *Implementation Science, 1*(3). Retrieved April 22, 2009, from http://www.implementationscience.com

Grimshaw, J. M., Eccles, M., Thomas, R., MacLennan, G., Ramsay, C., Fraser, C., & Vale, L. (2006). Toward evidence-based quality improvement: Evidence (and its limitations) of the effectiveness of guideline dissemination and implementation strategies 1966–1998. *Journal of General Internal Medicine: Official Journal of the Society for Research and Education in Primary Care Internal Medicine, 21*(Suppl. 2), S14–S20.

Grimshaw, J. M., Eccles, M. P., Walker, A. E., & Thomas, R. E. (2002). Changing physicians' behavior: What works and thoughts on getting more things to work. *Journal of Continuing Education in the Health Professions, 22*(4), 237–243.

Grimshaw, J. M., Shirran, L., Thomas, R., Mowatt, G., Fraser, C., Bero, L., Grilli, R., Harvey, E., Oxman, A., & O'Brien, M. A. (2001). Changing provider behavior: An overview of systematic reviews of interventions. *Medical Care, 39*(8, Suppl. 2), II2–II45.

Grimshaw, J. M., Thomas, R. E., MacLennan, G., Fraser, C., Ramsay, C. R., Vale, L., Whitty, P., Eccles, M. P., Matoue, L., Shirran, L., Wensing, M., Dijkstra, R., & Donaldson, C. (2004). Effectiveness and efficiency of guideline dissemination and implementation strategies. *Health Technology Assessment (Winchester, England), 8*(6), iii–iv, 1–72.

Grol, R. P., Bosch, M. C., Hulscher, M. E., Eccles, M. P., & Wensing, M. (2007). Planning and studying improvement in patient care: The use of theoretical perspectives. *Milbank Quarterly, 85*(1), 93–138.

Guihan, M., Bosshart, H. T., & Nelson, A. (2004). Lessons learned in implementing SCI clinical practice guidelines. *SCI Nursing: A Publication of the American Association of Spinal Cord Injury Nurses, 21*(3), 136–142.

Harvey, G., Loftus-Hills, A., Rycroft-Malone, J., Titchen, A., Kitson, A., McCormack, B., & Seers, K. (2002). Getting evidence into practice: The role and function of facilitation. *Journal of Advanced Nursing, 37*(6), 577–588.

Hendryx, M. S., Fieselmann, J. F., Bock, M. J., Wakefield, D. S., Helms, C. M., & Bentler, S. E. (1998). Outreach education to improve quality of rural ICU care. Results of a randomized trial. *American Journal of Respiratory and Critical Care Medicine, 158*(2), 418–423.

Horbar, J. D., Carpenter, J. H., Buzas, J., Soll, R. F., Suresh, G., Bracken, M. B., Leviton, L. C., Pisek, P. E., & Sinclair, J. C. (2004). Collaborative quality improvement to promote evidence based surfactant for preterm infants: A cluster randomised trial. *British Medical Journal (Clinical Research Edition), 329*(7473), 1004.

Hutchinson, A. M., & Johnston, L. (2004). Bridging the divide: A survey of nurses' opinions regarding barriers to, and facilitators of, research utilization in the practice setting. *Journal of Clinical Nursing, 13*(3), 304–315.

Hysong, S. J., Best, R. G., & Pugh, J. A. (2006). Audit and feedback and clinical practice guideline adherence: Making feedback actionable. *Implementation Science, 1*(9). Retrieved April 22, 2009, from http://www.implementation science.com/

The Improved Clinical Effectiveness through Behavioural Research Group (ICEBeRG). (2006). Designing theoretically-informed implementation interventions. *Implementation Science, 1*(4). Retrieved April 22, 2009, from http://www.implementationscience.com

Institute of Medicine. (2001). *Crossing the quality chasm: A new health system for the 21st century.* Washington, DC: National Academies Press.

Institute of Medicine. (2007a). *Advancing quality improvement research: Challenges and opportunities.* Workshop summary. Washington, DC: National Academies Press.

Institute of Medicine. (2007b). *The state of quality improvement and implementation research: Expert reviews.* Workshop summary. Washington, DC: National Academies Press.

Institute of Medicine. (2008). *Knowing what works in health care: A roadmap for the nation.* Committee on reviewing evidence to identify highly effective clinical services. Washington, DC: National Academies Press.

Jamtvedt, G., Young, J. M., Kristoffersen, D. T., O'Brien, M. A., & Oxman, A. D. (2006). Audit and feedback: Effects on professional practice and health care outcomes. *Cochrane Database of Systematic Reviews, 2,* CD000259.

Kirchhoff, K. T. (2004). State of the science of translational research: From demonstration projects to intervention testing. *Worldviews on Evidence-Based Nursing, 1*(Suppl. 1), S6–S12.

Kitson, A., Harvey, G., & McCormack, B. (1998). Enabling the implementation of evidence-based practice: A conceptual framework. *Quality in Health Care, 7*(3), 149–158.

Kitson, A., Rycroft-Malone, J., Harvey, G., McCormack, B., Seers, K., & Titchen, A. (2008). Evaluating the successful implementation of evidence into practice using the PARiHS framework: Theoretical and practical challenges. *Implementation Science, 3*(1). Retrieved April 22, 2009, from http://www.implementationscience.com

Lam, T. K., McPhee, S. J., Mock, J., Wong, C., Doan, H. T., Nguyen, T., Lai, K. Q., Ha-Iaconis, T., & Luong, T. N. (2003). Encouraging Vietnamese-American women to obtain Pap tests through lay health worker outreach and media education. *Journal of General Internal Medicine: Official Journal of the Society for Research and Education in Primary Care Internal Medicine, 18*(7), 516–524.

Leape, L. L. (2005). *Advances in patient safety: From research to implementation* (3rd ed.). Rockville, MD: Agency for Healthcare Research and Quality.

Lia-Hoagberg, B., Schaffer, M., & Strohschein, S. (1999). Public health nursing practice guidelines: An evaluation of dissemination and use. *Public Health Nursing (Boston, MA), 16*(6), 397–404.

Locock, L., Dopson, S., Chambers, D., & Gabbay, J. (2001). Understanding the role of opinion leaders in improving clinical effectiveness. *Social Science & Medicine, 53*(6), 745–757.

McCartney, P., Macdowall, W., & Thorogood, M. (1997). A randomised controlled trial of feedback to general practitioners of their prophylactic aspirin prescribing. *British Medical Journal (Clinical Research Edition), 315*(7099), 35–36.

McCormack, B., Kitson, A., Harvey, G., Rycroft-Malone, J., Titchen, A., & Seers, K. (2002). Getting evidence into practice: The meaning of "context." *Journal of Advanced Nursing, 38*(1), 94–104.

McGlynn, E. A., Asch, S. M., Adams, J., Keesey, J., Hicks, J., DeCristofaro, A., & Kerr, E. A. (2003). The quality of health care delivered to adults in the United States. *New England Journal of Medicine, 348*(26), 2635–2645.

McKenna, H., Ashton, S., & Keeney, S. (2004). Barriers to evidence-based practice in primary care: A review of the literature. *International Journal of Nursing Studies, 41*(4), 369–378.

Meijers, J. M., Janssen, M. A., Cummings, G. G., Wallin, L., Estabrooks, C. A., & Hal-fens, R. (2006). Assessing the relationships between contextual factors and research utilization in nursing: Systematic literature review. *Journal of Advanced Nursing, 55*(5), 622–635.

Meleis, A. (2005). *Theoretical nursing* (3rd ed.). Philadelphia, PA: Lippincott, Williams & Wilkins.

Michel, Y., & Sneed, N. V. (1995). Dissemination and use of research findings in nursing practice. *Journal of Professional Nursing: Official Journal of the American Association of Colleges of Nursing, 11*(5), 306–311.

Milner, M., Estabrooks, C. A., & Myrick, F. (2006). Research utilization and clinical nurse educators: A systematic review. *Journal of Evaluation in Clinical Practice, 12*(6), 639–655.

Nelson, E. C., Batalden, P. B., Huber, T. P., Mohr, J. J., Godfrey, M. M., Headrick, L. A., & Wasson, J. H. (2002). Microsystems in health care: Part 1. Learning from high-performing front-line clinical units. *Joint Commission Journal on Quality Improvement, 28*(9), 472–493.

Nieva, V., Murphy, R., Ridley, N., Donaldson, N., Combes, J., Mitchell, P., Kovner, C., Hoy, E., & Carpenter, D. (2005). From science to service: A framework for the transfer of patient safety research into practice. In K. Henriksen, J. Battles, E. Marks, & D. I. Lewin (Eds.), *Advances in patient safety: From research to implementation: Vol. 2, Concepts and methodology* (pp. 441–453, AHRQ Publication No. 05-0021-2). Rockville, MD: Agency for Healthcare Research and Quality.

O'Brien, M. A., Rogers, S., Jamtvedt, G., Oxman, A. D., Odgaard-Jensen, J., Kristoffersen, D. T., Forsetlund, L., Bainbridge, D., Freemantle, N., Davis, D. A., Haynes, R. B., & Harvey, E. C. (2007). Educational outreach visits: Effects on professional practice and health care outcomes. *Cochrane Database of Systematic Reviews, 4,* CD000409.

Pravikoff, D. S., Tanner, A. B., & Pierce, S. T. (2005). Readiness of U.S. nurses for evidence-based practice. *American Journal of Nursing, 105*(9), 40–51.

Randolph, W., & Viswanath, K. (2004). Lessons learned from public health mass media campaigns: Marketing health in a crowded media world. *Annual Review of Public Health, 25,* 419–437.

Rappolt, S., Pearce, K., McEwen, S., & Polatajko, H. J. (2005). Exploring organizational characteristics associated with practice changes following a mentored online educational module. *Journal of Continuing Education in the Health Professions, 25*(2), 116–124.

Rogers, E. (Ed.). (2003). *Diffusion of innovations* (5th ed.). New York, NY: Simon & Schuster.

Rosswurm, M. A., & Larrabee, J. H. (1999). A model for change to evidence-based practice. *Image—the Journal of Nursing Scholarship, 31*(4), 317–322.

Rubenstein, L. V., & Pugh, J. (2006). Strategies for promoting organizational and practice change by advancing implementation research. *Journal of General Internal Medicine: Official Journal of the Society for Research and Education in Primary Care Internal Medicine, 21*(Suppl. 2), S58–S64.

Rutledge, D. N., & Donaldson, N. E. (1995). Building organizational capacity to engage in research utilization. *Journal of Nursing Administration, 25*(10), 12–16.

Rutledge, D. N., Greene, P., Mooney, K., Nail, L. M., & Ropka, M. (1996). Use of research-based practices by oncology staff nurses. *Oncology Nursing Forum, 23*(8), 1235–1244.

Rycroft-Malone, J., Harvey, G., Seers, K., Kitson, A., McCormack, B., & Titchen, A. (2004). An exploration of the factors that influence the implementation of evidence into practice. *Journal of Clinical Nursing, 13*(8), 913–924.

Schouten, L. M., Hulscher, M. E., Akkermans, R., van Everdingen, J. J., Grol, R. P., & Huijsman, R. (2008). Factors that influence the stroke care team's effectiveness in reducing the length of hospital stay. *Stroke: A Journal of Cerebral Circulation, 39*(9), 2515–2521.

Scott, T., Mannion, R., Davies, H. T., & Marshall, M. N. (2003a). The quantitative measurement of organizational culture in health care: A review of the available instruments. *Health Services Research, 38*(3), 923–945.

Scott, T., Mannion, R., Davies, H. T., & Marshall, M. N. (2003b). Implementing culture change in health care: Theory and practice. *International Journal for Quality in Health Care: Journal of the International Society for Quality in Health Care, 15*(2), 111–118.

Silver, F. L., Rubini, F., Black, D., & Hodgson, C. S. (2003). Advertising strategies to increase public knowledge of the warning signs of stroke. *Stroke: A Journal of Cerebral Circulation, 34*(8), 1965–1968.

Soumerai, S. B., McLaughlin, T. J., Gurwitz, J. H., Guadagnoli, E., Hauptman, P. J., Borbas, C., Morris, N., McLaughlin, B., Gao, X., Willison, D. J., Asinger, R., & Gobel, F. (1998). Effect of local medical opinion leaders on quality of care for acute myocardial infarction: A randomized controlled trial. *Journal of the American Medical Association, 279*(17), 1358–1363.

Srinivasan, R., & Fisher, R. S. (2000). Early initiation of post-PEG feeding: Do published recommendations affect clinical practice? *Digestive Diseases and Sciences, 45*(10), 2065–2068.

Stetler, C. B. (2001). Updating the Stetler model of research utilization to facilitate evidence-based practice. *Nursing Outlook, 49*(6), 272–279.

Stetler, C. B. (2003). Role of the organization in translating research into evidence-based practice. *Outcomes Management, 7*(3), 97–103 (quiz 104–105).

Stetler, C. B., Legro, M. W., Rycroft-Malone, J., Bowman, C., Curran, G., Guihan, M., Hagedorn, H., Pineros, S., & Wallace, C. M. (2006). Role of "external facilitation" in implementation of research findings: A qualitative evaluation of facilitation experiences in the Veterans Health Administration. *Implementation Science, 1*(23). Retrieved April 22, 2009, from http://www. implementationscience.com

Sung, N. S., Crowley, W. F., Jr., Genel, M., Salber, P., Sandy, L., Sherwood, L. M., Johnson, S. B., Catanese, V., Tilson, H., Getz, K., Larson, E. L., Scheinberg, D., Reece, E. A., Slavkin, H., Dobs, A., Grebb, J., Martinez, R. A., Korn, A., & Rimoin, D. (2003). Central challenges facing the national clinical research enterprise. *Journal of the American Medical Association, 289*(10), 1278–1287.

Sussman, S., Valente, T. W., Rohrbach, L. A., Skara, S., & Pentz, M. A. (2006). Translation in the health professions: Converting science into action. *Evaluation & the Health Professions, 29*(1), 7–32.

Taylor, D. M., Auble, T. E., Calhoun, W. J., & Mosesso, V. N., Jr. (1999). Current outpatient management of asthma shows poor compliance with international consensus guidelines. *Chest, 116*(6), 1638–1645.

Titler, M. G. (2002). *Toolkit for promoting evidence-based practice.* Iowa City: University of Iowa Hospitals and Clinics.

Titler, M. G. (2004a). Methods in translation science. *Worldviews on Evidence-Based Nursing, 1*(1), 38–48.

Titler, M. G. (2004b). Translation science: Quality, methods and issues. *Communicating Nursing Research, 37,* 15, 17–34.

Titler, M. G. (2006). Developing an evidence-based practice. In G. LoBiondo-Wood & J. Haber (Eds.), *Nursing research: Methods and critical appraisal for evidence-based practice* (6th ed.). St. Louis, MO: Mosby.

Titler, M. G. (2008). The evidence for evidence-based practice implementation. In R. Hughes (Ed.), *Patient safety and quality—An evidence-based handbook for nurses* (1st ed.). Rockville, MD: Agency for Healthcare Research and Quality. Retrieved April 22, 2009, from http://www.ahrq.gov/qual/nurseshdbk

Titler, M. G., & Everett, L. Q. (2001). Translating research into practice. Considerations for critical care investigators. *Critical Care Nursing Clinics of North America, 13*(4), 587–604.

Titler, M. G., Everett, L. Q., & Adams, S. (2007). Implications for implementation science. *Nursing Research, 56*(4 Suppl.), S53–S59.

Titler, M., Herr, K., Brooks, J., Xie, X., Ardery, G., Schilling, M., Marsh, J. L., Everett, L. Q., & Clarke, W. R. (2009). Translating research into practice intervention improves management of acute pain in older hip fracture patients. *Health Services Research, 44*(1), 264–287.

Titler, M. G., Kleiber, C., Steelman, V. J., Rakel, B. A., Budreau, G., Everett, L. Q., Buckwalter, K. C., Tripp-Reimer, T., & Goode, C. J. (2001). The Iowa model of evidence-based practice to promote quality care. *Critical Care Nursing Clinics of North America, 13*(4), 497–509.

Tripp-Reimer, T., & Doebbeling, B. (2004). Qualitative perspectives in translational research. *Worldviews on Evidence-Based Nursing, 1,* S65–S72.

Vaughn, T. E., McCoy, K. D., BootsMiller, B. J., Woolson, R. F., Sorofman, B., Tripp-Reimer, T., Perlin, J., & Doebbeling, B. N. (2002). Organizational predictors of adherence to ambulatory care screening guidelines. *Medical Care, 40*(12), 1172–1185.

Wallin, L., Ewald, U., Wikblad, K., Scott-Findlay, S., & Arnetz, B. B. (2006). Understanding work contextual factors: A short-cut to evidence-based practice? *Worldviews on Evidence-Based Nursing, 3*(4), 153–164.

Wallin, L., Rudberg, A., & Gunningberg, L. (2005). Staff experiences in implementing guidelines for kangaroo mother care—A qualitative study. *International Journal of Nursing Studies, 42*(1), 61–73.

Wang, P. S., Berglund, P., & Kessler, R. C. (2000). Recent care of common mental disorders in the United States: Prevalence and conformance with evidence-based recommendations. *Journal of General Internal Medicine: Official Journal of the Society for Research and Education in Primary Care Internal Medicine, 15*(5), 284–292.

Wensing, M., & Grol, R. (1994). Single and combined strategies for implementing changes in primary care: A literature review. *International Journal for Quality in Health Care, 6*(2), 115–132.

Wensing, M., Wollersheim, H., & Grol, R. (2006). Organizational interventions to implement improvements in patient care: A structured review of reviews. *Implementation Science, 1,* (2). Retrieved April 22, 2009, from http://www.implementationscience.com

Wiecha, J. L., El Ayadi, A.M., Fuemmeler, B. F., Carter, J. E., Handler, S., Johnson, S., Strunk, N., Korzec-Ramirez, D., & Gortmaker, S. L. (2004). Diffusion of an integrated health education program in an urban school system: Planet health. *Journal of Pediatric Psychology, 29*(6), 467–474.

Zwarenstein, M., & Reeves, S. (2006). Knowledge translation and interprofessional collaboration: Where the rubber of evidence-based care hits the road of teamwork. *Journal of Continuing Education in the Health Professions, 26*(1), 46–54.

PART IV

Evaluating the Impact of EBP and Communicating Results

Cost as a Dimension of Evidence-Based Practice

Briana J. Jegier and Tricia J. Johnson

Cost is an important topic in health care today because the health care industry is facing increasing pressure to deliver higher-value care. Value can be broadly conceptualized as the balance between the quality of care a patient receives and the cost of the care. The cost component of value has received increased attention because health care spending represents roughly 17.9% of the gross domestic product of the United States and is one of the single most expensive budget items that businesses face today (Centers for Medicare & Medicaid Services [CMS], 2012; Congressional Budget Office [CBO], 2012). For example, the cost to the federal government of the United States for the Medicare, Medicaid, and State Children's Health Insurance Program (CHIP) accounts for 21% of the federal budget with future projections estimating that spending on these programs could reach as high as 25% of the budget by 2020 (CMS, 2012; CBO, 2012). Thus, it is important for health care researchers and practitioners to be conscious of the cost implications of their research and practice by including cost measurement in addition to quality-of-care measurement in their research and practice. Therefore, the purpose of this chapter is to introduce the concept of cost, to describe how to incorporate cost methodology into research and practice, and to improve the critical evaluation of cost findings published in research and practice publications.

THE DEFINITION OF COST

Before integrating cost into research and practice, one must determine how costs are defined and from what perspective they will be measured. Most people outside the field of economics refer to cost as the

---

Exhibit 17.1
Defining Cost

Cost is defined as the resources that are expended for goods or a service. The resources may or may not have an associated monetary value.

---

monetary value paid by a purchaser (e.g., a consumer, a provider, a payer, a government, or a society) for a good or service. The monetary value, referred to in economics literature as the price, is certainly one aspect of cost, but is not the only aspect. Cost is more accurately and broadly defined as the resources that are expended for a good or service (see Exhibit 17.1). These resources may or may not have an associated or measurable monetary value (Drummond, Sculpher, Torrance, O'Brien, & Stoddart, 2005; Gold, Siegel, Russell, & Weinstein, 1996). By defining cost in this broader sense of resource expenditure, it allows us to consider the fact that the acquisition of goods or services occurs within a complex, multiple-faceted environment where the resources that must be expended involve multiple parties. It also allows us to consider that not all goods and services include a price that is paid, in part or in full, by the individual or group receiving the good or service. For example, a patient rarely pays the full price of his or her medical care services, yet the patient is the one who benefits from those services.

A single good from a health care situation illustrates this complex relationship: what is the cost of 1 hour of nursing care for a hospitalized patient? To answer this question, you might start by asking yourself the cost to whom? One hour of nursing care could involve the participation of five different parties: the nurse, the hospital, the patient, the patient's family, and the insurance carrier. Table 17.1 demonstrates the resources that each party would expend for 1 hour of nursing care. These resources can be conceptualized into two primary categories: time (e.g., nurse, other health care professionals and staff, patient, patient's family, and insurance carrier employee) and resources (e.g., supplies, utilities, and space).

TYPES OF COST

The Cost of Time

The cost of time is usually characterized as opportunity cost. Opportunity cost can be conceptualized as the resource trade-off a person faces when deciding how to allocate his or her time. Most people face resource trade-off decisions to determine how to allocate their time every day. For example, a person chooses between watching a favorite television program and going to the gym, or chooses to work overtime instead of having dinner with a friend. In each instance, the person weighs the resources that would need to be expended for each choice. Perhaps the favorite television show is selected over the gym because the gym requires that the person drives 30 minutes, whereas the television program only requires that she or he walk to the den. Working overtime may be selected over dinner with a friend, because working overtime right now allows him or her to spend the whole weekend with the friend later. Each decision about how to allocate time incorporates the process of measuring and valuing the opportunity cost of each choice. The selected choice will have the most favorable opportunity cost to the individual making the decision.

Opportunity cost can present a measurement challenge given that every person has a complex decision process for how he or she spends time. In research and practice, researchers and providers also need to systematically measure opportunity cost using a standard unit of measure, and this is ideally reported in monetary terms. Therefore, economists define the measurement of opportunity cost as the monetary value of the next best alternative choice. The two alternatives that people decide between are paid work and leisure (e.g., reading a book and spending time with family and friends). The monetary value of an individual's opportunity cost is measured as the value of the wage from the paid work that one forgoes when choosing a leisure activity over paid work. Thus, in the "1 hour of nursing care" example, the nurse's opportunity cost was her decision to spend time at work versus some other activity she or he might enjoy (Table 17.1). The monetary value of that opportunity cost is the compensation she or he received for the additional hour she spent at work instead of pursuing another activity.

The Cost of Resources

The cost of resources is characterized as the cost of equipment, supplies, and other "objects" expended to provide the good or service. Using our example, the cost to provide the bed that a hospital uses for a patient is the monetary value they paid to purchase, install, maintain, and replace the bed so that it would be available for the patient for their 1 hour of nursing care. The cost of a resource is generally allocated over the life span of that object. Using the bed as an example, the cost for that 1 hour of the bed would be the total cost of purchase, installation, and maintenance for the bed divided by the number of hours the bed is expected to be in use. Thus if the bed cost $500 to purchase, $300 to install, and $400 to maintain over its life span then the total cost of the bed would be $1,200. If the bed was expected to be in use for 10,000 hours, then the cost of the bed for that 1 hour of care would be $1,200/10,000 or $0.12 per hour of use.

TABLE 17.1 Resources and Associated Monetary Value for the Delivery of 1 Hour of Nursing Care to a Hospitalized Patient

PERSPECTIVE	NURSE DELIVERING CARE	HOSPITAL WHERE THE CARE IS DELIVERED	HOSPITALIZED PATIENT	PATIENT'S FAMILY	INSURANCE CARRIER
Resources used	The nurse provides his or her time, knowledge, and expertise to the patient.	The institution provides the environment for the care to be delivered (e.g., bed, supplies, electricity, and nursing administration time).	The patient provides his/her time and presence during the care episode.	The patient's family members may also provide time during the care episode (e.g., waiting for patient).	The insurance carrier provides staff time to approve the hospitalization, process the payment for the hospital, and to answer any benefits questions the patient or family members have.
Monetary value	Measured monetarily as the compensation (salary and benefits) she or he accepts from the hospital for the time she or he spends with the patient. If she or he had not accepted this compensation, she or he could have done something else (e.g., spend time with friends/family, read a book, or watch a movie).	Compensation paid to the nurse as well as the amount paid for supplies, maintenance, utilities, and the space.	Wages and the monetary value of unpaid work (e.g., household work) forgone by the patient, because of the hospitalization as well as other out-of-pocket expenses incurred as a result of that hospitalization.	Wages and the monetary value of unpaid work (e.g., household work) foregone by other family members, because of the hospitalization and other out-of-pocket expenses incurred as a result of that hospitalization.	Compensation paid to the employee(s) who handle the claim, what the insurance carrier pays to operate their business, and what they pay to the hospital on behalf of their patient.

Direct and Indirect Cost

Once the time and resources used to provide a good or service are identified, then one can further classify each resource based on how they contribute to the delivery of that good or service. Costs can be classified as direct, indirect, or intangible costs. If the resource is absolutely integral to the delivery of the good or service, then that resource would be considered a direct cost. Using the example of 1 hour of nursing care, the cost of the bed would be a direct cost for a hospitalized patient, because the bed is absolutely necessary for the delivery of care to the hospitalized patient. If the resource is needed but not an integral part of the delivery of the good or service, then that resource would be considered an indirect cost. Using the example of 1 hour of nursing care, the cost of the hospital maintenance worker would be an indirect cost for a hospitalized patient. It is considered indirect because all patients must use the service of the maintenance worker in some way because he or she ensures that the beds are available; however, this work is not absolutely necessary for the delivery of care to any one individual hospitalized patient. Another indication of an indirect cost is if the cost is distributed equally regardless of the actual use by any given individual. For example, if a bed breaks during the care of one patient, that patient might use more maintenance resources than a patient whose bed continues to function properly. Both patients are allocated the same amount of maintenance worker resources, however, when the final costs of their respective stays are calculated. Another example is a hospital finance specialist who processes the patient's insurance claim. The time the finance specialist spends processing the claim does not change substantively based on the insurance provider. Thus, each patient receives the same charge for a finance specialist. Indirect costs in health care are sometimes called overhead costs.

Intangible Cost

The last type of cost is the intangible cost. An intangible cost is the cost for resources that do not have a clear and direct value, monetary or otherwise. Some examples of intangible costs include the cost of lost life due to a medical error and the cost of pain and suffering the patient experiences during care. It is clear that patients can experience pain and suffering during care, but there is not a uniform, straightforward way of placing value on that experience. For most intangible costs, there are standardized approaches to assign monetary values. These systems are most often developed by actuaries, but can also be products of process (such as the legal system) or by other types of professionals. For example, in legal cases the value of lost life due to a medical error might be valued at the lost wages estimated over one's life span.

MEASURING COST

In the nursing care example, time and resources from five different perspectives all contributed to the cost of 1 hour of nursing care. However, before measuring the monetary value of these costs, the decision over which perspective to use must be made. That decision is often dictated by who commissioned the measurement activity. The perspectives that might be used in any given cost analysis are the individual consumer, the corporation/business (e.g., hospital, health care provider, or health insurer), the government, and society as a whole. The cost to society as a whole is the most encompassing view of cost because it considers all of the potential perspectives. In the United States, a consensus was developed in the late 1990s by the Cost Evaluation Taskforce to use the societal viewpoint for all health care cost studies to maximize the ability to compare costs across studies (Weinstein, Siegel, Gold, Kamlet, & Russell, 1996). Thus, unless the cost measurement is commissioned from a distinct perspective (e.g., the provider), the societal perspective should be used when measuring costs or should be reported in conjunction with other perspectives. Once you have identified the perspective of the costs, all of the individual personnel time and resources are identified. The exact process of identification and measurement is determined by the type of cost analysis performed.

TYPES OF COST ANALYSIS

Drummond et al. (2005) identify eight types of cost analyses: cost description, cost–outcome description, cost, cost minimization, cost consequence, cost-effectiveness, cost–utility, and cost–benefit analysis (Drummond et al., 2005). The type of cost analysis that should be used depends on two factors: (1) whether a single activity or multiple alternative activities will be compared, and (2) whether costs alone or costs and their associated outcomes or consequences (e.g., improved health and reduced length of hospitalization) will be measured. Figure 17.1 presents a flow diagram for selecting the type of cost analysis. The next section explores each of the eight types of analyses in further detail.

Cost Description and Cost–Outcome Description

The cost description and the cost–outcome description analyses measure the cost of a single activity. The cost description solely measures the cost of the activity, whereas the cost–outcome measures both the cost and the outcome that results from the activity. The outcome of an activity is also referred to as the consequence, effect, or benefit. The cost and the cost–outcome descriptions are useful tools for researchers and practitioners, because they help quantify the cost implications of

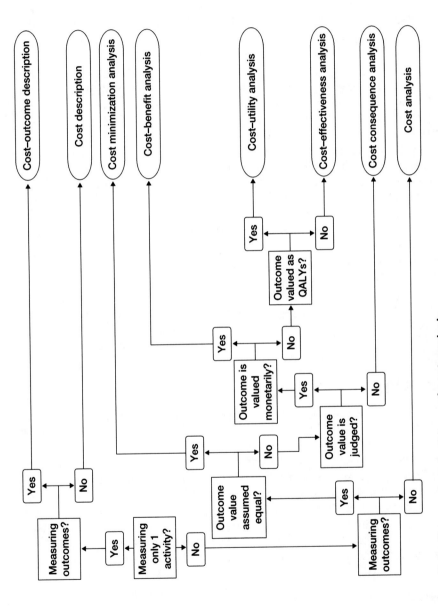

FIGURE 17.1 **Flow diagram to select type of cost analysis.**
QALYs, quality-adjusted life years.

a single type of activity. Both are used widely in health care to examine the economic magnitude of disease, because they can be used to answer questions such as: "How much does hospitalization for a heart transplant cost?" or "What is the hospital cost for stroke treatment and how long will I be hospitalized if I experience it?" The initial example of the cost of 1 hour of nursing care would be considered a cost description, because it measured a single activity—an hour of nursing care—and did not seek to identify any outcomes that might result from that activity (e.g., the patient living 1 day longer than she or he would without the care). Some examples of cost description and cost–outcome description from the published literature are Johnson, Patel, Jegier, Meier, and Engstrom (2012), American Diabetes Association (2013), and Gross et al. (2013).

Further, the cost and cost–outcome description analyses are so prevalent in health care that the Agency for Healthcare Research and Quality (AHRQ) has a free online tool, HCUPnet, that researchers and practitioners can use to identify the mean and median cost and length of stay for almost any type of inpatient hospitalization (HCUP Databases, 2012). The tool allows users to specify the cost they want by a specific diagnosis-related group (DRG), an individual diagnosis code (ICD [International Classification of Diseases]-9), and/or a procedure code (HCUP Databases, 2012). This is a particularly useful tool for researchers and practitioners to use when first examining which diseases are the largest contributors to overall health care costs at the national and/ or state level or when trying to present the "big picture" case for why developing interventions for a particular disease is important.

Cost Analysis

A cost analysis is an analysis that solely measures the monetary cost of two or more alternative activities. A cost analysis does not consider any consequences that may result from each activity. Cost analysis can be especially useful to researchers and practitioners when the cost implications of two or more alternative activities have not been previously measured. The cost analysis is the first step in exploring the cost implications of each alternative. These analyses are often followed by more comprehensive cost studies that compare the costs and consequences of each alternative activity. An example of cost analyses in the literature is Jegier, Meier, Engstrom, and McBride (2010).

Cost-Minimization Analysis

A cost-minimization analysis, like a cost analysis, also compares the monetary value of two or more alternative activities. However, cost minimization assumes that the consequences of each alternative activity are equal, whereas the cost analysis does not measure the consequences nor formulate any assumptions about them. Cost-minimization analyses are particularly useful when comparing two different treatment modalities for delivering the exact same treatment, for example, intravenous compared to oral delivery of a specific pain medication. In this example, the consequence of the pain medication (e.g., pain relief) should theoretically be equal; however, the cost to administer a drug orally versus intravenously would drastically differ. A cost-minimization analysis is also useful when effectiveness studies have already been completed to demonstrate that the outcomes are equal. This type of analysis identifies the lowest cost alternative, and it would be the recommended alternative. Some examples of cost-minimization analyses in the published literature are Dasta et al. (2010), Schuurman (2009), and Behera et al. (2012).

Cost-Consequence Analysis

A cost-consequence analysis also compares the costs and the consequences of two or more alternative activities. The cost-consequence analysis, however, does not assume that the consequences all have equal worth. Instead, the cost and each consequence are presented to the reader or audience. The audience or reader must then decide which alternative to choose using their own judgment regarding the balance between the cost and the consequences for each alternative activity. A cost-consequence analysis would be presented as follows— cost activity 1:consequences of activity 1. Cost consequence can be particularly helpful if there are multiple possible consequences and/ or if there is disagreement over the value of any consequence. The reader is allowed to weigh the relationship between the costs and consequences and consider that multiple consequences are possible. An example of a cost-consequence analysis in the published literature is Kroese et al. (2011).

Cost-Effectiveness Analysis

A cost-effectiveness analysis compares the monetary costs with the consequence of two or more alternative activities. The cost-effectiveness analysis measures the consequences of each alternative using a clinical outcome as the unit of measure. For example, if a new program claims to reduce length of hospital stay, a cost-effectiveness analysis would compare the costs and outcomes of the new program to other existing programs. Cost-effectiveness analysis is particularly useful for clinical providers, because it breaks down the costs to a cost per clinical outcome, and this clinical outcome is usually the most important outcome from a clinical or practice perspective. For example, a cost-effectiveness analysis might identify the cost per day of hospitalization saved. This can be quite powerful when presenting a business case for a new clinical program, because it ties the cost and clinical outcomes together. Some examples of cost-effectiveness analyses in the literature are Behl et al. (2012); Petrou, Taher, Abangma, Eddama, and Bennett (2011); and Patel et al. (2013).

PROMIS: The Future of QALY and DALY Measurement

The Patient Reported Outcomes Measurement Information System (PROMIS) is a U.S. federal initiative funded through the National Institutes of Health that provides standardized tools for measuring quality of life from the patient's perspective (Cella et al., 2007; Revicki et al., 2009). The tools are free for research use and provide researchers with a way to capture physical, mental, and social well-being using a series of validated and standardized questionnaires. These tools offer a unique opportunity to incorporate greater quality measures into research particularly because they include an electronic data collection system.

More information about PROMIS is available at www.nihpromis.org /default

Cost–Utility Analysis

A cost–utility analysis builds on the framework of a cost-effectiveness analysis. Specifically, cost–utility incorporates a standardized measure of quality of life as the consequence being measured. Thus, the typical consequence that is measured in cost–utility analysis is the quality-adjusted life year (QALY; pronounced KW-ALL-EE) or the disability-adjusted life year (DALY; pronounced DA-LEE). There are many different techniques for quantifying QALYs and DALYs; however, there are three scales that are typically used in clinical research. They are the Quality of Well-Being (QWB) Scale (Kaplan & Anderson 1988, 1996), the EuroQol 5-D (EuroQol Group, 1990; available at www.eurolqol.org), or the Short Form 36 (SF-36; Brazier, Roberts, & Deverill, 2002). The use of QALY and DALY in the cost–utility analysis can be very helpful to health care providers, particularly when counseling patients, because it allows the provider to present the quality of the life added by a treatment rather than just the raw time alone. This also allows comparison of the cost-effectiveness across different types of programs or interventions. Some examples of cost–utility analyses in the literature are Kaimal et al. (2011) and Smith et al. (2012).

Cost–Benefit Analysis

A cost–benefit analysis compares the cost and consequence of two or more alternative activities using monetary value for both the costs and the consequence. Cost–benefit analyses are helpful, because the cost and the consequences are measured using the same unit of measurement, which allows the reader to quantify the absolute monetary value of the activity. There is often controversy when consequences are measured in monetary value. If the consequence of an activity is that you live a year longer, how much is that additional year of life worth? Cost–benefit analysis requires assigning a monetary value to consequences, even if the consequence comes with an intangible cost. In addition to some of the standard approaches previously mentioned from certain professions (e.g., actuaries), there is a plethora of economic literature that explores how to apply monetary valuation to costs and consequences that typically are not measured monetarily. Good resources for monetary valuation are Viscusi and Zeckhauser (1994) and Viscusi and Aldy (2003). Further, some examples of cost–benefit analyses in the literature are Puzniak, Gillespie, Leet, Kollef, and Mundy (2004) and Kang, Mandsager, Biddle, and Weber (2012).

CONDUCTING THE COST ANALYSIS

Once the type of cost analysis planned is identified then measurement and analysis begin. There are five general steps for cost analyses: (1) defining the analysis assumptions, (2) measuring the resources used for each cost, (3) measuring the outcomes or consequences associated with each cost, (4) conducting a sensitivity analysis, and (5) comparing the cost and consequences of each alternative activity. Each of these steps is explored further below.

Defining the Analysis Assumptions

The first step of any type of cost analysis is to define the assumptions that will guide the analysis. Assumptions are a set of rules that the researcher will follow when conducting the analysis and in considering the costs and consequences of each activity. Assumptions typically fall into two categories: analysis standards and analysis scope. The analysis standards are the researcher's rules for the perspective that will be used (individual, business, and society) and how costs and consequences will be standardized. As previously described, the perspective is most often dictated by who commissioned the study. Standardization assumptions entail describing the way in which the researcher will measure all costs and consequences. Standardization involves the selection of a single year (e.g., 2012), to measure all costs and consequences. By selecting this year, the researcher is stating that all costs and consequences will be measured using the monetary value from 2012. If the study spans multiple years, then the researcher would inflate or deflate the costs from other years to match the value of money in 2012. It is important to standardize to a single year so that the costs and the consequences can be accurately compared. If the researcher does not standardize the costs and consequences, then any differences in costs and/or consequences may not be real, but rather reflect the fact that a dollar today is worth more than a dollar tomorrow (and a dollar yesterday is worth more than a dollar today). In the United States, a common method of standardizing the costs and consequences to a single year is to use the rate of inflation from the U.S. consumer price index for all goods or the consumer price index specifically for medical care (Bureau of Labor Statistics, 2012). Cost analysis in other countries may use those countries' comparable price indices.

The analysis scope assumptions generally include items that are similar to inclusion and exclusion criteria in a traditional research study. They are similar, because analysis scope assumptions frame the types of costs and consequences that will be measured. To illustrate an analysis scope assumption, let us examine a cost analysis that is comparing whether mothers who provide human milk for their premature infants have lower health care costs than mothers who do not provide it. In this analysis, one resource that the researcher might consider is travel time to bring the human milk to the neonatal intensive care unit (NICU). In this analysis, the researcher might assume that the travel time to bring the human milk to the NICU is zero because bringing the human milk typically occurs as a part of the mother's usual visit to the NICU. The researcher might support this assumption by providing data that demonstrates mothers who provide human milk visit their infants the same number of time as mothers who do not provide it.

Measuring the Resources Used for Each Cost

Once the assumptions have been identified, the researcher must identify all of the resources that will be used to create the total cost for each alternative that will be measured. These resources should include all time and resources expended, and ideally information about these resources is collected at the time that other data are collected during the study. During this step, it is often helpful to create a table that captures the name of each resource, how it is defined, how it is measured, how much it costs, what year the costs are measured, and where the cost data are obtained (Table 17.2). After all of the resources have been identified and the monetary value has been measured, the monetary value of all the resources used is summed to create a total cost for each activity in the analysis.

TABLE 17.2 A Guide to Measuring the Resources Used for Each Cost Using Selected Resources From the Example of 1 Hour of Nursing Care

RESOURCE NAME	DEFINITION OF RESOURCE	RESOURCE MEASUREMENT	TOTAL COST	COST YEAR	SOURCE(S) OF COST DATA
Nurse time	Nurse time reflects the time spent by the nurse directly with the patient and completing activities related to care for that patient (e.g., charting the activities that occurred and submitting a patient blood sample to the lab).	This resource was measured through direct observation of the nurse before, during, and after interaction with the patient by a research assistant (RA). The RA noted on a standardized time log the name and the total time in minutes for each distinct activity (e.g., interacting with patient and entering documentation into the health record). RAs followed the nurse for 2 weeks. The total cost per hour of care was measured as the nurse's hourly wage plus the hourly cost of the benefits the hospital provides. (Hourly wage = $25; hourly benefit cost = $1)	$26	2012	RA standardized time log; hospital human resource department
Supplies	Supplies reflect the actual supplies that were used during the care of the patient during a 1-hour time period.	This resource was measured through direct observation of the encounter with the patient by an RA. The RA noted each individual supply that was used and/or present in the room using a standardized supply log. These observations were cross-checked against the hospital supply system, which requires that a code unique to the patient room is entered before the supply can be sent to the room or is taken from the local supply system machine on the unit. The cost for each item was obtained from the hospital purchasing department. The total cost was the sum of the individual costs of each item.	$150	2012	RA standardized supply log; hospital supply system; hospital purchasing department
Space	Space reflects the total square footage of the room that the patient occupies during a 1-hour time period.	This resource was measured as the total square feet of the room. This measure was obtained from the hospital planning department. The total cost of the room for 1 hour was calculated by multiplying the total square feet of the room by the total hourly cost per square foot. (Total square feet = 100; total hourly cost = $1)	$100	2012	Hospital planning department

Measuring the Outcomes or Consequences Associated With Each Cost

After measuring the total cost of each activity, the same process is repeated to measure the outcomes or consequences associated with each activity. The outcomes or consequences can be measured for each individual resource used within the activity or for the activity as a whole. The monetary value of each outcome or consequence can be measured at the same time or immediately after each is identified, if the monetary value is required for the type of cost analysis selected. For most analyses, a single outcome or consequence is used to compare activities or programs. If multiple consequences/outcomes are needed, consider using a cost-consequence analysis.

Conducting a Sensitivity Analysis

Before comparing the costs and consequences of each alternative activity, it is important to determine which resources contribute the most to total costs. A sensitivity analysis is a technique that examines what happens to the total cost of each activity, if the underlying costs of the resources that are used change. Therefore, a sensitivity analysis is the process of recalculating the total costs by changing the underlying resource costs one at a time (i.e., "univariate" sensitivity analysis). Costs can be changed using a percentage method (e.g., changing each cost by 10%) or using a replacement method (e.g., replacing the actual hourly wage with a standard wage like the minimum wage for the location). As the cost of each resource is changed, the raw change in total cost and the percentage change in total cost are measured. The process of changing the cost of each resource is usually repeated until the total cost of the activity is doubled or tripled. The resource or resources that represent the largest or fastest change in total cost are the resources that a researcher would say the total cost of the activity is sensitive to or that drive the total cost of the activity. Knowing which resources drive the total cost of an activity allows the researcher to portray the potential cost range for the activity. Other more advanced methods of sensitivity analysis include multivariate sensitivity approaches that use bootstrapping, Monte Carlo, and/or Markov modeling methods. Bootstrapping methods are used to calculate 95% confidence intervals to evaluate uncertainty in cost-effectiveness ratios (Briggs, Wonderling, & Mooney, 1997; Polsky, Glick, Wilke, & Schulman, 1997; Tambour & Zethraeus, 1988). Monte Carlo and Markov approaches are used to evaluate uncertainty in analyses that examine costs and consequences over time. These more advanced methods should be performed in consultation with an expert in health economics as they require knowledge of advanced econometric modeling.

Comparing the Costs and Consequences of Each Alternative Activity

The final step in a cost analysis is to compare the costs and consequences of each alternative activity that was measured. The way in which the comparison of the cost and consequences is presented depends on the type of cost analysis used. Table 17.3 provides the presentation style for each type of cost analysis. Generally, the activity with the lowest cost and the best consequence is the activity that would be selected by the cost analysis as the optimal outcome.

SPECIAL CONSIDERATIONS

This section examines some considerations for common situations and scenarios that researchers and practitioners may encounter when conducting cost analysis. These considerations include selecting the standardization year, discounting, depreciation, and a brief description of some of the software programs that can assist with cost analysis.

Selecting the Standardization Year

Selecting what year to standardize all costs to can be a difficult decision, particularly when conducting the cost analysis long after the actual data were collected or when using a historical data set where considerable time has lapsed. There are two good options for selecting the standardization year: use the final year in which data were collected or use the present year. Using the final year the data were collected can be attractive because the costs are tied most closely to the time period the data were collected, and this limits the assumptions and decisions about the rate of inflation to use. The downside to using the final year is that the data may not reflect the costs of the present day, making interpretation for the reader more difficult. Using the present year can be attractive, because it ensures that the data are most relevant to the time period when the findings will actually be used. The downside to using the present year is that the researcher may have to make a number of assumptions regarding how to inflate the cost values to present-day dollars. Although the inflation can be complex, using the present year is preferable to the final study year, because the results will be most relevant to the present.

Discounting

Discounting is another topic that must be considered when conducting a cost analysis. Discounting is the process by which we standardize the value of any future costs, savings, or outcomes/consequences

TABLE 17.3 Presentation of the Comparison of Costs and Consequences by Type of Cost Analysis

TYPE OF COST ANALYSIS	PRESENTATION	FICTITIOUS EXAMPLES
Cost description	Total cost of single activity	A heart disease prevention program costs $50,000.
Cost–outcome description	Total cost of single activity per unit of the outcome	Lung cancer hospitalization costs $10,000 per hospitalization and each hospitalization is an average of 5 days in the hospital.
Cost analysis	Total cost of each individual activity	Heart disease program A costs $50,000. Heart disease program B costs $60,000.
Cost minimization	Total cost of each activity assuming constant consequence	Drug A and Drug B cure a bacterial infection in five treatment days. Drug A costs $1 per day of treatment; Drug B costs $2 per day of treatment.
Cost consequence	Total cost of each activity and total consequence of each activity	Heart disease program A costs $50,000. Heart disease program B costs $60,000 dollars.
		Heart disease program A saves $100,000 in hospital costs and reduces readmission by 10%. Heart disease program B saves $150,000 in hospital costs and reduces readmission by 10%.
Cost–benefit	Cost/savings of the unit of the outcome per total cost of each activity	Mammography screening saves $3 in cancer expenditure per $1 spent on screening. Teaching self-breast exam techniques saves $5 in cancer expenditure per $1 spent on teaching.
Cost–effectiveness	Total cost of each activity per unit of the outcome	Smoking-cessation program A saves $1,000 in annual primary care visits per patient who quits smoking. Smoking-cessation program B saves $1,500 in annual primary care visits per patient who quits smoking.
Cost–utility	Total cost of each activity per quality-adjusted unit of the outcome	Intramuscular injection flu immunization costs $10 per disability-adjusted life year gained. Nasal mist flu immunization costs $11 per disability-adjusted life year gained.

(Krahn & Gafni, 1993). Typically a 3% discount rate per year is applied to the value of any and all future costs, savings, or outcomes/consequences when comparing each alternative. Similar to inflation, discounting allows the researcher to ensure comparability of outcomes as well as avoid overstating the potential future implications.

Depreciation

Depreciation is an important consideration for cost analyses that examine resources that can be used for multiple years with substantial capital investments, such as expensive equipment. Depreciation allows the researcher to allocate the cost of that resource equally over the years of use that the resource will have rather than simply applying the total cost of the resource in the first year of its life. Depreciation is also a way to account for the cost of replacement for the resource at the end of its useful life. Typically, depreciation is allocated by equally dividing the total cost of the item over the expected total years of use. Sometimes a replacement investment percentage can be added to the total cost of the item to allow for the measurement of future resource expenses. To determine what depreciation, if any, should be included in your analysis, it is best to discuss how depreciation is accounted for with the organization that is commissioning the analysis. If the societal perspective is used, depreciation may not be specifically measured.

Programs That Assist With Cost Analysis

There are many software programs that can be used for cost analysis. Any basic or advance spreadsheet program (e.g. Microsoft Excel) can be used to capture costs and outcomes data. These programs also have formulas that will assist the researcher in standardizing costs and discounting to present value. These types of programs are likely all that is required for cost description, cost–outcome description, cost, cost minimization, and cost-consequence analyses. However, if you are pursuing cost-effectiveness, cost–utility, and cost–benefit analyses, a more sophisticated software package may be helpful. Software packages that are designed to allow decision tree construction and Markov modeling allow easy execution of cost-effectiveness, cost–utility, and cost–benefit analyses. One of the most user-friendly programs is TreeAge (Williamstown, MA). SPSS (Chicago, IL) and SAS (Cary, NC) can also be used to build more complex cost-analysis models.

SUMMARY

Throughout this chapter, we discussed the definition of costs, cost measurement, types of cost analysis, the process of conducting a cost analysis, and special considerations that should be taken into account when working with costs and undertaking a cost analysis. It is important that as researchers and practitioners, you apply the practices described in this chapter to critically evaluate the cost literature. This critical evaluation is important because cost analyses are another tool that can be used to support evidence-based practice. To integrate cost analyses, we must apply the same rigorous standards used to evaluate efficacy, effectiveness, and other clinical research. Cost analyses that do not clearly describe the resources they measured, the assumptions they made, or the year that their costs represent can lead the reader to erroneous conclusions that may hinder the implementation of valuable programs.

SUGGESTED ACTIVITIES

1. For each for the scenarios below identify what would be the appropriate type of cost analysis?

   a. A study that compares the cost of four different types of chemotherapy treatment for patients with lung cancer
   b. A study that measures the cost of a new enhanced discharge planning program
   c. A study that compares the cost and incidence of back injury among nurses following the implementation of new patient lift assist devices
   d. A study that measures the cost and health outcomes at 5 years of life for infants born preterm and term
   e. A study that compares the cost and quality of life for community health workers who undergo an academic training program versus an on-the-job program
   f. A study that compares the costs and length of stay for patients who receive open versus minimally invasive spinal surgery

2. For each of the scenarios above, what point of view would this study most likely use (individual, institution/corporation, government, society)?

3. Using a peer-reviewed article of your choosing or one of the exemplars listed in the chapter, review the article and identify the following:

   a. What is the main purpose of the article?
   b. What type of economic/cost analysis did they perform?
   c. What type of point of view did they use? Were they consistent in limiting their discussion to that point of view?
   d. How did they define costs and if appropriate outcomes/benefits?

e. Was the analysis comprehensive? Is there anything you think they should have added? Did they address any comprehensiveness issues in their limitations?

f. What were the main conclusions from the article?

g. Would you use the findings in the article to influence your practice? Why or why not?

REFERENCES

American Diabetes Association. (2013). Economic costs of diabetes in the U.S. in 2012. *Diabetes Care.*

Behera, M. A., Likes, C. E., III, Judd, J. P., Barnett, J. C., Havrilesky, L. J., & Wu, J. M. (2012). Cost analysis of abdominal, laparoscopic, and robotic-assisted myomectomies. *Journal of Minimally Invasive Gynecology, 19*(1), 52–57.

Behl, A. S., Goddard, K. A., Flottemesch, T. J., Veenstra, D., Meenan, R. T., Lin, J. S., & Maciosek, M. V. (2012). Cost-effectiveness analysis of screening for KRAS and BRAF mutations in metastatic colorectal cancer. *Journal of the National Cancer Institute, 104*(23), 1785–1795.

Brazier, J., Roberts, J., & Deverill, M. (2002). The estimation of a preference-based measure of health from the sf-36. *Journal of Health Economics, 21*(2), 271–292.

Briggs, A. H., Wonderling, D. E., & Mooney, C. Z. (1997). Pulling cost-effectiveness analysis up by its bootstraps: A nonparametric approach to confidence interval estimation. *Health Economics, 6*, 327–340.

Bureau of Labor Statistics. (2012). *Consumer price index for all urban consumers and all items.* Retrieved from http://www.bls.gov/cpi/#tables

Cella, D., Yount, S., Rothrock, N., Gershon, R., Cook, K., Reeve, B., . . . and On behalf of the PROMIS Cooperative Group. (2007). The Patient Reported Outcomes Measurement Information System (PROMIS): Progress of an NIH Roadmap Cooperative Group during its first two years. *Medical Care, 45*(5), S3–S11.

Centers for Medicare and Medicaid Services (CMS). (2012). *National health expenditure projections 2011–2021.* Baltimore, MD. Retrieved from https://www.cms.gov/Research-Statistics-Data-and-Systems/Statistics-Trends-and-Reports/NationalHealthExpendData/Downloads/Proj2011PDF.pdf

Congressional Budget Office (CBO). (2012). *The 2012 long-term budget outlook* (CBO Publication No. 4507). Washington, DC: U.S. Government Printing Office. Retrieved from http://www.cbo.gov/sites/default/files/cbo files/attachments/06-05-Long-Term_Budget_Outlook_2.pdf

Dasta, J. F., Kane-Gill, S. L., Pencina, M., Shehabi, Y., Bokesch, P. M., Wisemandle, W., & Riker, R. R. (2010). A cost-minimization analysis of dexmedetomidine compared with midazolam for long-term sedation in the intensive care unit. *Critical Care Medicine, 38*(2), 497–503.

Drummond, M. F., Sculpher, M. J., Torrance, G. W., O'Brien, B. J., & Stoddart, G. L. (2005). *Methods for the economic evaluation of health care programmes* (3rd ed.). New York, NY: Oxford University Press.

EuroQol Group. (1990). EuroQol—A new facility for the measurement of health-related quality of life. *Health Policy, 16*, 199–208.

Gold, M. R., Siegel, J. E., Russell, L. B., & Weinstein, M. C. (1996). *Cost-effectiveness in health and medicine*. New York, NY: Oxford University Press.

Gross, C. P., Long, J. B., Ross, J. S., Abu-Khalaf, M. M., Wang, R., Killelea, B. K., Gold, H. T., Chaqpar, A. B., & Ma, X. (2013). The cost of breast cancer screening in the medicare population. *JAMA Internal Medicine, 173*(3), 220–226.

HCUP Databases. (2012). *Healthcare cost and utilization project (HCUP): 2006–2011*. Rockville, MD: Agency for Healthcare Research and Quality. Retrieved from www.hcup-us.ahrq.gov/databases.jsp

Jegier, B. J., Meier, P. P., Engstrom, J. L., & McBride, T. M. (2010). The initial maternal cost of providing 100 mL of human milk for very low birth weight infants in the neonatal intensive care unit. *Breastfeeding Medicine, 5*(2), 71–77.

Johnson, T. J., Patel, A. L., Jegier, B. J., Meier, P. P., & Engstrom, J. L. (2013). The cost of morbidities in very low birth weight infants. *Journal of Pediatrics, 162*(2), 243–249.e1.

Kaimal, A. J., Little, S. E., Odibo, A. O., Stamilio, D. M., Grobman, W. A., Long, E. F., Owens, D. K., & Caughey, A. B. (2011). Cost-effectiveness of elective induction of labor at 41 weeks in nulliparous women. *American Journal of Obstetrics and Gynecology, 204*(2), 137.e1–137.e9.

Kang, J., Mandsager, P., Biddle, A. K., & Weber, D. J. (2012). Cost-effectiveness analysis of active surveillance screening for methicillin-resistant *Staphylococcus aureus* in an academic hospital setting. *Infection Control and Hospital Epidemiology, 33*(5), 477–486.

Kaplan, R. M., & Anderson, J. P. (1988). A general health policy model: Update and applications. *Health Services Research, 23*, 203–235.

Kaplan, R. M., & Anderson, J. P. (1996). The general health policy model: An integrated approach. In B. Spilker (Ed.), *Quality of life and pharmacoeconomics in clinical trials* (2nd ed., pp. 309–322). Philadelphia, PA: Lippincott-Raven.

Krahn, M., & Gafni, A. (1993). Discounting in the economic evaluation of health care interventions. *Medical Care, 31*(5), 403–418.

Kroese, M. E., Severens, J. L., Schulpen, G. J., Bessems, M. C., Nijhuis, F. J., & Landewé, R. B. (2011). Specialized rheumatology nurse substitutes for rheumatologists in the diagnostic process of fibromyalgia: A cost-consequence analysis and a randomized controlled trial. *Journal of Rheumatology, 38*(7), 1413–1422.

Patel, A. L., Johnson, T. J., Engstrom, J. L., Fogg, L. F., Jegier, B. J., Bigger, H. R., & Meier, P. P. (2013). Impact of early human milk on sepsis and health-care costs in very low birth weight infants. *Journal of Perinatology 33*(17), 514–519.

Petrou, S., Taher, S., Abangma, G., Eddama, O., & Bennett, P. (2011). Cost-effectiveness analysis of prostaglandin e2 gel for the induction of labour at term. *BJOG: An International Journal of Obstetrics and Gynaecology, 118*(6), 726–734.

Polsky, D., Glick, H. A., Wilke, R., & Schulman, K. (1997). Confidence intervals for cost-effectiveness ratios: A comparison of four methods. *Health Economics, 6*, 243–252.

Puzniak, L. A., Gillespie, K. N., Leet, T., Kollef, M., & Mundy, L. M. (2004). A cost-benefit analysis of gown use in controlling vancomycin-resistant Enterococcus transmission: Is it worth the price? *Infection Control and Hospital Epidemiology, 25*(5), 418–424.

Revicki, D. A., Kawata, A. K., Harnam, N., Chen, W. H., Hays, R. D., & Cella, D. (2009). Predicting EuroQol (EQ-5D) scores from the patient-reported outcomes measurement information system (PROMIS) global items and domain item banks in a United States sample. *Quality of Life Research, 18*(6), 783–791.

Schuurman, J., Schoonhoven, L., Defloor, T., van Engelshoven, I., van Ramshorst, B., & Buskens, E. (2009). Economic evaluation of pressure ulcer care: A cost minimization analysis of preventive strategies. *Nursing Economics, 27*(6), 390–400, 415.

Smith, K. J., Wateska, A. R., Nowalk, M. P., Raymund, M., Nuorti, J. P., & Zimmerman, R. K. (2012). Cost-effectiveness of adult vaccination strategies using pneumococcal conjugate vaccine compared with pneumococcal polysaccharide vaccine. *Journal of the American Medical Association, 307*(8), 804–812.

Tambour, M., & Zethraeus, N. (1988). Bootstrap confidence intervals for cost effectiveness rations: Some simulation results. *Health Economics, 7*, 143–147.

Viscusi, W. K., & Aldy, J. E. (2003). *The value of a statistical life: A critical review of market estimates throughout the world.* National Bureau of Economic Research (Working Paper 9487). Cambridge, MA. Retrieved from http://www.nber.org/papers/w9487

Viscusi, W. K., & Zeckhauser, R. J. (1994). The fatality and injury costs of expenditures. *Journal of Risk and Uncertainty, 8*(1), 19–41.

Weinstein, M. C., Siegel, J. E., Gold, M. R., Kamlet, M. S., & Russell, L. B. (1996). Recommendations of the panel on cost-effectiveness in health and medicine. *Journal of the American Medical Association, 276*, 1339–1341.

18

Evaluation of Outcomes

Leah L. Shever

Evaluation of outcomes in health care is drawing increasing attention from health care providers, consumers, regulatory bodies, and policy-makers. The shift in focus to health care outcomes has been driven by the fact that although health care costs continue to soar, reaching $1.6 trillion in 2003 (Cowan & Hartman, 2005), the quality of health care in the United States is dismally low compared to other nations (Anderson & Frogner, 2008; Nolte & McKee, 2008). Although there are a number of factors that contribute to the broken health care system in the United States, such as absent or lacking health care insurance, access to care, and appropriate use of limited resources (e.g., limiting the number of unnecessary tests, focusing on prevention, and limiting intensive care unit length of stay at the end of life), one of the most disturbing factors contributing to both health care cost and quality is the alarming number of errors and adverse events that are largely preventable (Institute of Medicine, 2000). Defining quality in health care is very difficult but examining health care outcomes is an essential part of the process.

Health care quality at the most basic level is keeping patients safe and not inflicting further harm. The Institute of Medicine (IOM) produced two reports, *To Err Is Human: Building a Safer Health System,* (Institute of Medicine, 2000) and *Crossing the Quality Chasm: A New Health System for the 21st Century* (Institute of Medicine, 2001) that illustrate that the current U.S. health care system too often does a poor job of keeping patients safe. In a more recent report, the IOM asserts that nurses are the health care providers most likely to not only prevent adverse events or complications but also to identify them and to activate the appropriate responses after a complication occurs (Institute of Medicine, 2004). It is therefore imperative that nurses monitor and evaluate health care outcomes beginning at the patient level and have an understanding of how aggregated patient outcomes are an indication of quality at the system or institution level.

EVOLUTION OF OUTCOMES EVALUATION

Agencies Impacting Health Care Outcomes and Quality

Outcomes in health care have always been important. Specific measures, their definitions, how they are collected, how they are reported, and the implications of those outcomes have evolved greatly over time. Although outcomes evaluation in nursing really started with one nurse, Florence Nightingale, during the Crimean War, there have been many organizations that have guided outcomes evaluation in the United States. A brief description of these organizations is provided in the following sections.

Specific to nursing, the American Nurses Credentialing Center offers Magnet recognition for hospitals that draw and retain nurses. This work began in the early 1980s when the American Academy of Nursing's (AAN) Task Force on Nursing Practice in Hospitals conducted a survey of approximately 160 hospitals in the United States and identified 41 hospitals where the environment attracted and retained nurses. In the early 1990s, the first U.S. hospital was given Magnet recognition and today this is an international recognition that is available in both acute care hospitals and long-term care facilities (American Nurses Credentialing Center, 2013).

In addition to attracting and retaining nurses, these hospitals have demonstrated high quality in specific outcomes that are nursing sensitive (Aiken, Havens, & Sloane, 2000a, 2000b; Scott, Sochalski, & Aiken, 1999). Magnet recognition identifies hospitals where the quality of nursing care is exceptional, unlike other accreditations, where accreditation demonstrates that a hospital has met the minimum requirements. Both *U.S. News Best Hospitals in America Honor Roll* and the *Leapfrog Hospital Survey* give institutions credit for being a Magnet-designated facility, indicating excellence in nursing care (American Nurses Credentialing Center, 2013).

The Magnet model was significantly modified in 2008 following an analysis of the 14 forces of Magnetism or standards of excellence. The analysis revealed that the 14 forces had five major themes or components: transformational leadership; structural empowerment; exemplary professional practice; new knowledge, innovations, and improvements; and empirical outcomes. Institutions that apply for Magnet recognition must demonstrate how they meet specific criteria under each of the five model components. Under the empirical outcomes model component, institutions must provide examples of the structures, processes, and outcomes they use for ongoing quality-improvement efforts and the people involved. In addition, institutions must show that they are outperforming their peer group (e.g., academic medical facilities, hospitals with similar bed capacity, etc.) on outcomes measures like pressure ulcers, falls, catheter-associated urinary tract infections, ventilator-associated events, central line blood stream infections, use of restraints, and pediatric intravenous (IV) infiltrations (American Nurses Credentialing Center, 2009).

Another influential agency that focuses on quality in U.S. health care is the Agency for Healthcare Research and Quality (AHRQ). AHRQ is a part of the U.S. Department of Health and Human Services (DHHS) and not only funds health services research but is also very active in disseminating research results and evidence-based practices, which greatly influence health care outcomes. AHRQ has many resources available to health care providers and health care consumers, such as evidence-based guidelines and outcomes evaluation tools to positively impact patient outcomes (Agency for Healthcare Research and Quality, 2013).

The National Quality Forum (NQF) is a nonprofit organization developed to set a strategy for measuring quality in health care. It was created in 1999 to address the need for valid and reliable health care performance indicators, and its members include a wide variety of public and private entities in roles such as health care consumer, health care provider, purchaser, community, supplier, and others. NQF works in partnership with key stakeholder groups to develop indicators for public reporting, to set and achieve priorities or goals for the nation, and to educate and disseminate information to reach established national goals (National Quality Forum, 2013).

The Centers for Medicare and Medicaid Services (CMS) is a federal agency that is charged with the administration of the Medicare and Medicaid programs within the United States. In 2011 Medicare alone covered 48.7 million Americans with expenditures close to $550 billion (The Boards of Trustees, Federal Hospital Insurance and Federal Supplementary Medical Insurance Trust Funds, 2012). Due to the high number of people and expenditures covered by Medicare and Medicaid, CMS is one of the single biggest influencers of health care quality in the United States; when they make a decision with respect to quality-related funding, it has a significant impact on hospitals across the country. The decisions of CMS not only impact patients covered by Medicare and Medicaid but also those covered by private insurance as many private insurance companies adopt policies for reimbursement that are in alignment with CMS policies.

One of the significant changes CMS made in quality-related reimbursement was to stop paying for certain complications patients incur while hospitalized, referred to as *hospital-acquired conditions* (HACs). Previously, if a patient covered by Medicare or Medicaid experienced an HAC that required additional care like surgical repair of a fracture from a fall, the hospital would be reimbursed by CMS for the costs associated with treating the fracture. The HACs that hospitals are no longer reimbursed to treat include foreign object retained after surgery; air embolism; blood incompatibility; stage III and IV pressure ulcers; falls and trauma (fractures, dislocations, intracranial injuries, crushing injuries, burns); complications associated with poor glycemic control; catheter-associated urinary tract infection (UTI); vascular catheter-associated infection; and surgical site infection mediastinitis after coronary artery bypass graft (CABG); surgical site infection after bariatric surgery for obesity; surgical site infection after orthopedic procedures of the spine, neck, shoulder, and elbow; surgical site infection after a cardiac implantable electronic device (CIED); deep vein thrombosis (DVT)/pulmonary embolism (PE) after a total knee or hip replacement; and iatrogenic pneumothorax with venous catheterization (Centers for Medicare and Medicaid, 2013). Part of the reason for not reimbursing for these HACs is because there is substantial evidence to support that these events can be prevented when the proper processes (e.g., adequate nurse staffing, proper risk assessment, and evidence-based interventions targeted to specific risk factors) are in place.

In October 2012, CMS took reimbursement for quality to the next level. Through a new program called *value-based purchasing* Medicare will provide financial incentives for hospitals to provide high-quality care. Starting in fiscal year 2013, Medicare reduced its prospective payments to hospitals by 1% across the board. This money is being redirected to fund the value-based purchasing program. Hospitals' performance on approximately 12 process measures and patients' experience of care received will be judged against the national average. Incentive payments will be based on that benchmark and the hospital's improvements over time in the metrics. The metrics being used were endorsed by NQF and it is anticipated that as the program evolves, more outcomes metrics will be added (U.S. Department of Health and Human Services, 2011).

Health care consumers are now able to go to the U.S. Department of Health and Human Services hospital comparison website (www.medicare.gov/hospitalcompare/search.html) and see how their local hospital performs in process measures, patient satisfaction, readmissions for specific conditions, mortality rates for certain conditions, use of imaging studies, and other metrics included in the value-based purchasing program to other hospitals and national averages. In theory, potential patients (i.e., consumers) can examine the data related to the specific health care problems and make an informed decision on what hospital provides the best care to fit their needs.

Current Trends in Reporting Outcomes Measures

More recently, patients, families, and communities have been engaged in setting research and quality agendas for the nation. The purpose in engaging health care consumers is to identify research questions and outcomes that are meaningful to patients, their families, and the community. Federal agencies like the Food and Drug Administration (FDA), the National Institutes for Health (NIH), and the AHRQ all have programs that include health care consumers as decision makers in identifying and setting priorities (Fleurence et al., 2013). The Patient Protection and Affordable Care Act of 2010 established funding for the Patient-Centered Outcomes Research Institute (PCORI), which has a mission to "help people make informed health care decisions, and improves health care delivery and outcomes, by producing and promoting high integrity, evidence-based information that comes from research guided by patients, caregivers and the broader health care community" (Patient-Centered Outcomes Research Institute, 2013).

PCORI put forward its first *National Priorities for Research and Research Agenda* in May 2012. The draft of research priorities was unchanged after a period of public review and comment. The five research priorities put forward included the following: (1) prevention, diagnosis, and treatment options for specific patient populations; (2) improving health care systems, including coordination of care; (3) communication and dissemination of information to health care consumers so that they can make informed decisions; (4) addressing disparities; and (5) accelerating patient-centered outcomes research (Fleurence et al., 2013; Patient-Centered Outcomes Research Institute, 2013).

DEFINITION AND INTRODUCTION OF TERMS

Health Outcomes Research

Health outcomes research evaluates the end result of specific health care treatments or interventions (Agency for Healthcare Research and Quality, 2013). The difference between outcomes research and other medical research is that the definition of the treatment is broader in health outcomes research. Typical medical research examines the impact of a specific surgical procedure or the effect of a medication, whereas outcomes research broadens the definition of *treatment* to include such things as counseling, staffing, or a care delivery model and how they impact outcomes (Kane & Radosevich, 2011). This is also sometimes referred to as *intervention research* (Grove, Burns, & Gray, 2013).

Efficacy Versus Effectiveness Research

Often when the general public hears "research" they think of randomized controlled trials (RCTs). RCTs are a type of *efficacy* research in which the *potential* benefits of the treatment or intervention are studied under ideal, controlled conditions (Brown, 2002; Shwartz & Ash, 2003; Sidani & Epstein, 2003; Sidani, Epstein, & Moritz, 2003; Whittemore & Grey, 2002). In comparison, *effectiveness* research refers to studying the impact of interventions or treatments on patient outcomes in a real-world situation where multiple other factors influence the outcome (Brown, 2002; Sidani & Epstein, 2003; Sidani et al., 2003; Titler, Dochterman, & Reed, 2004; Whittemore & Grey, 2002).

For a number of reasons, efficacy research in nursing poses many problems. One issue is the feasibility of conducting such research. It is difficult from a practical point of view to randomize patients to nursing treatments. From an ethical standpoint, it is difficult to randomize patients to treatment if there is evidence to suggest that the treatment will provide an improved outcome or comfort to the patient. Furthermore, it is rarely the case that only one specific nursing treatment is provided for a patient with any type of health concern. Typically, nursing takes a multifaceted approach to treating individuals with health care concerns, recognizing that each patient is an individual and therefore has a unique set of needs and wishes. Nursing is also only one health care discipline attempting to effectively treat a patient. Pharmacy, medicine, physical therapy, and others all work with nursing in a variety of settings to achieve desired patient outcomes. To conduct nursing efficacy research in a vacuum, thinking that only one specific nursing treatment is going to influence patient outcomes, appears to be a waste of time and resources given how nursing actually operates in collaboration with the patients, families, and other health care disciplines in a real-life setting. In short, the generalizability of nursing efficacy studies is very limited (Sidani et al., 2003).

Risk Adjustment

Risk adjustment refers to accounting, or controlling, for patient-specific factors that may impact outcomes (Iezzoni, 2003). If risk adjustment is not done, it is possible to reach a wrong conclusion about the treatment and/or outcome (Smith, Nitz, & Stuart, 2006). To illustrate the need for risk adjustment, consider two patients treated for a fracture of the tibia. Both require surgery to set the bone followed by weeks in a cast while the bone heals. The first patient is a 17-year-old healthy male who broke his leg playing football. He experiences no complications during or following surgery and is able to have the cast removed in the expected time frame. The second patient is an 83-year-old female who resides in a skilled nursing facility, has a history of diabetes and dementia, and broke her leg when she tripped over a footstool. This patient has her leg set surgically, has a cast applied but also develops pneumonia following surgery. She is hospitalized an additional 5 days, and never regains the mobility she had prior to the fracture. If no risk adjustment were done, we would evaluate the treatment (i.e., surgery and cast) based solely on the patients' outcomes—one regained full mobility and the other did not. An incorrect conclusion that the treatment is not effective may be made if the risk factors present in the second patient, such as her advanced age, comorbid conditions of diabetes, dementia, and pneumonia are not considered, or adjusted for.

There are varying methods of risk adjustment, and using the most appropriate method depends on which outcomes are being evaluated, the time period, the study population, and the purpose of the evaluation (Iezzoni, 2003). More common factors or variables, frequently used for risk adjustment include age, severity of illness, and comorbid conditions (Iezzoni, 2003; Smith et al., 2006).

CONSIDERATIONS FOR OUTCOMES EVALUATION

Whether conducting or evaluating an outcomes study or simply examining outcomes in a clinical setting, there are key components of outcomes measurement that must be considered to ensure valid and reliable data.

Conceptual Model

The first step in evaluating health care outcomes is to consider the conceptual model. This can sound like an intimidating process but it saves a lot of work if done at the beginning of the process. This first step is important whether conducting or evaluating an outcomes study, or when evaluating outcomes in a clinical setting. This first step is critical to ensure that relationships, and/or processes, that impact the outcome are considered (Kane & Radosevich, 2011). In a real-world clinical setting, it might be rare to spend time on considering a conceptual model but spending time considering the elements that impact an outcome will help delineate the structures and processes that contribute to the outcome and therefore make it easier to understand and explain. Consider infection rates on a nursing unit. It is clear from the literature that hand hygiene is the most effective way to reduce infection rates, and so if an evaluation of the infection rates on a unit did not include hand hygiene, that may be a potential flaw in the evaluation.

There are many conceptual models available to help guide outcomes evaluation and many are based, or influenced, by the work of Donabedian (2005). Donabedian created a model that describes how structures and processes influence outcomes. Examples of structure might include a hospital, a nursing unit, a patient's home, a clinic, an operating room, and more. Processes describe what is done within the structure. Processes could include such things as medical procedures, medication delivery, nursing treatments, and more. Outcomes are influenced by structures, processes, and the relationship among the two (Donabedian, 2005).

Data Sources and Measurement Issues

After the conceptual model with key relationships has been carefully developed, the next step is defining each variable or element of interest. Although defining variables may seem like an obvious step, it is sometimes minimized or overlooked. There are often many different ways to define the same variable or element of interest. A clinical example might be pain relief. If the question is whether the application of vibration therapy will provide pain relief associated with incisional pain, then clear definitions for both "vibration therapy" and "pain relief" would be needed. "Pain relief" might be defined as the patient's report that his or her pain is "better" compared to worse or no change or it could be the patient's self-report of pain intensity score that decreased by one measure (e.g., from 8/10 to 7/10). When defining variables, it is most important that the definition be clear and not open to interpretation because that will lead to inconsistency in measurement.

Very closely related to the definition of the variable is identifying the data source for each identified variable. The ideal data source is valid and reliable and lends itself well to precise, or detailed, measurement. In RCTs, the researcher has tighter control over the variables to ensure that they are valid and reliable. In research that uses clinical data, or data not collected for the purposes of research, identifying valid and reliable data sources is much more difficult because the data sources were not designed to be measurement tools used for research. They were designed for clinical purposes related to patient care. Although this problem does not exclude the data from being useful, it is certainly a limitation and must be taken into consideration when evaluating the data (Grove et al., 2013). In addition, there are multiple data sources for the same phenomenon. Pressure ulcers, for example, can be pulled from nursing documentation or provider (MD, PA, NP, etc.) documentation. Data from the two sources may vary significantly, which is why it is so important to pick the data source that is the most valid, reliable, and sensitive to the variable of interest.

The ease of data collection is another consideration when considering both the definition and the data source. When there are additional resources available for data collection and measurement, such as a funded research study, there is greater opportunity to use tools or measures that have greater sensitivity to the variable of interest. However, in the clinical setting, having another tool or measure that does not add clinical value is a challenge. Therefore, if conducting an outcomes evaluation in the clinical setting, first consider what measures are being collected for clinical or quality-improvement purposes to determine whether they would be appropriate.

Episode of Care or Time Period

The episode of care, or time period, is the designated time that the variables or elements (interventions and outcomes) will be monitored or collected. It is important to designate an episode of care that is in keeping with the conceptual model. The time frame for data collection needs to capture the phenomenon of interest, or when the intervention is going to achieve a measurable effect (Strickland, 1997). An example of this might be providing a congestive heart failure patient with targeted education on daily weight monitoring and proper diet, and expecting that education to reduce readmission to the hospital. If the time period for data collection is hospital admissions up to 30 days after discharge, the impact of the education intervention will probably not be captured because it would take longer than 30 days to see a change in a person's health as a result of diet and close monitoring of weight. A more realistic time period would be 6 months to 2 years.

Typically, the episode of care or time period of measurement for acute care settings is the patient's stay in the hospital. Often the focus is on interventions or treatments provided while the patient is in the hospital and the associated outcomes would be those that are observable while the patient is still in the hospital. For example, if the intervention of interest was whether or not hourly rounding by nursing personnel reduces fall rates, it would not be appropriate to continue to monitor patient falls after the patient has been discharged from the hospital. The designated episode of care would be the patient's stay on the care unit where hourly rounding is being conducted.

In the ambulatory or primary care setting, the episode of care could be a visit or a series of visits to a clinic until resolution of a problem. It is also common to include episodes of hospitalization and visits to the emergency department to determine whether interventions in primary care are leading avoidance of health care like hospitalization and emergency department visits. The time frame, or episode of care, for data measurement and collection is an important concept that should be carefully considered along with the key concepts in the conceptual model.

Level of Analysis

Health care is delivered in multiple environments, at multiple levels that are integrated, at various levels, with one another. Just like defining the episode of care, careful consideration of the level of analysis should be done in consideration of the conceptual model. The person conducting the outcomes evaluation needs to determine at what level the intervention, or treatment, of interest occurs. Using the same example of hourly rounding and falls can demonstrate this concept of being able to examine variables at multiple levels. If we wanted to know whether patients who received the treatment of interest (i.e., hourly rounding) had decreased probability of falling, the level of analysis would be the patient. We would collect data at the individual patient level on whether hourly rounding was done and whether a patient experienced a fall. If instead, we wanted to know whether nursing units that conducted hourly rounds had lower fall rates, the level of analysis would be the nursing unit. The intervention of interest (i.e., hourly rounding) would be calculated at the nursing unit level (e.g., hourly rounds were done 70% of the times expected) and the outcome of interest (i.e., fall rates) would also be measured at the nursing unit level (e.g., fall rate of 3.2 falls/1,000 patient days). If we changed our question to "Do hospitals that conduct hourly rounding have significantly lower fall rates?," then the level of analysis would be at the hospital level.

OUTCOMES MEASURES: NURSING, ORGANIZATIONAL, AND PATIENT SPECIFIC

Due to the extremely large number of potential health care outcomes, it is impossible to discuss them all. Therefore, outcomes more closely related to nursing care will be discussed. Outcomes that have been associated with nursing care are often referred to as "nursing sensitive."

Nursing-Sensitive Outcomes Measures

NQF breaks their health care performance measures into three categories: patient-centered outcomes, nursing-centered intervention measures, and system-centered measures, which can be seen in Table 18.1. It is important to note that there are very few *nursing-centered intervention* measures. The only nursing intervention that NQF has designated to impact patient outcomes is *smoking-cessation counseling* (National Quality Forum, 2004).

Before NQF, the American Nurses Association (ANA) produced the Nursing Care Report Card for Acute Care in 1995, which identified, defined, and measured nursing-sensitive quality indicators (American Nurses Association, 1995). This work evolved into the National Database of Nursing Quality Indicators (NDNQI), a database with more than 1,880 hospitals currently contributing data from all 50 states (American Nurses Credentialing Center, 2013). The NDNQI structure, process, and outcome indicators are shown in Table 18.2. There are multiple indicators that are the same between NQF and NDNQI, which can be seen in Table 18.2.

TABLE 18.1 National Voluntary Consensus Standards for Nursing-Sensitive Care

FRAMEWORK CATEGORY	MEASURE	DESCRIPTION
Patient-centered outcomes measures	1. Death among surgical inpatients with treatable serious complications (failure to rescue)	Percentage of major surgical inpatients who experience a hospital-acquired complication (i.e., sepsis, pneumonia, gastrointestinal bleeding, shock/cardiac arrest, deep vein thrombosis/pulmonary embolism) and die
	2. Pressure ulcer prevalence	Percentage of inpatients who have a hospital-acquired pressure ulcer (Stage 2 or greater)
	3. Falls prevalence	Number of inpatient falls per inpatient days
	4. Falls with injury	Number of inpatient falls with injuries per inpatient days
	5. Restraint prevalence (vest and limb only)	Percentage of inpatients who have a vest or limb restraint
	6. Urinary catheter-associated urinary tract infection (UTI) for intensive care unit (ICU) patients	Rate of UTI associated with use of urinary catheters for ICU patients
	7. Central line catheter-associated blood stream infection rate for ICU and high-risk nursery (HRN) patients	Rate of blood stream infections associated with use of central line catheters for ICU and HRN patients
	8. Ventilator-associated pneumonia for ICU and HRN patients	Rate of pneumonia associated with use of ventilators for ICU patients and HRN patients
Nursing-centered intervention measures	9. Smoking-cessation counseling for acute myocardial infarction (AMI)	Percentage of AMI inpatients with history of smoking within the past year who received smoking-cessation advice or counseling during hospitalization
	10. Smoking-cessation counseling for heart failure (HF)	Percentage of HF inpatients with history of smoking within the past year who received smoking-cessation advice or counseling during hospitalization
	11. Smoking-cessation counseling for pneumonia	Percentage of pneumonia inpatients with a history of smoking within the past year who received smoking-cessation advice or counseling during hospitalization

(continued)

TABLE 18.1 National Voluntary Consensus Standards for Nursing-Sensitive Care (*continued*)

FRAMEWORK CATEGORY	MEASURE	DESCRIPTION
System-centered measures	12. Skill mix (registered nurse [RN], licensed vocational/practice nurse [LVN/LPN], unlicensed assistive personnel [UAP], and contract)	▪ Percentage of RN care hours to total nursing care hours ▪ Percentage of LVN/LPN care hours to total nursing care hours ▪ Percentage of UAP care hours to total nursing care hours ▪ Percentage of contract hours (RN, LVN/LPN, and UAP) to total nursing care hours
	13. Nursing care hours per patient day (RN, LVN/LPN, and UAP)	▪ Number of RN care hours per patient day ▪ Number of nursing care hours (RN, LVN/LPN, and UAP) per patient day
	14. Practice Environment Scale–Nursing Work Index (PES-NWI) (composite and five subscales)	Composite score and mean presence scores for each of the following subscales derived from the PES-NWI ▪ Nurse participation in hospital affairs ▪ Nursing foundations for quality of care ▪ Nurse manager ability, leadership, and support of nurses ▪ Staffing and resource adequacy ▪ Collegial nurse–physician relations
	15. Voluntary turnover	Number of voluntary uncontrolled separations during the month for RNs and advanced practice nurses, LVN/LPNs, and nurse assistants/aides

TABLE 18.2   National Database for Nursing Quality Indicators

NATIONAL DATABASE FOR NURSING QUALITY INDICATORS	NATIONAL QUALITY FORUM ENDORSED MEASURE (YES OR NO)
Structure	
Nursing hours per patient day	Yes
Nursing skill mix	Yes
Nurse turnover rate	Yes
RN education/certification	No
RN survey with:	
▪ Practice environment scale	▪ Yes
▪ Job satisfaction scales	▪ No
Process	
Pain assessment/intervention/reassessment cycles completed	No
Outcomes	
▪ Assault/injury assault rates	No
Infection measures	
▪ Catheter-associated urinary tract infection rate	▪ Yes
▪ Central line-associated blood stream infection rate	▪ Yes
▪ Ventilator-associated pneumonia rate	▪ Yes
Fall rate	Yes
Fall injury rates	Yes
Hospital/unit-acquired pressure ulcer rates	Yes—hospital-acquired pressure ulcers
Peripheral IV infiltration rate	No
Physical restraint prevalence	Yes

Organizational Outcomes Measures

The indicators outlined above can be measured, or analyzed, at multiple levels that include the nursing unit, the hospital, the hospital system, and so on, depending on the level of analysis as discussed previously. There are, however, multiple indicators that would be inappropriate to measure and compare at a more discrete level than the hospital level due to their rare occurrence. Two of those measures, mortality and failure to rescue, are discussed below.

Mortality
This outcome is frequently examined when comparing quality across hospitals. Although death is typically dichotomous: death either

occurred or it did not; mortality (death) is typically reported as a rate. Mortality is a great example of an outcome in which careful risk adjustment must be done. What often varies when examining mortality is the episode of care. In other words, the outcome may be death during hospitalization, death during a specific medical treatment, death within 30 days after discharge from a hospital, and so on.

Failure to Rescue

Failure to rescue from a medical complication, usually referred to as "failure to rescue" in the literature, is defined as death following a complication during hospitalization. This variable was developed in 1992 at a time when hospitals were often ranked according to their complication and mortality rates, which may be a disadvantage for hospitals that treat more critically ill patients (Silber, Williams, Krakauer, & Schwartz, 1992). Failure to rescue from a medical complication was developed by the researchers as a measure of health care providers' recognition of a complication and their quick response to the complication.

Failure to rescue is typically reported as a rate. The denominator is a count of the number of patients who experienced one or more complications during hospitalization. The numerator is a count of deaths that occurred in patients included in the denominator (Silber et al., 1992). For example, if 1,200 patients in a hospital experienced a complication during 1 year and 200 of those 1,200 patients died, the failure to rescue rate would be 16.7% (200/1200). Examples of complications include DVT, pneumonia, gastrointestinal (GI) bleed, and others.

Failure to rescue is an example of a health care outcome in which it is very important to pay attention to how the variable is defined or calculated. In the previous paragraphs, failure to rescue was defined as death *occurring after a complication during hospitalization*, which may seem straightforward. However, there has been variability in how failure to rescue has been operationally defined and calculated. Although the operational definition of death may be clear, definitions of *complications* have varied greatly across failure-to-rescue studies.

A number of studies have used a broader definition of *complications* in which even if there were no documented complications, a death that occurred after surgery was counted as a failure to rescue (Aiken, Clarke, Cheung, Sloane, & Silber, 2003; Aiken, Clarke, Sloane, Sochalski, & Silber, 2002; Silber et al., 1992, 2000, 2002; Silber, Rosenbaum, Schwartz, Ross, & Williams, 1995). The rationale behind this definition is that a physician had deemed a patient as healthy or well enough to survive surgery, and therefore, when a patient dies following surgery, it is believed the patient experienced a complication, even if it is not documented.

In contrast, other researchers and organizations have defined failure to rescue as death that occurs after a patient experiences one of five *complications*: pneumonia, shock or cardiac arrest, upper GI bleed, sepsis, and DVT (National Quality Forum, 2004; Needleman, Buerhaus, Mattke, Stewart, & Zelevinsky, 2002). Needleman states that this newer definition of failure to rescue was "developed as a part of a project to identify nursing sensitive measures" (Needleman & Buerhaus, 2007). The original definition essentially included all deaths after surgery, whereas this later definition greatly limits the number of complications eligible for inclusion, and therefore also limits the number of deaths included.

Additional Patient Outcomes

Quality of Life

Recognizing that it is not always the goal to prolong life at the cost of the quality of life, there are tools that measure a patient's quality of life. Quality-of-life measures continue to gain importance as the number of people living with chronic illnesses grows. People with chronic illnesses may never be "cured" and it may be unrealistic to have the same health care outcomes expectations (e.g., avoiding hospitalization, lower cost, and lower length of stay) but it is still important to measure the quality of care provided. Measuring this phenomenon is more challenging as it is such a subjective measure. Some people would say that they have a high quality of life if they were able to do nothing more than communicate with their family. For others, a high quality of life would mean being able to care for themselves independently.

There are a great number of tools available to measure quality of life. When deciding what tool to use, consider the patients or subjects being surveyed. There are tools that have been tested or validated with people of specific ages (e.g., pediatric versus adult), who speak different languages and belong to different cultures, with disease-specific conditions (Coons, Rao, Keininger, & Hays, 2000).

Patient Satisfaction

Some of the key principles when evaluating patient satisfaction tools are to examine the reliability and validity, the specific concepts the tool is measuring, and the setting and sample on which it was tested. Most studies will include these items in the study description. Keep in mind that the reliability and validity are only applicable to the setting the tool was tested in. A tool highly valid and reliable in the acute care setting may not be valid and reliable in a home care setting (Grove et al., 2013; Lin, 1996).

One of the complaints, or drawbacks, to using patient satisfaction as an outcome is the difficulty in determining what care delivery process is affecting the patient's response. For example, patients are often asked to rate their overall hospital stay. When a patient states he or she was "not satisfied," it is often impossible to know whether he or she was dissatisfied with the nursing care received or with the lack of cleanliness of the room. Although it is important for patients and families to be satisfied with the overall hospital experience, it would not be possible to make process changes from this type of aggregated information.

As stated previously in this chapter, the patient experience and perceptions of care are becoming increasingly important. The Medicare value-based purchasing program provides incentives to hospitals that achieve higher levels of patient satisfaction (U.S. Department of Health and Human Services, 2011). The Magnet Recognition Program® also calls for hospitals to demonstrate how they are outperforming their peer groups in patient satisfaction measures that are relevant to nursing care (American Nurses Credentialing Center, 2009).

SUMMARY

A large part of outcomes evaluation is ensuring quality in health care. Quality in health care continues to be a priority for providers, consumers, regulatory agencies, and the U.S. government. Quality, and outcomes measurement and evaluation, will continue to be an important issue in the United States as costs remain astoundingly high. Nurses must be able to demonstrate how the care they provide impacts patient outcomes in order to ensure that their work is valued and appropriate resources are dedicated to ensure delivery of high-quality care. Outcomes evaluation helps guide practice change to achieve desired outcomes.

SUGGESTED ACTIVITIES

1. Go to the CMS Hospital Compare website (www.medicare.gov /hospitalcompare/search.html) and compare two hospitals in your area. Based on the information presented, how would you decide in which hospital one would receive the best care?
   - Develop a conceptual model that explains part, or all, of one of the reported outcomes. Consider the episode of care as defined on the Hospital Compare website and what processes could be measured and obtained that contribute to the outcome.
2. Develop a new nursing process measure for the National Quality Forum that is important to one or more patient outcomes. Define the process measure, the data source for the measure, and the rationale for including this measure.

REFERENCES

Agency for Healthcare Research and Quality. (2013). *About us*. Retrieved February 24, 2013, from http://www.ahrq.gov/about/index.html

Aiken, L. H., Clarke, S. P., Cheung, R. B., Sloane, D. M., & Silber, J. H. (2003). Educational levels of hospital nurses and surgical patient mortality. *Journal of the American Medical Association, 290*(12), 1617–1623.

Aiken, L. H., Clarke, S. P., Sloane, D. M., Sochalski, J., & Silber, J. H. (2002). Hospital nurse staffing and patient mortality, nurse burnout, and job dissatisfaction. *Journal of the American Medical Association, 288*(16), 1987–1993.

Aiken, L. H., Havens, D. S., & Sloane, D. M. (2000a). The Magnet nursing services recognition program. *American Journal of Nursing, 100*(3), 26–35 (quiz 35-26).

Aiken, L. H., Havens, D. S., & Sloane, D. M. (2000b). Magnet nursing services recognition programme. *Nursing Standard, 14*(25), 41–47.

American Nurses Association. (1995). *Nursing care report card for acute care.* Silver Spring, MD: American Nurses Association.

American Nurses Credentialing Center. (2009). *Application manual: Magnet recognition program.* Silver Spring, MD: American Nurses Credentialing Center.

American Nurses Credentialing Center. (2013). *History of the magnet program.* Retrieved February 21, 2013, from http://www.nursecredentialing.org/MagnetHistory.aspx

Anderson, G. F., & Frogner, B. K. (2008). Health spending in OECD countries: Obtaining value per dollar. *Health Affairs, 27*(6), 1718–1727.

The Boards of Trustees, Federal Hospital Insurance and Federal Supplementary Medical Insurance Trust Funds. (2012, April 23). *2012 Annual report of the Boards of Trustees, Federal Hospital Insurance and Federal Supplementary Medical Insurance Trust Funds.* Retrieved February 21, 2013, from http://www.cms.gov/Research-Statistics-Data-and-Systems/Statistics-Trends-and-Reports/ReportsTrustFunds/Downloads/TR2012.pdf

Brown, S. J. (2002). Nursing intervention studies: A descriptive analysis of issues important to clinicians. *Research in Nursing and Health, 25*(4), 317–327.

Centers for Medicare and Medicaid. (2013). *Hospital acquired conditions.* Retrieved February 21, 2013, from http://www.cms.gov/Medicare/Medicare-Fee-for-Service-Payment/HospitalAcqCond/Hospital-Acquired_Conditions.html

Coons, S. J., Rao, S., Keininger, D. L., & Hays, R. D. (2000). A comparative review of generic quality-of-life instruments. *Pharmacoeconomics, 17*(1), 13–35.

Cowan, C. A., & Hartman, M. B. (2005). *Financing health care: Businesses, households, and governments, 1987–2003.* Retrieved March 30, 2013, from http://www.cms.gov/Research-Statistics-Data-and-Systems/Research/HealthCareFinancingReview/Downloads/Cowan2.pdf

Donabedian, A. (2005). Evaluating the quality of medical care. 1966. *Milbank Quarterly, 83*(4), 691–729.

Fleurence, R., Selby, J. V., Odom-Walker, K., Hunt, G., Meltzer, D., Slutsky, J. R., & Yancy, C. (2013). How the patient-centered outcomes research institute is engaging patients and others in shaping its research agenda. *Health Affairs, 32*(2), 393–400.

Grove, S. K., Burns, N., & Gray, J. (2013). *The practice of nursing research: Appraisal, synthesis, and generation* (7th ed.). St. Louis, MO: Elsevier Saunders.

Iezzoni, L. I. (2003). Getting started and defining terms. In L. I. Iezzoni (Ed.), *Risk adjustment for measuring health care outcomes* (3rd ed., pp. 17–32). Chicago, IL: Health Administration Press.

Institute of Medicine. (2000). *To err is human: Building a safer health system.* Washington, DC: National Academies Press.

Institute of Medicine. (2001). *Crossing the quality chasm: A new health system for the 21st century.* Washington, DC: National Academies Press.

Institute of Medicine. (2004). *Keeping patients safe: Transforming the work environment of nurses.* Washington, DC: National Academies Press.

Kane, R. L., & Radosevich, D. M. (2011). *Conducting health outcomes research.* Sudbury, MA: Jones and Bartlett.

Lin, C. C. (1996). Patient satisfaction with nursing care as an outcome variable: Dilemmas for nursing evaluation researchers. *Journal of Professional Nursing, 12*(4), 207–216.

National Quality Forum. (2004). *National voluntary consensus standards for nursing-sensitive care: An initial performance measure set.* Washington, DC: Author.

National Quality Forum. (2013). *About NQF.* Retrieved February 21, 2013, from http://www.qualityforum.org/About_NQF/About_NQF.aspx

Needleman, J., & Buerhaus, P. I. (2007). Failure-to-rescue: Comparing definitions to measure quality of care. *Medical Care, 45*(10), 913–915.

Needleman, J., Buerhaus, P., Mattke, S., Stewart, M., & Zelevinsky, K. (2002). Nurse-staffing levels and the quality of care in hospitals. *New England Journal of Medicine, 346*(22), 1715–1722.

Nolte, E., & McKee, C. M. (2008). Measuring the health of nations: Updating an earlier analysis. *Health Affairs, 27*(1), 58–71.

Patient-Centered Outcomes Research Institute. (2013). *Patient-centered outcomes research institute.* Retrieved March 3, 2013, from http://www.pcori.org

Scott, J. G., Sochalski, J., & Aiken, L. (1999). Review of magnet hospital research: Findings and implications for professional nursing practice. *Journal of Nursing Administration, 29*(1), 9–19.

Shwartz, M., & Ash, A. S. (2003). Estimating the effect of an intervention from observational data. In L. Iezzoni (Ed.), *Risk adjustment for measuring health care outcomes* (3rd ed., pp. 275–295). Chicago, IL: Health Administration Press.

Sidani, S., & Epstein, D. R. (2003). Enhancing the evaluation of nursing care effectiveness. *Canadian Journal of Nursing Research, 35*(3), 26–38.

Sidani, S., Epstein, D. R., & Moritz, P. (2003). An alternative paradigm for clinical nursing research: An exemplar. *Research in Nursing and Health, 26*(3), 224–255.

Silber, J. H., Kennedy, S. K., Even-Shoshan, O., Chen, W., Koziol, L. F., Showan, A. M., & Longnecker, D. E. (2000). Anesthesiologist direction and patient outcomes. *Anesthesiology, 93*(1), 152–163.

Silber, J. H., Kennedy, S. K., Even-Shoshan, O., Chen, W., Mosher, R. E., Showan, A. M., & Longnecker, D. E. (2002). Anesthesiologist board certification and patient outcomes. *Anesthesiology, 96*(5), 1044–1052.

Silber, J. H., Rosenbaum, P. R., Schwartz, J. S., Ross, R. N., & Williams, S. V. (1995). Evaluation of the complication rate as a measure of quality of care in coronary artery bypass graft surgery. *Journal of the American Medical Association, 274*(4), 317–323.

Silber, J. H., Williams, S. V., Krakauer, H., & Schwartz, J. S. (1992). Hospital and patient characteristics associated with death after surgery. A study of adverse occurrence and failure to rescue. *Medical Care, 30*(7), 615–629.

Smith, M. A., Nitz, N. M., & Stuart, S. K. (2006). Severity and comorbidity. In R. L. Kane (Ed.), *Understanding health care outcomes research* (2nd ed.). Boston, MA: Jones and Bartlett.

Strickland, O. L. (1997). Challenges in measuring patient outcomes. *Nursing Clinics of North America, 32*(3), 495–512.

Titler, M., Dochterman, J., & Reed, D. (2004). *Guideline for conducting effectiveness research in nursing and other health services.* Iowa City, IA: The University of Iowa, College of Nursing, Center for Nursing Classification & Clinical Effectiveness.

U.S. Department of Health and Human Services. (2011). *Administration implements new health reform provision to improve care quality, lower costs.* Retrieved February 24, 2013, from http://www.healthcare.gov/news/factsheets/2011/04/valuebasedpurchasing04292011a.html

U.S. Department of Health and Human Services. (2013). Hospital compare. Retrieved February 24, 2013, from http://www.medicare.gov/hospital compare/search.html

Whittemore, R., & Grey, M. (2002). The systematic development of nursing interventions. *Journal of Nursing Scholarship, 34*(2), 115–120.

19

Ethical Aspects of a Study

Marcia Phillips, Julie Johnson Zerwic,
and Marquis D. Foreman

The process of obtaining approval to conduct a research study varies among clinical settings. Many organizations now favor a *nursing research committee* (Fowler, Leaton, Baxter, McTigue, & Snook, 2008; Kirchhoff & McGuire, 1985) that promotes the integration and acculturation of evidence-based practice generating nursing research. The research proposals are then submitted to the *institutional review board* (IRB) or the hospital research committee to examine issues related to the protection of subjects from the risks of participating in research. At institutions without a nursing research committee, research proposals go directly to the IRB for review with all of the other research protocols.

REVIEW COMMITTEES

Whether a nursing research committee or an IRB exists, the research investigator must also consider the following:

- *Frequency of the committee meetings.* Some organizations schedule meetings on an as-needed basis if the volume of clinical studies is small. If both a nursing research committee and an IRB exist, the institution's policies state whether a proposal for review can be submitted to both simultaneously or whether one must approve the proposal before it can be submitted to the other for review. It is important to know the structure and timeline of your institution's review process so that the investigator can factor this into the timeline of his or her study.

- *Composition of the review committees.* It cannot be assumed that all review committees include a member who is familiar with nursing research. Therefore, it is important to write the proposal for readers who may not have expertise in that particular content area and may not be familiar with nursing research.
- *The presence of site-specific idiosyncrasies.* Some institutions require that an employee or physician be listed as principal investigator (PI) in a submission. This may require that the researcher set up collaborations in advance. Institutional review boards require the PI and other research team members to complete initial training in research ethics before a protocol can be submitted. The Collaborative Institutional Training Initiative (CITI) provides online training for participating institutions and may be transferable. Although these issues may seem trivial, such things can delay the process of approval while the committees seek additional information. By dealing directly and proactively with these issues, the investigator establishes credibility and demonstrates professionalism.

Nursing Research Committees

Nursing research committees were initiated for the review of (a) scientific merit of a proposal for which an investigator is seeking support from nursing services and (b) the nature and magnitude of the resources required of nursing services to implement the proposed research.

The nature and magnitude of resource consumption can range from minimal (e.g., a request merely to access subjects for the study) to significant (e.g., an expectation that nursing staff will both implement various elements of an intervention and collect data regarding the feasibility and efficacy of the intervention).

Nursing research committees should be composed of members who have sufficient education and training in research to be able to examine the scientific merit of the study. Many institutions have PhD-prepared nurses lead these committees. A goal of these committees would be to advance nursing science and, where possible, provide the research team with feedback that will improve the study.

Institutional Review Boards

IRBs, also called human subject review committees, exist to provide fair and impartial review of research proposals and are responsible for the critical oversight of the research conducted on human subjects to protect them from any unnecessary risks associated with participation in research. In the United States, the Food and Drug Administration (FDA) and Department of Health and Human Services (specifically Office for Human Research Protections [OHRP]) regulations have empowered federally funded IRBs to approve, modify planned research prior to approval, or disapprove research. Institutions may not have a formal review structure if they do not receive federal funding, are small, or produce a limited volume of research. However, they can negotiate an agreement with a larger institution or external review committee to provide the required oversight.

In organizations in which a large volume of research is conducted, there may be more than one IRB (e.g., biomedical committee, a social-behavioral committee, and a biobehavorial committee). In the absence of federal funding and a formal review structure, the review may be done informally by an administrator of the institution. However, in this instance, the investigator should obtain a review from an external human subjects committee to document that the researcher has adhered to federal guidelines concerning the protection of human subjects from risk. Several independent IRBs can be found on the Internet. Having approval from some type of IRB may be a journal or organizational requirement for publication of the results.

Guidelines for Review

IRBs usually have a set of guidelines or principles that govern their procedures and reviews. Institutions that receive federal funding must follow 45 CFR 46. This section of the Code of Federal Regulations can be obtained at www.hhs.gov/ohrp/humansubjects/guidance/45cfr46.html.

Some small IRBs may use the principles set forth in the Belmont report, which can be accessed at www.hhs.gov/ohrp/humansubjects /guidance/belmont.html. International review committees tend to use principles from the World Medical Association codified in the Declaration of Helsinki, found at http://history.nih.gov/research/downloads/helsinki .pdf.

Federal code stipulates the composition of the IRB (U.S. Department of Health and Human Services, 2009). An IRB must consist of a minimum of five members with varying backgrounds to ensure a complete and adequate review of the research activities commonly conducted by the institution. Furthermore, by regulation, an IRB may not consist entirely of members of one profession, gender, or racial group. Collectively, the IRB must be sufficiently qualified through the experience and expertise of its membership to have knowledge of and sensitivity to prevailing attitudes. If the particular IRB routinely reviews research involving vulnerable subjects, then the composition of the board must include one or more individuals knowledgeable about and experienced working with these vulnerable populations. Also, the IRB must include at least one member whose primary concerns are in non-scientific areas and one who is not otherwise affiliated with the institution. One of the members should be able to discuss issues emanating from the perspective of the community and its values. No IRB member shall participate in the review if that person has a conflict of interest affiliated with the project. Lastly, an IRB may invite additional individuals with special areas of expertise to participate in the review and discussion of research proposals to enable the IRB to fulfill its purpose. Please see the regulations at 45 CFR 46.107 for complete information on all of the required qualifications to properly compose an IRB.

Jurisdiction of an IRB

The jurisdiction of an IRB is determined by answering two fundamental questions: "Is the activity research?" and "Does the activity involve human subjects?" For health care professionals, the first question may not be so easily answered because the distinction between research and therapy is not always readily apparent. Federal policy defines research as a "systematic investigation, including research development, testing and evaluation designed to develop or contribute to generalized knowledge" (U.S. Department of Health and Human Services, 2009, 45 CFR 46.105[d]). Furthermore, research itself is not inherently therapeutic in that the therapeutic benefits of experimental interventions are unknown or may prove to be ineffective (Office for Human Research Protections, 1993, pp. 1–3). If the focus of the proposed activity is currently accepted as standardized methods of care or if the research addresses institutional or patient-specific case issues, then the activity is generally not considered research and consequently does not require IRB reporting and review. However, if there is any uncertainty as to whether the activity is research, the activity should be treated as research and reported to the IRB. An activity is research if the answers to the following two questions are "yes": "Does the activity employ a systematic approach involving predetermined methods for studying a specific topic, answering a specific question, testing a specific hypothesis, or developing a theory?" and "Is the activity intended to contribute to generalizable knowledge by extending the results (e.g., publication of presentation) beyond a single individual or internal unit?" (45CFR 46.102 [d]).

There is one caveat. If the activity is to be disseminated (i.e., reported in a publication or presentation), the general practice is to consider the activity research and report it to the IRB. An activity that causes great confusion as to whether or not it constitutes research is continuous quality improvement. Quality improvement is considered an essential component of responsible professional health care (Cretin et al., 2000) and a means for improving the processes, efficiencies, safety, and quality of care while preventing substandard care (Bellin & Dubler, 2001; Casarett, Karlawish, & Sugarman, 2000; Johnson, Vermeulen, & Smith, 2006). However, quality-improvement activities frequently consist of methods traditionally associated with randomized clinical trials, blurring the distinction between quality-improvement activities and research (Johnson et al., 2006). Some observers suggest that all activities should be reviewed by the IRB to ensure that the activity, research, or quality improvement does not compromise patient autonomy or safety (Bellin & Dubler, 2001; Miller & Emanuel, 2008). Those who advocate the review of all activities contend that once the activity receives IRB approval, it is sanctioned, thereby ensuring all that the activity complies with commonly accepted ethical practices and involves a minimal level of risk for all participating parties, the human subjects, investigators, and the institution. However, many in the health care community believe that review of all activities would stall the research enterprise (e.g., Casarett et al., 2000; Johnson et al., 2006). According to Johnson et al. (2006), if any of the following apply to the activity, it should be considered research and submitted to the IRB for review:

- Results are to be disseminated
- Results contribute to generalized knowledge
- Conditions are systematically assigned to patients
- Conditions are other than a standard of care
- Risks of participation exceed those of usual care
- Information collected goes beyond routine patient care
- Personal health information will be sent outside institution
- Risks to privacy and confidentiality exist

Only if all of these points do not apply should the activity be considered quality improvement.

Once the activity has been deemed research, the investigator should ask whether the research activity involves human subjects. A human subject is a living individual about whom an investigator obtains data through intervention or interaction with the individual or obtains identifiable private information (45 CFR 46 102(f)). For example, an investigator whose research activities involve accessing health records of only patients who have died is not conducting research with human subjects.

LEVELS OF REVIEW

Once it has been established that the activity falls within the jurisdiction of the IRB, the level of IRB reporting and review must be identified. There are three levels of review, determined on the basis of the degree of risks inherent in the proposed research. Risk is defined by federal policy as "the probability of harm or injury (physical, psychological, social or economic) occurring as a result of participation in research. Both the probability and magnitude of risk can vary from minimal to significant" (Office for Human Research Protections, 1993, pp. 1–3). The three levels of review are exempt, expedited, and full. It is important to determine which level of review is required because the extent of information required, the forms to be completed, and the time necessary for the review are determined by the type of review. For any questions about the level of review or the submission process you should consult your IRB.

Exempt From Review

Research activities that are *exempt* from review by the IRB are those that pose no risks to subjects, have no means by which a subject can be identified, and use human subjects who are capable of freely consenting to participate (U.S. Department of Health & Human Services, 2009). Even though a research activity falls into the exempt category, it still must be submitted to the IRB for affirmation. Examples of activities that are exempt from review are listed in Exhibit 19.1.

Copies of surveys, interview guides, or questionnaires and the exact introductory remarks and consent forms to be used must be submitted. If advertisements for subjects are used, copies of the text for the planned advertisement must also be submitted. Although these materials are not formally reviewed in the committee, a member of

---

Exhibit 19.1
Research Activities Exempt From 45 CFR 46

A. Research conducted in established or commonly accepted educational settings, involving normal educational practices, such as
   1. research on regular and special education instructional strategies, or
   2. research on the effectiveness of or the comparison among instructional techniques, curricula, or classroom management methods.

B. Research involving the use of educational tests (cognitive, diagnostic, aptitude, achievement), survey procedures, interview procedures, or observation of public behavior, unless:
   1. information obtained is recorded in such a manner that human subjects can be identified, directly or through identifiers linked to the subjects; and
   2. any disclosure of the human subjects' responses outside the research could reasonably place the subjects at risk of

criminal or civil liability or be damaging to the subjects' financial standing, employability, or reputation.

C. Research involving the use of educational tests (cognitive, diagnostic, aptitude, achievement), survey procedures, interview procedures, or observation of public behavior that is not exempt above, if:
  1. the human subjects are elected or appointed public officials or candidates for public office; or
  2. federal statute(s) require(s) without exception that the confidentiality of the personally identifiable information will be maintained throughout the research and thereafter.

D. Research involving the collection or study of existing data, documents, records, pathological specimens, or diagnostic specimens, if these sources are publicly available or if the information is recorded in such a manner that subjects cannot be identified, directly or through identifiers linked to the subjects.

E. Research and demonstration projects that are conducted by or subject to the approval of department or agency heads, and that are designed to study, evaluate, or otherwise examine:
  1. public benefit or service programs;
  2. procedures for obtaining benefits or services under those programs;
  3. possible changes in or alternatives to those programs or procedures; or
  4. possible changes in methods or levels of payment for benefits or services under those programs.

F. Taste and food-quality evaluation and consumer acceptance studies:
  1. if wholesome food without additives is consumed or
  2. if food is consumed that contains an ingredient at or below the level and for a use found to be safe, or agricultural chemical or environmental contaminant at or below the level found to be safe, by the Food and Drug Administration or approved by the Environmental Protection Agency or the Food Safety and Inspection Service of the U.S. Department of Agriculture.

Adapted from U.S. Department of Health and Human Services (2009).

the IRB will assess the materials to verify that the activity meets the stipulations for exemption. This verification usually requires a few days (but may take a few weeks), after which the investigator receives a document from the IRB indicating the exact criteria used to judge whether the activity does or does not meet the requirements for an exemption. If the initial assessment determines that the activity does not fulfill the requirements for exemption, the investigator may be asked to submit an additional justification or the appropriate materials for an expedited review.

Expedited Review

There are two types of activities that receive an expedited review:

1. Activities that pose no more than a minimal risk to subjects for participation in the activity. Minimal risk is defined as "a risk where the probability and magnitude of harm or discomfort in the proposed research are not greater, in and of themselves, than those ordinarily encountered in daily life or during the performance of routine physical or psychological examinations or tests" (U.S. Department of Health and Human Services, 2009, 45 CFR 46.102[i]). If the risks are greater than minimal and if precautions, safeguards, or alternatives cannot be incorporated into the research activity to minimize the risks to such a level, then a full review is required.
2. Activities requiring minor changes in previously approved research, during the period for which approval is authorized (1 year or less) (U.S. Department of Health and Human Services, 2009, 45 CFR 46.110[b]).

Activities that are considered within the exempt category but that provide a means by which the individual subjects can be identified must be reviewed at the expedited level because of the potential risk resulting from loss of anonymity and confidentiality. Materials required for an expedited review generally consist of an abbreviated research protocol that presents the objectives, methods, subject selections, criteria, theoretical or potential risks and benefits, precautions and safeguards, and a sample of the informed consent. The proposal may be reviewed by a member of the IRB.

As with all levels of review, the investigator receives a document from the IRB, indicating the exact criteria used to determine that the activity fulfills the requirements for an expedited review. If the initial assessment determines that the activity does not fulfill the requirements, the investigator may be asked for justification or to submit the appropriate materials for a full review. Federal policy requires that all members of the IRB be advised of all proposals that have been approved under the expedited review process (U.S. Department of Health and Human Services, 2009, 45 CFR 46.110[c]).

Full Review

A full review of any proposed research activity involving human subjects must occur in all other situations, such as those in which participation in the activity poses greater than minimal risk, those for which the subject cannot freely consent, and those involving vulnerable populations as subjects. Materials required for a full review are identical to those required for an expedited review. It is the review process that differs. A full review requires at least 1 month from the submission of materials to the notification of the disposition of the proposal. The proposal is reviewed by at least three members of the IRB. (A member cannot participate in the discussion and determination of disposition of a project in which the member is an investigator. In such cases, the investigator member must be absent from the discussion and this absence must be reflected in the minutes of the meeting.)

The review of the proposed research activity, which is to focus on the aspects listed in Exhibit 19.2 and Exhibit 19.3, must occur at a convened meeting at which a majority of the members of the IRB are

---

Exhibit 19.2

Criteria for IRB Approval of Research

All of the following requirements must be satisfied for approval of research.

1. Risks to subjects are minimized.
2. Risks to subjects are reasonable in relation to anticipated benefits.
3. Selection of subjects is equitable.
4. Informed consent is sought to the extent required.
5. Informed consent is documented.
6. There is adequate provision for monitoring the data collected to ensure the safety of subjects.
7. There are adequate provisions to protect the privacy of subjects and to maintain the confidentiality of data.
8. If any subject is vulnerable to coercion or undue influence, for example, children, prisoners, pregnant women, mentally disabled persons, or economically or educationally disadvantaged persons, additional safeguards have been included in the study to protect the rights and welfare of these subjects.

Adapted from U.S. Department of Health and Human Services (2009).

Exhibit 19.3
Basic Institutional Review Board Review

In the review of research proposals, the members of the IRB must follow the guidelines listed below:

1. Identify the risks associated with participation in the research.
2. Determine that the risks will be minimized to the extent possible.
3. Identify the probable benefits to be derived from the research.
4. Determine that the risks are reasonable in relation to the benefits to the subjects and the importance of the knowledge to be gained.
5. Ensure that potential subjects will be adequately informed as to the risks or discomforts and anticipated benefits.
6. Determine the intervals for periodic review.
7. Determine the adequacy of the provisions to protect privacy and maintain confidentiality of the data.
8. In the case of vulnerable population, determine that appropriate additional safeguards are in place to protect their rights and welfare.

Adapted from U.S. Department of Health and Human Services (2009).

present. The impartial review conducted by the IRB typically focuses on the mechanisms within the proposed research by which the subjects are safeguarded or protected from any undue risks of participation, and the process and content of informed consent, that is, the ethics of the research. However, scrutiny of the research methodology also falls within the purview of the IRB because research that is poorly designed could identify and expose the subjects, the investigator, and the institution to unnecessary risks. Although a proposal may be deemed ethically sound, if it is methodologically unsound, the IRB must disapprove the application. For proposed research to be approved, it must receive the approval of a majority of those members present at the meeting (U.S. Department of Health and Human Services, 2009, 45 CFR 46.108[b]).

A research proposal must receive approval from the IRB before the collection of data can be initiated. Once permission has been granted by the IRB, the researcher is obligated to conduct the study as proposed. Any changes or alterations to the IRB-approved research must be reviewed and approved by the IRB before proceeding with the changes. For example, if the investigator wants to enroll more subjects than originally requested, this step needs to be approved in advance. The IRB defines a subject as anyone who has consented even if the individual did not participate in research activities. Any changes in the method of recruitment or changes in questionnaires must also receive IRB approval. Investigators are required to provide at least an annual progress report (see Exhibit 19.4). The IRB may require more frequent progress reports for high-risk protocols. Also, any increased risks or unforeseen problems should be reported to the IRB immediately. The individual study participants' data should not be identifiable. Protected health information is listed in Exhibit 19.5 (U.S. Department of Health and Human Services, 2004).

Exhibit 19.4
Elements of a Periodic Review

Periodic reviews of research should include:

1. Any amendment to the currently approved research (e.g., the addition of research personnel, or a change in funding, research protocol, consent documents, Health Insurance Portability and Accountability Act [HIPPA] authorization, or any other change to the research)
2. Preliminary results, especially those that might suggest one intervention is better or worse than the other with respect to risks, benefits, alternatives, or willingness to participate
3. Subject enrollment and demographics
4. Information about any subject complaints, refusals or withdrawals from participation, and safety
5. Reportable events (e.g., study-related adverse events) and protocol violations
6. Review by other IRBs
7. Suspension of research activity
8. Presentations and publications
9. Conflicts of interest

Note: Periodic reviews are mandatory for all ongoing studies; the intervals between the reevaluations are to be appropriate to the degree of risk but are to take place not less than once a year (IRB guidebook).

Adapted from U.S. Department of Health and Human Services (2009).

Exhibit 19.5
Protected Health Information

1. Names
2. Any geographic subdivision smaller than a state (including street names, city, county, precinct, ZIP code)
3. Any element of dates directly related to an individual (e.g., birth date, admission date, date of death)
4. Telephone numbers
5. Facsimile numbers
6. Electronic mail addresses
7. Social Security numbers
8. Medical record numbers
9. Health plan beneficiary numbers
10. Account numbers
11. Certificate/license numbers
12. Vehicle identifiers
13. Device identifiers
14. Web universal resource locators (URLs)
15. Internet protocol (IP) address numbers
16. Biometric identifiers (e.g., fingerprints and voiceprints)
17. Full-face photographic images
18. Any other unique identifying number, characteristic, or code

Adapted from U.S. Department of Health and Human Services (2004).

Informed Consent

Informed consent is one of the primary ethical requirements related to research with human subjects. It reflects the basic principle of *respect for persons*. Informed consent ensures that prospective human subjects have a clear understanding of the nature of the research and can knowledgably and *voluntarily* decide whether to participate in the research being proposed. "Voluntary" is defined as acting of one's own free will. The process of providing informed consent is not a distinct moment in time at which the subject simply signs a form. It is an ongoing educational process between the investigator and the subject. Consequently, informed, voluntary participation of the subject should be verified at every interaction between the investigator or a representative of the research team and the subject. Because of the nature and complexity of some studies (e.g., longitudinal, multiphase studies), informed consent may be required for various phases of the study.

Although some IRBs require the use of standardized format for consent procedures, modifications are usually permitted as long as the process provides for full disclosure, adequate comprehension, and voluntary choice—elements easy to enumerate but not so easy to achieve (see Exhibit 19.6) (U.S. Department of Health and Human Services, 2009). Usually any element may be omitted that is not relevant to the study. However, a statement that the subject understands what will occur as a result of his or her participation in the study and affirming that the subject freely agrees to participate must be included at the end of the form, followed by a place for the subject's and witness' signatures and date (see Exhibit 19.7). When a parent or guardian signs for a subject, the subject's name should be clearly identified, as should the signatory's relationship to the subject. If the research is complex or poses a significant risk, the IRB may encourage the investigator to develop a "patient information sheet" that presents the information from the formal consent form in simple, unambiguous language that is devoid of all "legalese." Copies of the consent and information sheets are given to the subject, and the investigator should retain the originals for at least 5 years. Guidelines for developing a consent form as well as sample consents can usually be obtained from the IRB.

When the research involves a vulnerable population, there is a greater challenge for consenting. Vulnerable populations are those that may lack knowledge or understanding (i.e., children, pregnant women, fetuses, mentally impaired or seriously ill persons, and economically or educationally disadvantaged individuals). These populations may require special protection and abide by different guidelines. It is important that investigators working with these populations become familiar with subparts B, C, and D of 45 CFR 46 (see U.S. Department of Health and Human Services, 2009, 45 CFR 46.201Sub B, C & D).

Few circumstances allow for the waiver of consent. Situations in which waivers may be approved include the following: (a) the research involves no more than minimal risks to subjects; (b) the waiver or alteration will not adversely affect the rights and welfare of the subjects; (c) the research cannot practically be carried out without the waiver or alteration; and (d) whenever appropriate, the subjects will be provided with additional pertinent information after they have participated (U.S. Department of Health and Human Services, 2009, 45 CFR 46.116[d]). An example of a situation in which a waiver of consent is granted is a study that uses only data that have been previously collected for nonresearch purposes, such as the medical record. The investigator must demonstrate that it would not be practicable to go back and obtain consent from the individuals whose records are to be used. It may be the case that a large number of individuals cannot be reached because their contact information has changed, because the patients are no longer affiliated with the medical center, or because they are deceased.

Exhibit 19.6
General Requirements for Informed Consent

In seeking informed consent the following information shall be provided to each subject:

1. A statement that the study involves research, including an explanation of the purposes, expected duration and procedures, especially if they are experimental
2. A description of any reasonably foreseeable risks or discomforts to the subject
3. A description of any benefits to the subject or to others that may reasonably be expected from the research
4. Disclosure of appropriate alternative procedures or course of treatment that might be advantageous to the subject
5. A description of how confidentiality of records will be maintained
6. If research is greater than minimal risk, a description of compensation for participation and what is to occur with injury from participation
7. An explanation with contact information for persons who can provide additional information regarding questions about the research and research subjects' rights, and research-related injury
8. A statement that participation is voluntary and that refusal has no consequent penalties or loss of benefits to which the subject is otherwise entitled
9. Additional elements when appropriate:
   a. Acknowledgment if procedure may involve currently unforeseeable risks to the subject, or to the embryo or fetus, *if* the subject is or may become pregnant
   b. Circumstances under which the subject's participation may be terminated by the investigator without regard to the subject's consent
   c. Additional costs to the subject from participation in the research
   d. Consequences of withdrawal and procedures for orderly termination of participation
   e. Provision of new information that may influence the subject's willingness to continue to participate
   f. The approximate number of subjects involved in the research

Adapted from U.S. Department of Health and Human Services (2009).

Exhibit 19.7
A Sample Consent Form

You are being asked to be a subject in research under the direction of Dr. _____, a professor in the College of Nursing at the University of _____. Many older patients get confused while in the hospital. This confusion can affect their recovery from illness. Although you are not now confused, confusion may occur while you are in the hospital. You are being told about this research and may be able to take part because of your current illness and hospitalization. Before you agree to be in this research, please read this form. Your participation is completely voluntary. Your decision will not affect your relations with the university, your physicians, the hospital staff, or your care. If you decide to participate, you are free to quit at any time.

The purpose of the research is to study the effects of confusion on the health of older patients who are in the hospital. Approximately 720 patients may take part in this research. We are interested in looking at the effects of confusion on bathing and eating; memory and thinking; the use of health care services; and the severity, length, and return of any confusion.

If you agree to take part, I, or another member of the research team, will visit you daily while you are in the hospital to ask you questions about your thinking and your ability to perform daily activities. The first interview will last about 20 minutes. All other daily visits will last about 10 minutes. These visits will be scheduled at a time that is convenient for you and your care. Each day, we would like to review your hospital record to obtain information about your care, medications, and any tests and their results. We would also like your permission to talk with a relative, friend, or caregiver about your recent illness. When you leave the hospital, we would like to get a copy of your hospital bill.

The risks of being in this research include possible inconvenience of interviews and possible breach of privacy and confidentiality.

There is no direct benefit to you. This research will not help in your current care or treatment. We hope that what we learn from this research will help to improve the care to patients like you in the future.

(continued)

(*continued*)

If you decide to take part, we will be careful to keep all information about you strictly confidential. Only members of the research team will have access to this information. All information about you will be kept under lock and key in the research office of Dr. _____. When results are published or discussed, no information will reveal your identity.

There is no payment for your participation.

You may ask questions now. If you have questions later, you may contact Dr. _____ at XXX.XXX.XXXX or by e-mail at _____.

If you have questions about your rights as a research subject, you can call the Office for Protection of Research Subjects at the _____ at XXX.XXX.XXXX.

Your participation in this research is entirely voluntary. Your decision will not affect your care. You can refuse to answer any question or stop answering altogether. You can quit the research at any time without consequences of any kind. You will be given a copy of this form for your information and to keep for your records.

I have read (or someone else has read to me) the above information. I have been given a chance to ask questions, and my questions have been answered to my satisfaction. I have been given a copy of this form.

Signature of the Researcher _____

Date _____

For individuals experiencing health emergencies, there is a provision by the Federal Drug Administration (FDA) and the Department of health and Human Services (DHHS) that allows emergency research to proceed without voluntary prospective informed consent by the patient (21 CFR 50.24). However, these health emergencies must render the patient incapable of providing informed consent. Examples of such health emergencies include patients who are experiencing life-threatening illnesses or trauma and those requiring resuscitation in which research is clearly necessary to identify safe and effective therapies (Sugarman, 2007). These health emergencies may occur out of the hospital or in the emergency department or intensive-care unit.

According to 21 CFR 50.24, "Exception from informed consent requirements for emergency research" (FDA, 2007), requires that the potential subject must be in a life-threatening situation and current treatments must be either unproven or unsatisfactory. Obtaining informed consent is not feasible, because the subject is unable to consent as a result of the health emergency, a surrogate is not readily available, and there is a limited window of opportunity to intervene. Participation may provide direct benefit to the subject, and the project must have been prospectively reviewed and approved with waiver of consent by an IRB. Additional protections of the rights and welfare of the subjects also must be ensured; for example, either the patient or his or her surrogate must provide informed consent as soon as practicable (21 CFR 50.24). However, research in which participation does not hold the potential for "therapeutic benefit" continues to require informed consent of either the patient or a legal surrogate (Chen, Meschia, Brott, Brown, & Worral for the SWISS Investigators, 2008).

At the end of subject recruitment as approved by the IRB, the researcher may need to complete a form telling the IRB how many subjects were taken in, any adverse events that occurred, when the data collection ended, and when the study will conclude with IRB supervision. The de-identification of the data may be considered the last step in reporting, required by the IRB.

RESEARCH MISCONDUCT

Research misconduct occurs when a researcher fabricates or falsifies data and/or the results, or plagiarizes information within a research report (42 CFR Parts 50 & 93). The misconduct must be committed intentionally, knowingly, or recklessly and the allegation must be proven with sufficient evidence. Research misconduct does not include honest error or differences of opinion. All institutions that receive Public Health Service (PHS) funding are required to have written policies and procedures for addressing any allegations of the misconduct. Research misconduct involving National Institutes of Health (NIH) awards ultimately falls under the authority of Office of Research Integrity (ORI), which has specific procedures to handle allegations of the misconduct.

An individual found guilty of misconduct can lose federal funding, be restricted to supervised research, or even lose his or her job. One may also be required to submit a correction or retraction of published articles. Thorough investigation of an allegation is extremely important considering the serious penalty that can be inflicted.

An excellent resource for further reading on research conduct is available at http://ori.hhs.gov/documents/rcrintro.pdf.

SUMMARY

Obtaining ethical review and approval of a study is an essential preliminary step for conducting research. It can consume large amounts of time and provide numerous opportunities for success or failure. The recommendations offered are intended to facilitate development of a partnership in pursuing knowledge that results in a positive research experience for all, as well as the successful completion of the research.

SUGESTED ACTIVITIES

Persons who sustain a mild brain injury (MTBI) have been reported to experience difficulties with memory. It has been reported in the literature that using a handheld personal digital assistant (PDA) might help persons with MTBI with their memory. On the basis of your review of the literature, you decide to recruit participants for a study. Participants will be randomly assigned to times when they are scheduled to call a research voicemail. A 2-week predetermined call schedule will be assigned to each participant. Half of the participants will use a PDA as a reminder, and half will not.

Before conducting the study, you are required to obtain IRB approval.

1. Acquire and complete the IRB forms at your institution.
2. Write an informed consent form for potential participants to complete.
3. Write a script that will be used when recruiting a participant.

REFERENCES

Bellin, E., & Dubler, N. N. (2001). The quality improvement–research divide and the need for external oversight. *American Journal of Public Health, 91*(9), 1512–1517.

Casarett, D., Karlawish, J. H. T., & Sugarman, J. (2000). Determining when quality improvement initiatives should be considered research. *Journal of the American Medical Association, 283*(17), 2275–2280.

Chen, D. T., Meschia, J. F., Brott, T. G., Brown, R. D., & Worrall, B. B., for the SWISS Investigators. (2008). Stroke genetic research with adults with impaired decision-making capacity. A survey of IRB and investigator practices. *Stroke, 39*, 2732–2735.

Cretin, S., Keeler, E. B., Lynn, J., Batalden, P. B., Berwick, D. M., & Bisognano, M. (2000). Should patients in quality-improvement activities have the same protections as participants in research studies? [Letter]. *Journal of the American Medical Association, 284*(14), 1786.

Fowler, S., Leaton, M. B., Baxter, T., McTigue, T., & Snook, N. (2008). Evolution of nursing research committees. *Journal of Neuroscience Nursing, 40*(1), 60–63.

Johnson, N., Vermeulen, L., & Smith, K. M. (2006). A survey of academic medical centers to distinguish quality improvement and research activities. *Quality Management and Health Care, 15*(4), 215–220.

Kirchhoff, K. T., & McGuire, D. B. (1985). The nursing review process in a clinical setting. *Journal of Professional Nursing, 1,* 311.

Miller, F. G., & Emanuel, E. J. (2008). Quality-improvement research and informed consent. *New England Journal of Medicine, 358*(8), 765–767.

Office for Human Research Protections (OHRP). (1993). *National Institutes of Health: Protecting human research subjects: Institutional Review Board Guidebook.* Retrieved January 11, 2013, from http://www.hhs.gov/ohrp /archive/irb/irb-guidebook.htm

Sugarman, J. (2007). Examining the provisions for research without consent in the emergency setting. *Hastings Center Report, 37*(1), 12–13.

U.S. Department of Health and Human Services. (2004). *Protecting personal health information in research: Understanding the HIPAA privacy rule* (revised July 13, 2004). Retrieved January 11, 2013, from http://www.priva cyruleandresearch.nih.gov/pr_02.asp

U.S. Department of Health and Human Services. (2009). Protection of human subjects: Title 45, Code of Federal Regulations, Part 46 (revised January 15, 2009). Washington, DC: Office of Protection from Research Risks. Retrieved January 11, 2013, from www.hhs.gov/ohrp/policy/ohrpregulations.pdf

U.S. Food and Drug Administration. (2007). *Exception from informed consent requirements for emergency research. 21 CFR 50.24.* Retrieved January 11, 2013 from, http://www.fda.gov/RegulatoryInformation/Guidance/ucm126482.htm

WEB RESOURCES

General Resources

Office for Human Research Protections (OHRP): http://www.ohrp/index.html

Office for Human Research Protections (OHRP) *IRB guidebook*: http://www .hhs.gov/ohrp/archive/irb/irb_guidebook.htm

U.S. Department of Veterans Affairs, Human Subjects Protection: http://www .va.gov/oro/Human_Subjects_Protection.asp

U.S. Food and Drug Administration, Guidance, Compliance and Regulatory Information: http://www.fda.gov/drugs/guidancecomplianceregulatoryin formation/default.htm

For Information About the Registration of Clinical Trials

"Is this clinical trial fully registered?": http://www.icmje.org/update_may05.html

FDAAA 801 requirements: http://www.clinicaltrials.gov/ct2/manage-recs/fdaaa

Guidance on public law 110-85 enacted to expand the scope of clinicaltrials .gov registration: http://grants.nih.gov/grants/guide/notice-files/not-od-08-014 .html

Registration of clinical trials as required by Public Law 110-85, Title V: http:// www.clinicaltrials.gov

For Online Ethics Training

Collaborative Institutional Training Initiative (CITI): https://www.citiprogram.org

20

Communicating Research Through Oral Presentations

Diane L. Stuenkel

The dissemination of research findings is a key step in the translational research continuum (Grady, 2010) and provides the foundation for nursing's evidence-based practice. Clearly and concisely communicating information about a completed study or a study in progress is vital to the growth of the profession's body of evidence. As the profession moves toward increasing the numbers of doctorally prepared nurses (American Association of Colleges of Nursing, 2012), it will be imperative for advanced practice nurses (APNs) to disseminate research findings in order to transform patient care. Numerous opportunities to share research exist, including oral presentations in the clinical setting, events sponsored by an organization, poster or podium sessions at conferences, use of Internet sites, and via traditional and social media. The growing availability of technology such as webcasting, broadcasting, and blogging has led to the expedited dissemination of information, thereby reaching a larger and varied audience quickly.

PREPARING THE PRESENTATION

Ideally, dissemination of a study's findings is considered during the planning phase of the study. The Agency for Healthcare Research and Quality (AHRQ) has a guideline for planning one's dissemination of research results (www.ahrq.gov/qual/advances/planningtool.htm). This guideline may assist researchers to think through their dissemination plans and suggest appropriate modes and venues for sharing findings early in the research process. An initial step is identifying opportunities for presentations at research, clinical, or educational conferences. Conference sponsors solicit presenters by announcing a call for papers or call for abstracts. Reviewing the conference focus to determine whether your study fits the focus of the conference is crucial. An abstract topic that is timely, congruent with conference objectives, and aligns with the interests of the anticipated target audience, will have a greater likelihood of being accepted for presentation. After determining that your study is a good fit, carefully review the detailed requirements for submitting an abstract as outlined in the conference brochure or online.

Abstracts of completed research usually are considered for oral or poster presentations. Research in progress is considered only for a poster session. The abstract, typically 200 to 500 words in length, is used by reviewers to determine the worthiness of a study. Thus, it is imperative that submission guidelines are followed precisely. Most guidelines for research abstracts require the inclusion of these major aspects of the study (Burns & Grove, 2011):

1. Title—should include key variables, participants, and setting
2. Purpose of the study
3. Brief description of sample—number of subjects and distinct characteristics such as diagnosis, age range, and gender
4. Methods—design of the study; setting; procedure for collecting data; instruments, including reliability and validity information
5. Findings—data and significant statistical (level of significance) or clinical differences
6. Conclusions—summary of the results in relation to the purpose of the study and meaning of the data

In addition, an organization may require a brief author biography. Criteria used to evaluate abstracts may include originality, scientific merit, clinical relevance, soundness of findings, overall quality, relevance to conference theme and objectives, and clarity (for examples of abstract submission guidelines and criteria, see the International Council of Nursing's website at www.icn.ch or Sigma Theta Tau International's website at nursingsociety.org). It is important to keep the organization's evaluative criteria in mind when writing the abstract.

Presentation of research-related activities may be included in scientific conferences. The format of an abstract meant for clinical presentations includes the following (Happell, 2007):

1. Why? Relevance and importance of topic
2. Where? Setting and clients (specific needs)
3. How? Overview of initiative, preparation, issues, challenges, and strategies in achieving goals of a program
4. What? Observed outcomes
5. What now? Structured evaluation findings; implications for practice; lessons learned

Acceptance of an abstract for either paper (oral) or poster presentation triggers the need to start preparing for a successful event. The letter of acceptance usually includes presentation guidelines. Although organizations' guidelines vary, most paper presentations are scheduled for 20 minutes with 15 minutes for content delivery and 5 minutes for questions. Poster presentations may occur over several days with designated times when presenters need to be at the poster to interact with conference participants.

Things to keep in mind when developing a paper presentation include the target audience—researchers, clinicians, and lay people; setting—size of the room and seating arrangement; and time (Sawatzky, 2011). Adapt the language to match the audience's level of sophistication and expertise (e.g., use research language if the audience is primarily researchers). Also keep in mind that conferences are becoming more interdisciplinary.

Identifying the Content

Develop a detailed outline to serve as a roadmap when you write your script to practice the presentation. Include the key aspects of the study that were included in the abstract you submitted. Remember your time frame. It is important to "get to the punch line" (findings and implications for practice) and not spend too much time on background information. A sentence or two to set up the problem and purpose of the study is sufficient for most audiences.

Developing Visual Aids

An important aspect of your preparation is determining the audio-visual aids you will use to convey your information. Most presentations call for the use of slides and some presenters also distribute handouts.

The purpose of slides is to enhance the presentation of your content. As you develop your presentation, determine the types and number of slides that will be used—word, pictorial, or a combination. There are numerous computer software programs (e.g., Harvard Graphics, PowerPoint, or Presentation) that can be used for making slides. The most commonly used software at conferences is PowerPoint. Users of iPads are advised to check with the venue to see whether alternate presentation software such as Keynote will be supported. Information is available from various websites that can be used to help you develop slides for effective presentations (http://presentationsoft.about.com /od/powerpointtips/qt/planningppt.htm; www.microsoft.com/atwork /skills/presentations.aspx#fbid=fdRVXGU_W-P).

Developing slides on a computer allows easy preview and reordering of the slides. Color combinations can be previewed before producing the slide. The choice of colors is vital for readability. For example, light pink when used for words on a light-blue background is difficult to read. Combinations with higher contrast improve readability and enhance recall. Keep in mind that venues often have silver projection screens that can make colors appear murkier than they do on the computer screen. Other considerations when developing slides are: (a) use a consistent simple template, (b) use an easy-to-read font type such as Arial or Times consistently, (c) use text size 40 to 44 for main headings and 28 to 32 for text, (d) use the 5–7–7 rule, five words in title, seven words per line, and seven lines per slide, left-justify text. When using graphs, you must orient the audience to essential aspects of the graph (Hardicre, Coad, & Devitt, 2007; Shepherd, 2006; Vollman, 2005).

Slide presentations can be saved on a USB flash drive and easily transported. Experienced presenters recommend saving more than one version of the file to be safe. Sending the presentation file to oneself via e-mail or uploading it to a file hosting service such as Dropbox are other means of retrieving a file if the unthinkable and unexpected happens. Always bring a flash drive (Sawatzky, 2011, suggests bringing two) with a copy of your presentation file to the event even if it has been uploaded by the technical team beforehand. In addition, always bring a print copy of your file; this ensures that you can give your presentation effectively in the event of technical or electrical power malfunction. If at all possible, preview your slides using the equipment that will be used during the presentation and practice delivering your presentation. Be sure to time yourself.

Strategies for Public Speaking

Nurses have much to say that will positively impact health care delivery in our society. The opportunity for nurses to speak publicly will escalate in the coming years. The vast amount of nursing research that is currently under way in clinical, educational, and administrative practice will necessitate nurses sharing their findings to transform patient care. Another factor that will contribute to our mandate to present research publicly is the changing focus of health care to wellness, prevention, and delivery of care in community settings. Whereas nurses have always played an important role in teaching self-care to patients, the demand will increase as the population ages and the demand for quality care increases. Nurses must continue to engage in research and seek appropriate opportunities to present their findings publicly.

Despite the anxiety most people feel when speaking publicly, the experience can be rewarding and exciting. Public speaking, like any skill, requires preparation and practice (Sawatzky, 2011). There are several websites that provide a good overview of presentation skills. Examples of both good public speaking skills and, frankly, terrible public speaking skills abound on YouTube (www.youtube.com).

Tutorials to aid in the development of presentation skills are available at the following websites:

- http://web.mit.edu/urop/resources/speaking.html
- www.kumc.edu/SAH/OTEd/jradel/effective.html
- www.aresearchguide.com/3tips.html
- www.toastmasters.org/tips.asp

There are many strategies that you can use to help make this experience exciting and worthwhile (Barton, Reichow, & Wolery, 2007; McConnell, 2002; Heinrich, 2012):

- Know your audience. Speak their language and present your material in a way that is meaningful to them.
- Organize your thoughts.
- Use audiovisual aids.
- Use charts and graphs—most often, research findings can best be displayed with the use of tables, charts, graphs, figures, and so on. These tools help to better organize the findings for the audience.
- Speak to the audience and maintain eye contact.
- Rehearse your presentation and know the time it takes so that you can fit the schedule.
- Dress appropriately—if you are doing a presentation during working hours on site at your organization, everyday work clothes may be appropriate. In other instances, when presenting off-site, business clothing is the appropriate attire.
- Elicit audience participation by asking questions or presenting a concept, idea, or finding, and then ask: "What does this mean to you," or "What do you think about this study result?"
- Vary your tone of voice.
- Allow time for questions. The nature of research stimulates inquiry, so people will likely have questions. Hence plan time for the audience to ask questions.
- Always repeat the question so that everyone can hear it.
- Use tact in responding to criticism to your research and keep an open mind.
- Recognize people who have made significant contributions to the research.
- Thank the audience and let them know where you may be reached by e-mail or phone. Provide your business card for those who wish to follow up with you.

CONDUCTING THE PAPER PRESENTATION

Review your notes on the day of your presentation. Arrive early at the room where you are scheduled to present so that you can meet the moderator and any fellow speakers. This gives you time to acquaint yourself with the podium and audiovisual setup and to practice advancing and backing up slides. As you begin your presentation, take time to briefly introduce yourself to the audience. This helps establish your credibility with the participants. Sometimes an interesting or humorous anecdote related to the conference location or focus or your content serves to relax both you and the audience. Presentations scheduled after lunch, late in the afternoon or evening, or at the end of a conference can be challenging because audience energy may be low. Including humor or using strategies that frequently encourage audience participation, such as nonthreatening questioning, may enliven your presentation (Goldman & Schmalz, 2007; McConnell, 2002).

Although most presentations are delivered to a live audience in the same location, you may be offered the opportunity to present via a satellite teleconference or web-based platform. Virtual conferences are being offered with increasing frequency. Webinars may consist of the audience viewing slides and listening to the audio portion of the presentation or they may use an interactive format with video and audience participation. Conducting face-to-face oral presentations gives you the opportunity to see your audience, interact with them, and receive verbal and nonverbal feedback during the presentation. On the other hand, you only reach a small number of people. Web-based presentations may be viewed by large numbers of people, but limit your ability to read your audience and interact with them. Regardless of the medium used, strategies for preparing the presentation are the same.

Presenting via a teleconference or web-based format requires extra attention to clothing, fielding questions, and dealing with technical issues. Attire should be professional, clean, and solid colored. Patterns, particularly stripes, should be avoided to prevent the "spatial aliasing effect" (resulting in a moiré pattern—that shimmery, jumpy movement noted on screen when weathermen wear skinny-striped ties). Large, bright prints may be distracting. Wear some color near your face. If the background is white and you are presenting in a white dress shirt, the effect is that of a "talking head." Long necklaces may rub against a microphone attached to your lapel and produce a scratchy noise. Clipping the microphone to your nondominant side may decrease interference from head movement as well (Longo & Tierney, 2012).

Discuss how the audience will be able to ask questions prior to your presentation. If they can call in, you may want to ask that questions be held until the end. If attendees can e-mail or instant message questions, an assistant is often available to collect these questions, group them by theme, and pose the questions to you at the end of the session. Be sure to provide your e-mail, telephone, or other contact information at the end for follow-up. Webinars may be available asynchronously, so it is important that people viewing your presentation at a later time will be able to contact you.

Technical assistance is a must. Technical support is needed initially to load your presentation, ensure that your microphone is working, and that you and your slides appear centered in the screen shots. Technical assistance may also be needed to troubleshoot issues arising from the attendees' end of the computer. Audio issues and visual issues may require adjustments from the technical support person. As you begin your presentation, ask the audience to e-mail or phone the technical support line if they have difficulty accessing your presentation. A resource for additional tips and guidelines may be found at www.dianehoward.com/Dr._H._teleconferencing_videoconferencing _streaming_webcasting.htm.

CONDUCTING THE POSTER PRESENTATION

Like the paper presentation, the poster includes the major categories included in the abstract. Because the primary purpose of a poster is to visually communicate research in a simple way, it is necessary to be concise and clear in presenting the information (Hardicre, Coad, & Devitt, 2007; Briggs, 2009). A poster should be easily understood within 5 minutes. Readability is enhanced when the text is concise, the flow of the segments is logical, and font is readable from a distance of at least 4 to 6 feet. Conference sponsors often have specific guidelines for preparing the poster; size, type of display (free standing or wall), and how to sequence content (left to right horizontally versus a vertical flow) are often stipulated. Presenters are reminded to check the conference website or information provided in the acceptance letter for exact specifications.

Several authors have suggested methods for preparing for poster presentations (http://people.eku.edu/ritchisong/posterpres.html; www .kumc.edu/SAH/OTEd/jradel/Poster_Presentations/PstrStart.html; www .pitt.edu/~etbell/nsurg/PosterGuide.html). Poster preparation generally includes:

1. Information gathering
   - Conference date and location
   - Length of time for poster session and requirement for being present at poster
   - Type of display—table or board, usually 4 feet by 8 feet. When a table is provided, use a stand-alone table-top display. A stand-alone display can be constructed by using a foam board or a portable commercial stand in which Velcro fasteners can be used to mount segments of the poster. A cork board requires a method for mounting the poster such as the use of pins.

2. Types of information to be included
   - Title—Heinrich (2012) suggests finding the "sexy slant" of your presentation and using this as the focus for a catchy title.
   - Author names and affiliation
   - Problem and a brief background
   - Method—design, sample, setting, and data collection process
   - Data analysis
   - Results and implications
   - Acknowledgment—sources of funds

3. Poster assembly
   - Layout of poster—consider the sequence of ideas, and use headings, arrows, or broken lines to guide the reader
   - Use of color—pictures and title of sections. A descriptive, concise, and "eye-catching" poster (Briggs, 2009, p. 36) will convey your topic and attract viewers.
   - Self-explanatory graphs or tables
   - Available resources
     Self-assembly involves using your personal computer to lay out the poster (using PowerPoint or other software) and a printer to print texts of sections. Make use of any in-house audiovisual department resources. Many hospitals and universities have the capability to produce posters. Check with the marketing, education, or media services department in your institution. Office supply stores (e.g., Staples and FedEx Office) can help produce your poster for a fee.
   - Portability—Consider the use of poster boards in separate pieces for portability as a hand-carry. If traveling by air, check with the airline ahead of time to determine whether a poster tube can be carried on the plane or if it must be checked. Be forewarned that an additional baggage charge may be levied if you are required to check the poster tube. Consider sending a poster "overnight" via FedEx or another carrier to the hotel or conference site. Be sure to call ahead to determine whether this is a viable option and inquire as to how to address the package (e.g., "future hotel guest"). A painful lesson learned by this author is that if you are sending a poster to another country, your package may be held up in customs (sadly, my poster was cleared the day *after* the conference ended!).

4. Other Considerations
   - Availability of handouts: Have copies of the abstract, which includes authors, affiliation, address, e-mail, and telephone number available. If you were given a proof copy of your poster prior to printing, consider making color copies available to those interested in your study.

■ Use of display items such as data collection tools: Mark these as "for display only" and put them in a plastic sleeve or have them laminated.

5. Poster Session
   ■ Dress professionally and appropriately for conference/venue. Wear comfortable shoes as you will be standing for the entire poster session.
   ■ Set up the poster and take it down at designated times. Allow time to set up the poster and bring extra pushpins, Velcro fasteners, and binder clips (these come in handy for a variety of display challenges). Be collegial—help your co-presenters with their display and they will assist you. Attempting to tack up a 6-foot poster alone is futile.
   ■ Be at the poster and interact with participants. Introduce yourself and ask attendees their research interests. Answer questions and accept constructive criticism gracefully. Do not become defensive if challenged about "why didn't you do xyz?" Provide your rationale or respond with "that's a good suggestion for future research in this area."
   ■ Note participant requests for information by asking individuals to write on the back of their business cards their request or on a clipboard at the poster. Respond to these inquiries within 2 weeks of the conference.
   ■ Look at other posters and seek permission from authors to take a picture of posters you find attractive.
   Offer your business card to attendees who are interested in your area of research or who request one.

6. Evaluation
   Immediately following the presentation, jot down things you would do differently—format, colors, written content, type, and number of handouts. Consider the following criteria when evaluating posters that you viewed:
   ■ Overall appearance—attractiveness, accuracy of information, color combination, readability, inclusion of only necessary information, and uncluttered appearance
   ■ Content—current, logical, and grammatically correct words, and inclusion of components of the research
   ■ Presentation—author's knowledge of the study, professional appearance of the presenter, and availability of presenter to participants

Poster presentations have distinct advantages over oral presentations or publications when disseminating research. By conducting a poster presentation, findings are communicated by authors to participants in an informal way. The informal exchange of ideas between the author and the participant promotes immediate feedback to the author, which may be useful in future presentations, preparation of manuscripts, clarification of unclear or confusing aspects of the study, and networking. Editors of nursing journals often solicit manuscripts after viewing posters and talking to the presenter.

Posters are excellent vehicles for disseminating research findings to the community as well as to the profession. They can easily be used at community health fairs, at local professional meetings, and seminars, and can be developed for display in shopping malls, physicians' offices, and community and social service agencies. When the plan is to use a poster for different types of audiences, it is helpful if the entire poster is not developed as a whole piece. Develop separate segments for sections such as the research methods and conclusions so that these sections can be adapted for each audience.

Computer poster sessions and digital poster sessions are two additional means of presenting research. A computerized poster may be presented during a standard poster viewing session. The poster typically is designed to be viewed on a laptop screen. Formats include a PowerPoint slide show, video clips, or other multimedia. Key elements remain the same as for a static poster. Digital poster sessions are web based and usually asynchronous. They may be accessed by many people over time. Digital poster sessions may incorporate PowerPoint slides, video clips, audioclips or other media. One digital poster session (De Simone, Rodrian, Osswald, Sack, De Simone, & Hagl, 2001) involved 2-minute videotaped segments of each of the presenters sharing highlights and key aspects of their posters. These video clips accompanied the digitally formatted posters. Digital presentations should adhere to the principles of universal design to meet accessibility standards. References and contact information must be included.

A sample digital poster session available on the web may be accessed at http://kairos.technorhetoric.net/praxis/index.php/Doing _Digital:_a_production-focused_pedagogy. Resources and web-based tutorials on digital poster design may be found at http://elearning facultymodules.org/index.php/Digital_Posters_and_Digital_Poster _Sessions.

Disseminating Research Findings Through the Media

The media—television, radio, and the Internet—are powerful vehicles for disseminating nursing research. Before considering the media as an outlet for disseminating information, check with your employer about existing policies. There may be a staff member who is charged with assisting those who wish to communicate research findings to the media. Some organizations submit press releases—a written overview of events that are occurring. If this is being done, find out how you could submit your research findings.

Professional organizations often invite reporters from local television stations to conferences so that research of interest to the public can be identified. Because of this possibility, many organizations will ask you to sign a document indicating your willingness to share the study with the media. A website that is useful in preparing researchers to disseminate their study findings is A Communications Toolkit for Health Researchers, which can be accessed at www.ruralhealthresearch.org/pdf/toolkit.pdf.

Television and Radio

Television, radio, and newspaper reporters often search the Internet for evidence-based research reports on topics of current interest. If you have disseminated research in any way, always do an Internet search on your topic and see if you find mention of yourself and your work. If you do, be prepared for the possibility of being contacted by a reporter. Develop key talking points related to your topic to manage the interview and make sure your message is heard. Also, always know and be ready to talk about the implications of your topic to the public. The University of Arizona's Media Interview Guide (http://cals.arizona.edu/pressrelease/interviewguide.pdf) provides an overview of how to work effectively with media representatives while keeping the focus on your research. Press releases from the National Institute for Nursing Research (www.ninr.nih.gov) serve as examples for sharing scientific information in a concise format. Television remains a powerful medium for disseminating research.

Nurses can be proactive and seek out this medium by contacting local television stations to arrange a meeting with producers. Local stations often have a health segment that may be an appropriate fit with your research. Before contacting the local station, ensure that your institution is supportive. Have a clear idea of the type of local show that might broadcast your findings, know the type of people who watch particular shows, determine the fit between your topic and the show, and maintain confidentiality of study participants. If an interview is granted, inquire whether the interview will be live or taped and if you are the only person being interviewed or if there are other participants. If there are other participants, find out the background of each participant. Start preparing by doing an outline, a script, and practicing with a colleague or by videotaping your presentation and reviewing the tape. The guidelines for preparing an oral presentation and public speaking strategies presented in this chapter are useful.

Carefully preparing for an interview with the media is important. Preparing for an interview with the media includes familiarity with the mechanics that will be used (i.e., face to face, by telephone, and video/audio taping for television or radio). There are several strategies for preparing for the various stages (prior to, during, and after the interview), which are presented at www.cals.arizona.edu/pressrelease /interviewguide.

1. Be clear on ground rules related to topics you will and will not address and the opportunity to review and correct misstatements.
2. Identify possible questions that support and do not support your study and formulate a 10- to 30-second response.
3. Respond directly to a question, use citations, and do not predict when hypothetical situations are presented and an answer is being sought.
4. Determine the key points of your interview and emphasize the points each time you have the opportunity.
5. Look at the interviewer during the taping or when you are not being interviewed. See www.bottomlinemediacoaching.com/5-mistakes -to-avoid-during-a-tv-interview for more tips, including knowing the pronunciation of the interviewer's name.
6. Use terms that lay people will understand.
7. Limit your movements during the interview.
8. Immediately correct the interviewer when something that is said is incorrect.
9. Communicate enthusiasm and smile.
10. Wear a solid-color outfit.
11. Write a thank-you note to the host and the producer.

A local news channel is likely to be open to allowing a short segment presentation when the topic is one that is of great interest to its viewers. Also, consider a national channel if your research findings have major implications for the health of society. Reading newspapers and magazines that the public reads will give you an idea of topics that are relevant and interesting to the public as well as how this information is presented.

Radio is also a powerful medium for research dissemination. Most people invest some amount of time listening to the radio on a daily basis. The radio audience potential is vast. Many local stations host special-interest shows and talk shows and invite people to participate. It would be wise to invest time in searching out these likely opportunities.

There are advantages and disadvantages for the use of the media in disseminating research findings. Distinct advantages are that this type of medium has a greater potential for reaching a larger audience and influencing the public's perception of nurses' contributions to their health. On the other hand, the short time allotment for the presentation increases the possibility of misinterpretation of your message. Thus, researchers must provide a comprehensive presentation of the research methodology, findings, and implications in an understandable and concise manner. To help counter the simplicity and brevity of this type of research presentation, provide your name and a work e-mail, phone number, or address where you can be reached so that community members may contact you to learn more about your study. Do not give out home or personal contact information. Providing contact information is also a helpful way to solicit participants for future studies.

Electronic Media Options

Technology plays a major role in providing opportunities for the further dissemination of our research. The Internet offers a fast and convenient means to not only obtain information but to effectively share new research findings. Web-based venues are transforming how we transfer knowledge and influence global health care. As an example, YouTube.com is a video-sharing website where users can upload, view, and share video clips. A quick search of YouTube with the keywords "nursing research" provides many ideas for disseminating your research findings to the world. More and more frequently, journal websites are technology enabled, allowing authors of articles to post supplemental content, such as a video clip discussing research. Social media and professional networking sites such as LinkedIn, blogs, Twitter, and listservs are more informal ways of sharing ideas, obtaining feedback from others, and identifying potential colleagues with whom to collaborate. Posting your research interests and a brief summary of research completed on appropriate sites may lead to further opportunities to share your findings. In order to keep postings very concise (Twitter has a 140-character limit) yet meaningful, judicious editing is needed.

A cautionary note is warranted. Postings to electronic media are in the public domain, even if the site is password protected or accessible by subscription only. Nurses are advised to re-acquaint themselves with the Healthcare Insurance Portability and Accountability Act (HIPAA) regarding patient privacy and confidentiality rights. Likewise, state boards of nursing (BRNs; NCSBN, 2011) and the American Nurses Association (ANA, 2011) have developed guidelines to assist nurses in determining what content can be shared electronically. Nurses whose web postings (on blogs, Facebook, LinkedIn, etc.) violate HIPAA standards face professional and legal sanctions.

Videotaping

Most laptops and computer monitors now include web camera (webcam) capability. In addition to allowing individuals to participate interactively in web-based conferences or seminars, a webcam can be used to record video and audio. A software program, such as Microsoft Move Maker for the PC, may already be loaded on your computer or can be downloaded/purchased from the Internet. After recording yourself discussing your research or presenting your poster, you may save it to a digital video disc (DVD), save it as a media file for viewing as a podcast, or post it on YouTube.com or another appropriate website. Podcasts may be an audio file only, audio with video clips, or even a pdf file (Digitalpodcast.com). Videocasting may be done in real time as well. Software can be downloaded to assist you in editing your digital recording and to post it to a server on the web.

DVDs can be made and given to colleagues, patient care units in the hospital, television stations, community agencies, and professional organizations. In addition, all or just segments of the DVD can be broadcast through select Internet venues.

Professional DVDs offer a polished finished product that controls for lighting, noise level, and background. Disadvantages include the cost, the difficulty, and length of time needed for production. When planning any video recording, consider the target audience, desired outcomes, and content. Identify the most effective ways to communicate your message and use visual aids that support the script or photography.

Writing a script is important to ensure that the message is succinct and will be delivered within the allotted time. During the recording, it is helpful to consider the camera as the audience and to pretend that you are in your living room speaking to guests. A researcher could market a DVD by giving a copy to professional organizations who may find utility for its members.

SUMMARY

The mode of disseminating research findings is varied. The goal is effective communication with the target audience. Oral and poster presenters must conform to the guidelines set forth by the sponsoring organization to contribute to the success of the event. Taking the time to reflect and evaluate your poster or oral presentation is essential to further developing one's professional presentation skills.

SUGGESTED ACTIVITIES

1. After reviewing your research findings and the University of Arizona's Media Interview Guide (http://cals.arizona.edu/pressre lease/interviewguide.pdf), complete these steps in preparation for a mock interview:

   ■ What is new or unique about your findings?
   ■ Why are your findings important? In what way will they add to safe, quality nursing care?

- Who or what benefits as a result of your findings?
- How do your findings advance the cause of health care reform?

2. Based on the context of your oral presentation content and your desire to maintain audience attention:

- Develop an analogy that illustrates complex content (e.g., childbirth process as analogy for the thesis/dissertation process).

- Identify a few key points in your talk that might be illustrated with humor (an anecdote, a cartoon, or a poem).

- Identify and mark areas in your presentation notes where you want to (a) pause, (b) remind yourself to look at audience and smile, and (c) ask questions or otherwise engage your audience (e.g., If you had a patient with X, what would you do? Why would you think it was a problem?).

ACKNOWLEDGMENTS

The author would like to acknowledge the work done by this chapter's original authors Dr. S. Smith and Dr. M. Mateo.

REFERENCES

American Association of Colleges of Nursing. (2012). Fact Sheet: The Doctor of Nursing Practice (Revised 10/22/2012).

American Nurses Association (ANA). (2011). *Principles for social networking and the nurse.* Silver Spring, MD: ANA.

Barton, E. E., Reichow, B., & Wolery, M. (2007). Guidelines for graphing data with Microsoft PowerPoint. *Journal of Early Intervention, 29*(4), 320–336.

Briggs, D. J. (2009). A practical guide to designing a poster for presentation. *Nursing Standard, 23*(34), 35–39.

Burns, N., & Grove, S. K. (2011). *Understanding nursing research: Building an evidence-based practice* (5th ed., pp. 55 – 57). Maryland Heights, MO: Elsevier.

De Simone, R., Rodrian, J., Osswald, B., Sack, F., De Simone, E., & Hagl, S. (2001). Initial experience with a new communication tool: The "Digital Interactive Poster Presentation." *European Journal of Cardio-Thoracic Surgery, 19*(6), 953–955.

Goldman, K. D., & Schmalz, K. J. (2007). Speech righting: Presentation preparation principles for potent performances. *Health Promotion Practice, 8*(2), 114–118.

Grady, P. A. (2010). Translational research and nursing science. *Nursing Outlook, 58*(3), 164–166.

Happell, B. (2007). Hitting the target! A no tears approach to writing an abstract for a conference presentation. *International Journal of Mental Health Nursing, 16*(6), 447–452.

Hardicre, J., Coad, C., & Devitt, P. (2007). Ten steps to successful conference presentations. *British Journal of Nursing, 16*(7), 402–404.

Hardicre, J., Devitt, P., & Coad, C. (2007). Ten steps to successful poster presentation. *British Journal of Nursing, 16*(7), 398–401.

Heinrich, K. T. (2012). Four steps to preparing irresistible presentations. *American Nurse Today, 7*(3), 22–24.

Longo, A., & Tierney, C. (2012). Presentation skills for the nurse educator. *Journal for Nurses in Staff Development, 18*(1), 16–23.

McConnell, E. A. (2002). Making outstandingly good presentations. *Dimensions of Critical Care Nursing, 21*(1), 28–31.

National Council of State Boards of Registered Nursing (NCSBN). (2011). *A nurse's guide to the use of social media.* Chicago, IL: NCSBN

Sawatzky, J. V. (2011). My abstract was accepted—Now what? *Canadian Journal of Cardiovascular Nursing, 21*(2), 37–41.

Shepard, M. (2006). How to give an effective presentation using PowerPoint. *European Diabetes Nursing, 3*(3), 154–158.

Vollman, K. M. (2005). Enhancing presentation skills for the advanced practice nurse. *AACN Clinical Issues, 16*(1), 67–77.

21

Reporting Results Through Publication

Norma G. Cuellar

As the value and quality of clinical research in nursing have improved, more and more nurses are making concerted efforts to disseminate their findings though multiple channels. As well, more clinicians are going back for their Doctorate of Nursing Practice, which often requires dissemination of scholarly projects. Because disseminating findings is an integral part of the research/scholarly process, the plan for communicating findings must be developed at the time a research study (research doctorate) or scholarly project (clinical doctorate) is proposed.

One factor that may influence dissemination of findings from a research study or scholarly project includes requirements of the funding agency and organization that supported the project. Some funding agencies and organizations require a review of results before findings are disseminated and expect to be listed in acknowledgments. To ensure scientific integrity, it is expected to report who funded the study when appropriate, to control for bias. The funders may also require approval of submission of manuscript before it is submitted. Because these reviews may delay the dissemination process, it is important to be familiar with requirements of funding agencies and the organization where you are employed before plans for presentations or publications are initiated.

Although the traditional approach to publishing research findings and scholarly projects is through professional journals, other publication options are cyberspace, electronic journals, newsletters, professional societies, and newspapers. This chapter examines strategies for successfully disseminating your research findings through publications. Emphasis is placed on the process and strategies to adequately develop high-quality, professional presentations of your work. Although strategies pertinent to different types of publications are delineated, the principles apply to most types of publications.

PRINT JOURNALS

According to the Citations in Nursing and Allied Health website (www .cinahl.com), there are 763 journals and magazines in nursing; however, only a small percentage are exclusively research journals. Publishing in research journals allows nurse researchers to report the conduct of their investigation using a standard, structured-research-report format: background, review of the literature, methods, findings, and implications (Tornquist, 1999). The credibility of publishing in a research journal is based on the "peer-review" process intended to evaluate the quality of work by peers who are expert in the field. The process is intended to maintain standards, improve performance, and provide credibility, thereby making it suitable for publication (Baker, 2012).

Publishing a Research Article

Publishing in a research journal signifies an important contribution to the science of nursing. It is the highest level of publishing in scholarship. A series of publications in research journals or high-impact journals can move your career to the next level. The primary focus of review for the research journal is scientific merit, be it quantitative or qualitative research.

Choosing a journal of high quality is important to publish your manuscript. One determinant of the quality of a journal is the impact factor. The impact factor is an objective indicator of the relative importance and quality of the paper and the journal in which it was published. The higher the impact factor, the greater the importance of the journal in its field. The impact factor measures the number of times an article has been cited in a certain time frame (Sonuga-Barke, 2012). The more times an author is cited, the greater the increase in impact the author has had on the profession. These reports are available at the Institute of Scientific Information (ISI). An author can find out how many times he or she was cited and in which journals. Unfortunately, nursing journals have low impact factors, so, if you want to be cited and read by other professions to increase your scholarship visibility, you may want to consider publishing outside of nursing. There are a variety of other measures for the quality of journals, that is, the usage measure, which measures how many times the article is used or read through the Internet (Pesch, 2012; Sonuga-Barke, 2012). The criteria remain debatable in the publishing world.

Research journals use the IMRAD format, which includes introduction, methods, result, and discussion. The introduction includes a brief background of the topic and the study purpose(s). Methods comprise the design, setting, sample description, intervention, and outcome measures. Results include the primary findings. Finally, the discussion is the section where conclusions and implications for practice and research are presented. A structured abstract format is suggested because it helps readers to select articles that are appropriate to their topic (Nakayama, Hirat, Yamazaki, & Naito, 2005).

A more exact process to standardize reports of research is the Consolidated Standards of Reporting Trials (CONSORT), which was developed to decrease inadequate reporting of randomized controlled trials (RCTs) and develop consistency among articles to improve evidence-based practice (Altman, Moher, & Schulz, 2012). The CONSORT statement is used to report the minimum set of recommendations for reporting clinical trials. This standardization of publication allows facilitation of complete and transparent reporting with critical appraisal and interpretation. A checklist and diagram are provided to assist the authors to organize the text of the manuscript. Although the CONSORT statement is used for clinical trials, other CONSORT statements have developed because of CONSORT's success in publications. There are a variety of reporting guidelines as described in Table 21.1.

After you complete publication of your research findings, you may also publish in a nonresearch or clinical journal (Tornquist, 1999; Webb, 2007). Clinical articles may include problem-solving skills, clinical decision making, and discussion and debate regarding professional issues in nursing. Although not oriented toward data, the clinical article can focus on a variety of practice topics that improve nursing practice, including examining clinical guidelines in practice, innovative clinical practice, new ways of clinical practice, case studies, health care outcome evaluations, and clinical scholarly projects. This article may be a more labor-intensive effort as you cannot follow the traditional research report format. Guidelines for writing clinical articles are more available (Happell, 2012). The nonresearch journal will require a less formal language, a process approach to your topic (what was the problem you faced, how did you go about solving it, and what did you discover?), and creative, interesting headings.

Editors are critically aware of the need to have a data-driven practice base and are eagerly seeking research-based information that holds the potential for transforming nursing practice. So whatever type of journal you choose to publish your research findings, you will find editors are receptive.

CYBERSPACE PUBLICATIONS

Cyberspace is the electronic medium of computer networks in which online communication takes place (www.thefreedictionary.com/cyber space). By using the Internet, vast amounts of information can be "published" and retrieved. Every day more and more businesses and people establish websites to promote themselves, supply information, and sell their products. Because of its great use and unlimited potential,

TABLE 21.1 Research Reporting Guidelines and Initiatives

ORGANIZATION/GUIDELINE	DESCRIPTION
ASSERT: A Standard for the Scientific and Ethical Review of Trials	Standard for the review and monitoring of randomized clinical trials by research ethics committees. Checklist incorporates certain elements of CONSORT, to ensure fulfillment of the requirements for scientific validity in the ethical conduct of clinical research (18-item checklist).
CDISC: Clinical Data Interchange Standards Consortium	Standards supporting the acquisition, exchange, submission, and archive of clinical research data and metadata. Develops and supports global, platform-independent data standards that enable information system interoperability to improve medical research and related areas of health care.
COPE: Committee on Publication Ethics	Forum for editors of peer-reviewed journals to discuss issues related to the integrity of the scientific record. Supports and encourages editors to report, catalogue, and instigate investigations into ethical problems in the publication process. All Elsevier journal editors are COPE members.
CONSORT: Consolidated Standards of Reporting Trials	Evidence-based, minimum recommendations for reporting RCTs. Offers a standard way for authors to prepare reports of trial findings, facilitating their complete and transparent reporting, and aiding their critical appraisal and interpretation (25-item checklist). See CONSORT 2010 Statement (Update) Extensions of the CONSORT statement for specific types of RCT journals that support CONSORT.
CONSORT Plus	Extension of CONSORT requirements that imposes data integrity constraints not possible in text-based reporting.
CSE: Council of Science Editors	Organization that promotes excellence in the communication of scientific information. Fosters networking, education, discussion, and exchange. Authoritative resource on current and emerging issues in the communication of scientific information. CSE Editorial Policies and Endorsement

EASE: European Association of Science Editors	Internationally oriented community of individuals who share an interest in science communication and editing. Offers the opportunity to stay abreast of trends in the rapidly changing environment of scientific publishing, whether traditional or electronic.
EQUATOR: Enhancing the QUAlity and Transparency Of health Research	Umbrella organization that brings together developers of reporting guidelines, medical journal editors and peer reviewers, research funding bodies, and other collaborators with mutual interest in improving the quality of research publications and of research itself. EQUATOR Network Plan: 2007–2012 Additional Resources and pages of other Reporting Guidelines Vandenbroucke, J. P. (2009, January 30). STREGA, STROBE, STARD, SQUIRE, MOOSE, PRISMA, GNOSIS, TREND, ORION, COREQ, QUOROM, REMARK... and CONSORT: For whom does the guideline toll? *Journal of Clinical Epidemiology* [Epub ahead of print]. PubMed PMID: 19181482 Simera, I., Altman, D. G., Moher, D., Schulz, K. F., & Hoey, J. (2008, June 24). Guidelines for reporting health research: The EQUATOR network's survey of guideline authors. *PLoS Medicine*, 5(6), e139. PubMed PMID: 18578566; PubMed Central PMCID: PMC2443184
FAME Editorial Guidelines: Forum for African Medical Editors	68-page guidelines
GNOSIS: Guidelines for Neuro-Oncology: Standards for Investigational Studies	Guidelines to standardize the reporting of surgically based Phase 1 and Phase 2 neuro-oncology trials. The guidelines are summarized in a checklist format that can be used as a framework from which to construct a surgically based trial. Chang, S., Vogelbaum, M., Lang, F. F., Haines, S., Kunwar, S., Chiocca, E. A., . . . and American Association of Neurological Surgeons and Congress of Neurological Surgeons (AANS/CNS). (2007). GNOSIS: Guidelines for neuro-oncology: Standards for investigational studies – reporting of surgically based therapeutic clinical trials. *Journal of Neuro-Oncology, 82*(2), 211–220 [Epub 2006, December 5]. PubMed PMID: 17146595 Chang, S. M., Reynolds, S. L., Butowski, N., Lamborn, K. R., Buckner, J. C., Kaplan, R. S., et al. (2005). GNOSIS: Guidelines for neuro-oncology: Standards for investigational studies – reporting of phase 1 and phase 2 clinical trials. *Journal of Neuro-Oncology, 7*(4), 425–434. PubMed PMID: 16212807; PubMed Central PMCID: PMC1871726

(continued)

435

TABLE 21.1 Research Reporting Guidelines and Initiatives (*continued*)

ORGANIZATION/GUIDELINE	DESCRIPTION
GPP2: Good Publication Practice	Guidelines that encourage responsible and ethical publication of the results of clinical trials sponsored by pharmaceutical companies. *BioMed Central* and *BMJ* ask authors of industry-sponsored studies, or of papers in industry-sponsored supplements, to follow GPP. Graf, C., Battisti, W. P., Bridges, D., Bruce-Winkler, V., Conaty, J. M., Ellison, J. M., . . . International Society for Medical Publication Professionals. (2009, November 27). Research methods & reporting. Good publication practice for communicating company sponsored medical research: The GPP2 guidelines. *British Medical Journal, 339*, b4330. doi: 10.1136/bmj. b4330. PubMed PMID: 19946142
GLISC: Grey Literature International Steering Committee	Guidelines for the production of scientific and technical reports and writing/distributing grey literature.
Herbal Consort Statement	CONSORT Extension: Given that herbal medicinal products are widely used, vary greatly in content and quality, and are actively tested in randomized controlled trials (RCTs), recommendations were developed to improve reporting RCTs of herbal medicine interventions.
ICMJE: International Committee of Medical Journal Editors	Uniform Requirements for Manuscripts Submitted to Biomedical Journals Vancouver Group Journal list.
INANE: International Academy of Nursing Editors	International collaborative whose primary mission is to promote best practices in publishing and high standards in the nursing literature.
Instructions to Authors in the Health Sciences: Mulford Library, University of Toledo HSL	Journal titles listed in alphabetical order. Contains publishing guidelines for some journals. Indicates which journals follow CONSORT and/or other guidelines.
Mayfield Handbook of Technical & Scientific Writing	A handbook.

MIAME: Minimum Information About a Microarray Experiment	Describes the minimum information about a microarray experiment that is needed to enable the interpretation of the results of the experiment unambiguously and, potentially, to reproduce the experiment.
	Brazma, A., Hingamp, P., Quackenbush, J., Sherlock, G., Spellman, P., Stoeckert, C., et al. (2001, December). Minimum information about a microarray experiment (MIAME)–toward standards for microarray data. *Nature Genetics*, 29(4), 365–371. PubMed PMID: 11726920
	Knudsen, T. B., & Daston, G. P. (2005). Teratology Society. MIAME guidelines. *Reproductive Toxicology, 19*(3), 263. PubMed PMID: 15686863
MIBBI: Minimum Information for Biological and Biomedical Investigations	Aims to increase the visibility of projects developing guidance for the reporting of aspects of biological and biomedical science. Finds MIBBI-registered reporting guidelines for various domains in the life sciences through the portal: www.biosharing.org/standards/mibbi
MOOSE: Meta-analysis of Observational Studies in Epidemiology	Proposal for reporting meta-analyses of observational studies in epidemiology.
	Stroup, D. F., Berlin, J. A., Morton, S. C., Olkin, I., Williamson, G. D., Rennie, D., et al. (2000). Meta-analysis of observational studies in epidemiology (MOOSE) group. *Journal of the American Medical Association, 283*(15), 2008–2012 (Review). PubMed PMID:10789670
Nonpharmacological Interventions	CONSORT extensions for the reporting of trials of nonpharmacologic treatments (NPT) such as surgery, technical interventions, rehabilitation, psychotherapy, behavioral interventions, implantable and non-implantable devices, and complementary medicine.
Ophthalmology Study Design Worksheet #6 [no longer available on website]	Checklist for cross-sectional studies submitted to the journal, *Ophthalmology* (42-item checklist).
ORION Statement: Guidelines for Transparent Reporting of Outbreak Reports and Intervention studies Of Nosocomial infection	Items to include when reporting an outbreak or intervention study of a nosocomial organism (22-item checklist). Endorsed by a number of professional special interest groups and societies including the Association of Medical Microbiologists (AMM), British Society for Antimicrobial Chemotherapy (BSAC), and the Infection Control Nurses' Association (ICNA) Research and Development Group.

(continued)

TABLE 21.1 Research Reporting Guidelines and Initiatives (*continued*)

ORGANIZATION/GUIDELINE	DESCRIPTION
Practihc: Pragmatic Randomized Control Trials in Healthcare	European Union-funded converted action that provides open-access tools, training, and mentoring to researchers in developing countries that are interested in designing and conducting pragmatic RCTs of health care interventions.
PRIMER Collaboration: Presentation and Interpretation of Medical Research	Group that aims to improve the design of studies, their presentation, interpretation of results and translation into practice.
PRISMA: Preferred Reporting Items for Systematic Reviews and Meta-Analyses	Evidence-based minimum set of items for reporting in systematic reviews and meta-analyses. PRISMA has "focused on randomized trials, but ... can also be used as a basis for reporting systematic reviews of other types of research, particularly evaluations of interventions. PRISMA may also be useful for critical appraisal of published systematic reviews, although it is not a quality assessment instrument to gauge the quality of a systematic review."
QUOROM: QUality Of Reporting Of Meta-analyses	Checklist that describes the group's preferred way to present the abstract, introduction, methods, results, and discussion sections of a report of a meta-analysis. Moher, D., Cook, D. J., Eastwood, S., Olkin, I., Rennie, D., & Stroup, D. F. (1999). Improving the quality of reports of meta-analyses of randomised controlled trials: The QUOROM statement. Quality of reporting of meta-analyses. *Lancet, 354*(9193), 1896–1900 (Review). PubMed PMID: 10584742
RedHot: Reporting Data on Homeopathic Treatments (A Supplement to CONSORT)	Standard for reporting details of homeopathic treatments. Eight-item checklist designed to be used by authors and editors when publishing reports of clinical trials. Dean, M. E., Coulter, M. K., Fisher, P., Jobst, K. A., & Walach, H. (2007). Reporting data on homeopathic treatments (RedHot): A supplement to CONSORT. *Journal of Alternative and Complementary Medicine, 3*(1), 19–23. PubMed PMID: 17309373

The REFLECT Statement: Reporting guidElines For randomized controLled trials for livEstoCk and food safeTy	Evidence-based minimum set of items for trials reporting production, health, and food-safety outcomes (22-item checklist).
	Sargeant, J. M., O'Connor, A. M., Gardner, I. A., Dickson, J. S., Torrence, M. E., Dohoo, I. R., et al. (2010). The REFLECT statement: Reporting guidelines for randomized controlled trials in livestock and food safety: Explanation and elaboration. *Journal of Food Protection, 73*(3), 579–603. PubMed PMID: 20202349
	Sargeant, J. M., O'Connor, A. M., Gardner, I. A., Dickson, J. S., Torrence, M. E., & Consensus Meeting Participants: Dohoo, I. R., Lefebvre, S. L., Morley, P. S., Ramirez, A., Snedeker, K. (2010, January 12). The REFLECT statement: Reporting guidelines for randomized controlled trials in livestock and food safety: Explanation and elaboration. *Zoonoses Public Health* [Epub ahead of print] PubMed PMID: 20070652
REMARK: REporting recommendations for tumor MARKer prognostic studies	Guidelines for reporting of tumor marker studies.
	McShane, L. M., Altman, D. G., Sauerbrei, W., Taube, S. E., Gion, M., Clark, G. M., & Statistics Subcommittee of NCI-EORTC Working Group on Cancer Diagnostics. (2006). REporting recommendations for tumor MARKer prognostic studies (REMARK). *Breast Cancer Research and Treatment, 100*(2), 229–235 [Epub 2006 Aug 24]. PubMed PMID: 16932852
SMRS: Standard Metabolic Reporting Structures	Summary recommendations for standardization and reporting of metabolic analyses.
	Lindon, J. C., Nicholson, J. K., Holmes, E., Keun, H. C., Craig, A., Pearce, J. T., et al. (2005). Standard Metabolic Reporting Structures Working Group. Summary recommendations for standardization and reporting of metabolic analyses. *Nature Biotechnology, 23*(7), 833–838. PubMed PMID: 16003371
STARD: STAndards for the Reporting of Diagnostic accuracy	Aims to improve the accuracy and completeness of reporting of studies of diagnostic accuracy, to allow readers to assess the potential for bias in the study (internal validity) and to evaluate its generalizability (25-item checklist).
	Adopters of STARD: (1) Visit homepage; (2) Click "Adopters of STARD."

(continued)

439

TABLE 21.1   Research Reporting Guidelines and Initiatives (*continued*)

ORGANIZATION/GUIDELINE	DESCRIPTION
STREGA: STrengthening the REporting of Genetic Associations	The purpose of the workshop was to develop evidence-based guidelines to promote clear reporting of genetic-association studies, and reduce gaps in the evidence regarding potential methodological biases in such studies.
STRICTA: STandards for Reporting Interventions in Controlled Trials of Acupuncture	Designed as a supplement to CONSORT, which has led to improved reporting of trial design and conduct in general. Current plans are to revise STRICTA in collaboration with the CONSORT Group, such that STRICTA becomes an "official" extension to CONSORT. STRICTA journals.
STROBE: STrengthening the Reporting of OBservational studies in Epidemiology	The STROBE Statement is referred to in the Uniform Requirements for Manuscripts Submitted to Biomedical Journals by the International Committee of Medical Journal Editors. www .strobe-statement.org
	These journals refer to STROBE in their Instructions for Authors.
Structured Abstracts	National Library of Medicine (NLM) description of structured abstracts and how they are formatted for MEDLINE.
Trial Bank Project: University of California, San Francisco.	The Trial Bank Project has moved away from pursuing trial bank publishing to explore new research avenues.
WAME: World Association of Medical Editors	Group that aims to publish original, important, well-documented peer-reviewed articles on clinical and laboratory research. WAME journals.

Adapted from the U.S. National Library of Medicine. Retrieved from http://www.nlm.nih.gov/services/research_report_guide.html

the Internet is an easy, quick, and inexpensive way to disseminate research findings. Visiting sites, such as a nursing journal publisher (www.nursingcenter.com), or simply using any search engine (google .com for example) for keywords such as "nursing listserv or "nursing blog" produces hundreds of possible venues (lists, bulletin boards, user groups, and wikis) on which you might disseminate ideas related to your research. The limitation to publishing in nonpeer-reviewed websites is the lack of peer review. There is no one controlling the quality of what is published; therefore, the research is not given as much credit in academia and may not be considered as prestigious as publishing in a peer-reviewed journal.

Publishing in Cyberspace

YouTube.com, founded in 2005, is an increasingly popular site for nurses to watch and share original videos that can be viewed through websites, mobile devices, blogs, and e-mail. A simple YouTube search using keywords "nursing research" produced a plethora of narrated videos about all aspects of nursing research conducted by faculty, students, and practitioners. Use of the search term "writing for publication" had the same type of result. So if you learn best through visual representations, YouTube may be for you.

A wiki, a mass communication mechanism that allows open editing by anyone of all posted content, is rapidly being used in health care to share common work and ideas, including research. Go to http:// en.wikipedia.org/wiki/Nursing_research or http://en.wikipedia.org /wiki/Nursing. Click various links to learn about its potential to assist you as you proceed through the nursing research process (from idea generation to dissemination). If you are not finding what you need related to your research, it is easy to start your own wiki and get all the assistance you desire from around the world. To see how a cardiovascular service line administrator set up a wiki in her health system to connect key nurses, physicians, managers, and support staff regarding specific issues, see Clancy's (2007) article.

What you post to any open-access website can easily be taken and used by someone without your knowledge. Likewise, what you post has the potential to exist forever. So make sure that what you post today will not be an embarrassment to you years later when seen by a potential employer or school admissions officer.

Internet Dissemination of Information

Numerous health care organizations have their own websites, which are copyrighted and where nurse researchers may post their studies.

Another possibility is developing your own dedicated website. Almost every Internet service provider (Google, Yahoo, AOL, etc.) provides free website space with building instructions, as does FreeWebs (http://members.freewebs.com). Almost every journal publisher is converting originally published print-journal content to an electronic format. This process gives an author who is published in the print version exposure to readers who prefer to search the Internet for information rather than use a library indexing reference. Electronically search the Internet addresses given previously to find print journals that also have an electronic version.

Electronic Journals

Almost all publishers are using web-based systems to acquire, review, edit, and produce their journals' content. Publication in an electronic peer-reviewed journal has the advantage of almost immediate publication—material is submitted electronically to an editor, forwarded by the editor to reviewers electronically, and revised and published electronically. There is little delay in generating knowledge to disseminating it to those who can use it. Another advantage is that resources are conserved—no paper, no discs, no photocopying, and no postage. In addition, your content can also easily be updated with new information and hypertext links to other sites related to your topic. Readers can enter into a dialogue with you and the editor through electronic mail, which can be appended to the electronic article. With the increase in online journals, revenues have decreased, thereby passing the cost of publishing to the author. Some journals may charge the author to publish in the journal to offset the costs of publishing.

CRITICAL SUCCESS FACTORS FOR PUBLISHING

Journal publication is the most frequent method for research dissemination because many nurses can be reached by one effort—writing a high-quality, focused manuscript. To increase the chance of having your manuscript accepted for publication (Happell, 2005; Smith, 2010), the following guidelines are recommended (Table 21.2).

Select the Appropriate Audience

The first step in any writing project is selecting the appropriate audience: To whom do you wish to convey your findings? Who would benefit most from your research findings? When writing your paper, be specific in the introduction as to your intended audience. By focusing on a particular audience, you can present your research findings to meet that audience's needs. For example, if your research findings

TABLE 21.2   Critical Success Factors for Publishing

■ Select the appropriate audience
■ Select the appropriate journal
■ Query the editor
■ Conform to submission guidelines
■ Adhere to copyright laws
■ Include implications for practice
■ Use recent references
■ Maintain organization
■ Use tables and graphs
■ Determine authorship entitlement
■ Acknowledge appropriately
■ Conform to ethical practices

suggested a cost-effective way to deliver nursing care, practitioners and administrators would be interested in the topic. However, practitioners would be interested in the clinical implications, whereas administrators would be interested in the management aspects.

Select the Appropriate Journal

The most innovative, well-written manuscript will be rejected if it is submitted to the wrong journal (Smith, 2010). Having identified your audience allows you to select the journals that are edited for that group. Consider the impact factor of the journal and how often your manuscript will be read by others to impact nursing practice. Publishing in a high-impact journal may be more difficult but worth the effort. Once your potential journals are selected, obtain the guidelines for authors that most journals publish in each issue. Frequently included is a short mission statement highlighting the major focus of the journal, the intended readership profile, and types of topics that are appropriate for submission. In addition to seeking this information to make the appropriate journal choice, examine several recent issues to assess the preferred format approach of the journal.

Query the Editor

When you plan your writing project, it is a good idea to first query editors of potential journals that might be appropriate for your topic. Although queries can be by mail, telephone, or e-mail, almost all editors prefer electronic queries. They are fast and can be answered at the editor's convenience. Do not attach files to your queries; place your query in the e-mail message area. Information for authors' guidelines often include which approach the editor prefers. Figure 21.1 shows an acceptable format for an e-mail query. Please note that although an e-mail query has a more casual format than a formal mailed letter, it is still professional. Figure 21.2 illustrates a query to a consumer journal on the same topic as that in Figure 21.1. Note the change in language and tone.

Querying the editor can save you time and effort. Although it is acceptable to query several editors at the same time, it is not acceptable to send a manuscript to more than one journal at the same time.

Editors are professionals and experts in writing for publication. Editors know the types of manuscripts they would like to obtain for publication. When querying an editor, explain in detail your research and plans for the manuscript's content (Smith, 2010). The editor may discuss your thoughts and approach for organizing the manuscript content. The editor may persuade you to use a different focus to increase your chances of acceptance of the manuscript for publication. And, the editor may inform you that the particular journal is not interested in your manuscript because of its similarity to already published or soon-to-be published papers. Receiving this type of information allows you to tailor your manuscript to the journal whose editor has expressed the most interest in your topic.

Dear (name of editor)

     I wish to submit a manuscript to (*name of publication*). Our research examined processes of change used in smoking cessation by 190 smokers and former smokers selected through random-digit dialing. A mailed cross-sectional survey had an 84% response rate. Multivariate analysis of variance of 10 processes of change across 5 stages of smoking cessation (precontemplation, contemplation, relapse, recent, and long-term quitting) was significant, $F(40,590) = 5.02$, $p = .0001$. Post hoc analysis revealed statistically significant differences on 7 of the 10 processes of change ($p < .05$). The readers of your journal can apply our study findings in their practice to help clients stop smoking.

    (Optional to add content outline here if above paragraph is not self-explanatory as to approach.)

    (Optional brief paragraph here indicating your qualifications to write on your topic if that is not obvious in your ending signature information.)

    The manuscript will be ready for submission within 6 weeks of receiving your positive reply. I look forward to hearing from you.

(Contact Person)

(Work or home address and telephone number; work information preferred)

FIGURE 21.1   Sample e-mail query letter for nursing journal.

Dear (name of editor)

Smoking is an addiction with severe consequences—cancer, emphysema, circulatory problems, to name a few. Despite the widely known negative effects of smoking, people have great difficulty quitting, spending millions to beat their addiction.

As a nurse expert with years of helping people stop smoking, I would like to write a manuscript for your (insert magazine name). The manuscript will present 10 significant strategies, shown in a recent nursing research study to assist people advance successfully through the 5 stages of smoking cessation.

This practical manuscript to assist your readers to stop smoking can be submitted now according to your requirements. I look forward to hearing from you.

(Your Name)

(Address and telephone number)

FIGURE 21.2   Sample e-mail query letter for consumer magazine.

Include Implications for Practice

Often a good manuscript is rejected for publication because the author does not discuss the implications of the research findings for the journal's readership. As the topic expert, readers expect a discussion of the utility of findings to practice. The length of the implications section will vary depending on the journal's purpose. The implications section in a research journal is often short compared to a clinical journal's focus on application.

When discussing implications for the study, present your findings in relation to similar studies. Highlight how your findings support as well as differ from those of others if similar studies have been reported. Finally, suggest directions for future research that are needed to further apply your research to practice.

Conform to the Submission Requirements

All journals have requirements for formatting and submitting your manuscript. Although these requirements are not often printed in the journal, they can usually be found on the journal's website. Journal editors have a bias toward manuscripts that are correctly formatted. An incorrectly formatted manuscript can be a "red flag." Often, editors assume that if the author of a paper was serious about its publication in the journal, the author would have made an effort to send it properly formatted. A lingering thought in the editor's mind will be, "If the author did not pay attention to simple formatting requirements, what attention has been paid to ensure the integrity of the research and the manuscript?"

Adhere to Copyright Laws

Once a manuscript is accepted for publication, authors are required by the publisher to sign an agreement that transfers copyright of the author's material to the publisher (Dames, 2012; Rhoads & White, 2008). Once signed, the agreement renders the manuscript the copyrighted work of the publisher. The author must have the publisher's written permission to use a significant part of the article in another publication, oral, written, or electronic. When in doubt about using copyrighted work, call and/or write the copyright holder (Dobbins, Souder, & Smith, 2005; Rhoads & White, 2008).

Use Recent References

References used in your manuscript should be current and relevant to your topic. The definition of current varies from editor to editor, but, generally, a 3-year range is acceptable. Obvious exceptions to this rule of thumb might be "classic" works related to your topic. Use of older references is also acceptable when you are replicating a study. Using current references conveys to the editor and your readers that your research has been placed in the context of contemporary concerns and that you are making a new contribution to the health care literature.

Maintain Organization

A manuscript with a logical flow of ideas is easy to read and understand. Developing an organized, orderly paper, however, requires work, particularly when presenting a complex research protocol that was not necessarily linear. Facilitate order and clarity by outlining your content and using headings and subheadings. Always have a colleague read a draft of your paper solely for the logical progression of its content.

Use Tables and Graphs

Tables, graphs, and illustrations add significantly to the overall sophistication of your manuscript. They also serve to clarify concepts and present research findings and outcomes in a more easily understood way. The use of tables and graphs also assists in organizing your information. Before writing the paper, decide which concepts lend themselves to display in a graphic form. When discussing table or graph information in text, do not restate every piece of information. Highlight one or two key points and refer the reader to the table or graph. Refer to Chapter 8 for further information on using tables to present results.

Develop tables that are self-explanatory by keeping in mind the following guidelines (American Psychological Association, 2009; Rice University, 2008).

- Keep the title clear and concise
- Label each row and column and provide units of measure for the data
- Include notes (general, specific, and probability notes) below the table: general—provides information applicable to the table (e.g., abbreviations and symbols); specific—refers to an entry, column, or row; probability—indicates results of tests of significance

Graphs are used to synthesize data and show the relationship between two or more variables. Effective graphs are accurate, simple, clear, neat, professional, and attractive. There are several considerations when developing graphs (American Psychological Association, 2009; Rice University, 2008). These considerations include using a frame to establish a boundary between the data and other information, prominent symbols to plot data, and a scale appropriate to the data.

Determine Authorship Entitlement

Authorship implies significant involvement in writing a paper and in the work that led to that writing. It implies "substantial intellectual contribution" (Nativio, 1993, p. 358). The reality is that authorship is often given to (or insisted on by) people with minimal involvement in the writing project—perhaps a supervisor, a data collector, or a statistician. Guidelines for authorship make it clear that "Authorship credit should be based on (1) substantial contributions to conception and design, or acquisition of data, or analysis and interpretation of data; (2) drafting the article or revising it critically for important intellectual content; and (3) final approval of the version to be published. Authors should meet conditions 1, 2, and 3. Acquisition of funding, collection of data, or general supervision of the research group, alone, does not justify authorship" (ICMJE, 2008). In large, multisite research projects, it is becoming common to list the research group as the author, with individuals mentioned in a footnote. When this is the case, all members of the group still must meet the stringent requirements for authorship.

There is no rule for order of authorship (Bosch, Pericas, Hernandez, & Torrents, 2012; Cleary, Jackson, Walter, Watson, & Hunt, 2012). The order of authorship should be discussed before writing begins. The joint decision of the coauthors, after analysis of each author's contribution to the work, can further determine whether adjustments should be made. This analysis is best done at the start of a project so that expectations are clear and conflicts are later avoided. Order of authorship in nursing journals often indicates greatest to smallest contribution. This order might be based on the amount of time given or on the importance of the contribution. In other journals, it may be alphabetical listing. Some put the senior investigator as the last author instead of the first. You can never assume that being the first author is better than being the last author unless you know the journal's guidelines to authorship. The authorship must be decided before the manuscript is written, during the planning stages of writing the manuscript.

Acknowledge Appropriately

If not everyone who contributed to a research project is entitled to authorship, then certainly each person who contributed should be acknowledged. But there is almost as much controversy about who is entitled to acknowledgment as there is to authorship entitlement. Although some editors feel that authors who blindly acknowledge family, friends, and colleagues are frivolous, others feel generous acknowledgments reflect the humanity of authors (Mundy, 2002). As a rule of thumb, acknowledgments are reserved for those who have made a substantial contribution to the project being reported in a paper, including editorial and writing assistance (Flanagin & Rennie, 1995). People who might be acknowledged are data collectors, a project director, an editorial assistant, or a faculty advisor. Be aware that not everyone wishes to be acknowledged publicly. For this reason, obtain written permission from those named in an acknowledgment to ensure that they approve your use of their name in material that will be published and widely disseminated. This must be done before including people's names in the manuscript. Some journals require a signed statement from those acknowledged.

Conform to Ethical Practices

Adhering to ethical practices when publishing is vital; unethical practices can ruin your chances for future publication. Two easily avoided unethical practices are submitting the same manuscript to different journals at the same time and plagiarism.

It is unethical to submit a manuscript to more than one journal at the same time. Every journal's Information for Authors' guidelines has a statement to the effect that the author warrants that he or she is submitting original, unpublished material, under consideration by no other publisher. So, although it is acceptable to query as many editors as desired about interest in your manuscript, it can only be submitted to one journal at a time. If your manuscript is rejected, it is permissible then to send it to another journal.

Plagiarism is claiming someone's ideas and work, published or unpublished, as your own. The four common types of plagiarism are

(1) verbatim lifting of passages, (2) rewording ideas from an original source as an author's own style, (3) paraphrasing an original work without attribution, and (4) noting the original source of only some of what is borrowed (American Medical Association, 2007). Be acutely aware of when your writing reflects the ideas of others and appropriately reference the original source. If you borrow a significant amount of material (copyright law does not define "significant") through paraphrasing or direct quotation, write the copyright holder, which is usually the publishing company, and obtain written permission. Likewise, any published item, no matter how large or small that is complete unto itself, such as a table, figure, chart, graph, art work, poem, or picture requires that you have permission from the copyright holder to reproduce the item. For further discussion of the intricacies of copyright in order to avoid plagiarism or copyright law violation, see publications such as Rhoads and White (2008), American Medical Association (2008), or visit the federal government copyright office's website (www.lcweb .loc.gov/copyright).

MANUSCRIPT REVIEW PROCESS

Peer review, also called the referee process, is the process that editors use to help ensure the professional integrity of nursing knowledge through an unbiased, (usually) blinded critique (Ludwig & Wood, 2012). This process has three main purposes—detection of errors, fair and impartial treatment of authors' ideas, and identification and publication of innovative and new ideas to advance the profession (Clarke, 2006; Miracle, 2008; Spear, 2004; Swartz, 2008). To accomplish these purposes, editors assume the responsibility of selecting reviewers who have demonstrated advanced knowledge or practice in a particular nursing role (administrator, researcher, or educator) or patient care specialty. Manuscripts then are reviewed by at least two reviewers, often three. Reviewers screen the manuscripts for quality, accuracy, timeliness, relevance, and appropriateness prior to the editor's consideration of the paper for publication.

Peer review has been criticized as not always being an effective means to ensure the validity of content published or the fairness of the manuscript selection process (Miracle, 2008). Despite its potential weaknesses, peer review is the most appropriate means for selecting manuscripts for publication It gives readers assurance that the journal's content meets acceptable standards of scholarship, conferring validity and credibility on an author's work (Dougherty, 2006; Froman, 2006).

A nonpeer-reviewed publication is one that does not have an editorial board and is not considered credible for research or scholarly projects. Nonpeer-reviewed publications include many Internet sites that report news or health care information, magazines, and newspapers

(Ludwig & Wood, 2012). When journals are not peer reviewed, the editor reviews manuscripts and decides which manuscripts will be published, using similar criteria to that used by peer-reviewed journals. Although the articles in such journals may be excellent, the lack of peer review lessens their credibility. Journals that are peer reviewed will state so somewhere within the issue. If such a statement is not found, contact the journal's editorial office and seek clarification.

Because of promotion and tenure criteria, faculty in institutions of higher education and some major academic health science centers receive credit only for publications in peer-reviewed journals. Although the quality of material published in a nonpeer-reviewed journal may not be any different from that in a peer-reviewed journal, your choice of journal should be made in light of current job requirements as well as your planned career track.

DEALING WITH REJECTION OF A MANUSCRIPT

If your manuscript is not accepted for publication by your first-choice journal, do not give up. Many published authors have had their works rejected for publication. The art of writing requires practice and study. Receiving feedback about your manuscript's strengths and weaknesses from reviewers and editors helps you focus on developing the skills you need to successfully publish.

If your manuscript is rejected, there are two options (neither of which is never writing again!). First, you could call and speak to the editor personally. Ask what you can do to revise the work to have it published. Editors are very quick to acknowledge such requests and most will work with you to recommend suggestions for revision and resubmission. A good editor will be honest about the quality of your manuscript and may recommend other journals that may be more appropriate for your work.

The second option is to revise and submit the manuscript to another journal. Remember to focus your revised content to the new journal's readership and editorial purpose. Many excellent manuscripts are needlessly rejected because the author did not target content for a journal's readership or conform to its style.

There are advantages and disadvantages to publishing research findings in a print journal, with the advantages outweighing the disadvantages. Some of the advantages include the following:

- Enhanced self-esteem
- National recognition of work
- Achievement of professional goals
- Identification as an expert in topic area
- Ability to appropriately disseminate research
- Contribution to the nursing profession

Some disadvantages are as follows:

- Inability to interact with the audience
- Inability to personally answer questions
- Inability to provide clarification of content without additional effort on the part of the reader
- Limited space in which to present your work
- Rarely is an honorarium or royalty paid
- Copyright, and thus subsequent unlimited use, of the manuscript content is transferred to another party

SUMMARY

Nursing research contributes positively to the health care delivery system. As more nurses are prepared at the graduate and doctoral levels, more and more nursing research is being conducted in clinical, administrative, and education settings. Nurses who conduct research have a professional obligation to share their findings. This is how a profession grows and matures. In the past, we have been shy about presenting our findings (Winslow, 1996), but this is changing. Nurses are making outstanding contributions to the future health of the world.

SUGGESTED ACTIVITIES

Website: http://owl.english.purdue.edu/owl/resource/681/01
    The Owl (Online Writing Lab) at Purdue is an excellent site at which to hone your writing and research skills.

1. Go to http://owl.english.purdue.edu/owl/resource/629/02 and complete an "Audience Analysis."
2. Go to http://owl.english.purdue.edu/owl/resource/567/01 and identify your blocks to writing and try two of the suggested intervention strategies.
3. Go to http://owl.english.purdue.edu/owl/resource/553/02 and evaluate the value of the next three sources of information you plan to use in your research.

REFERENCES

Altman, D., Moher, D., & Schulz, K. (2012). Improve the reporting of randomized trials: The CONSORT statement and beyond. *Statistics in Medicine, 31*(25), 2985–2997.

American Medical Association. (2007). *AMA manual of style* (10th ed.). New York, NY: Oxford University Press.

American Psychological Association. (2009). *Publication manual of the American Psychological Asociation* (6th ed.). Washington, DC: Author.

Baker, J. (2012). The quid pro quo of peer review. *AORN, 96*(4), 356–360.

Bosch, X., Pericas, J., Hernandez, C., & Torrents, A. (2012). A comparison of authorship policies at top-ranked peer-reviewed biomedical journals. *Archives of Internal Medicine, 172*(1), 70–72.

Clancy, T. R. (2007). Organizing: New ways to harness complexity. *Journal of Nursing Administration, 37*(12), 534–536.

Clarke, S. P. (2006). Reviewing peer review: The three reviewers you meet at submission time. *Canadian Journal of Nursing Research, 38*(4), 5–9.

Cleary, M., Jackson, D., Walter, G., Watson, R., & Hunt, G. (2012). Location, location, location—The position of authors in scholarly publishing. *Journal of Clinical Nursing, 21*(5/6), 809–811.

Dames, K. (2012). The coming copyright clash in higher education. *Information Today, 29*(7), 24–25.

Dobbins, W. N., Souder, E., & Smith, R. M. (2005). Living with fair use and TEACH: A quest for compliance. *Computers Informatics Nursing (CIN), 23*(3), 120–124.

Dougherty, M. C. (2006). The value of peer review. *Nursing Research, 55*(2), 73–74.

Flanagin, A., & Rennie, D. (1995). Acknowledging ghosts. *Journal of the American Medical Association, 273*(1), 73.

Froman, R. D. (2006). The importance of peer review. *Research in Nursing and Health, 29*(4), 253–255.

Happell, B. (2005). Disseminating nursing knowledge: A guide to writing for publication. *International Journal of Psychiatric Nursing Research, 10*(3), 1147–1155.

Happell, B. (2012). Writing and publishing clinical articles: A practical guide. *Emergency Nurse, 20*(1), 33–38.

International Committee of Medical Journal Editors (ICMJE). (2008). *Authorship and contributorship*. Retrieved January 10, 2009, from http://www.icmje.org

Ludwig, R., & Wood, B. (2012). The difference between peer review and non-peer review. *Radiologic Technology, 84*(1), 90–92.

Miracle, V. A. (2008). The peer review process. *Dimensions in Critical Care Nursing, 27*(2), 67–69.

Mundy, D. (2002). A question of missing acknowledgement. *Science Editor, 25*(2), 58–59.

Nakayama, T., Hirat, N., Yamazaki, S., & Naito, M. (2005). Adoption of structured abstracts by general medical journals and format for a structured abstract. *Journal of the Medical Library Association, 93*, 237–242.

Nativio, D. G. (1993). Authorship. *IMAGE: Journal of Nursing Scholarship, 25*, 358.

Pesch, O. (2012). Usage factor for journals: A new measure for scholarly impact. *Serials Librarian, 63*(3–4), 261–268. DOI: 10.1080/0361526X.2012.722522

Rhoads, J., & White, C. (2008). Copyright law and distance nursing education. *Nurse Educator, 33*(1), 39–44.

Rice University. (2008). *Displaying data in written documents*. Retrieved January 10, 2009, from http://www.owlnet.rice.edu/~cainproj/courses/comp482/Data_Written_Docs.doc

Smith, S. P. (2010). The manager as published author: Tips on writing for publication. In M. Harris (Ed.), *Handbook of home health care administration* (5th ed.). Sudbury, MA: Jones and Bartlett.

Sonuga-Barke, E. (2012). "Holy grail" or "siren's song"?: The dangers for the field of child psychology and psychiatry of over-focusing on the journal impact factor. *Journal of Child Psychology & Psychiatry, 53*(9), 915–917.

Spear, H. J. (2004). On ethical peer review and publication: The importance of professional conduct and communication. *Nurse Author & Editor, 14*(4), 1–3.

Swartz, M. (2008). The importance of peer review. *Journal of Pediatric Health Care, 22*(60), 333–334.

Tornquist, E. M. (1999). *From proposal to publication: An informal guide to writing about nursing research.* Menlo Park, CA: Addison Wesley.

Webb, C. (2007). Publishing from a research thesis. *Nurse Author & Editor, 17*(3). Retrieved December 30, 2008, from http://www.nurseauthoreditor.com/article.asp?id=86

Winslow, E. H. (1996). Failure to publish research: A form of scientific misconduct? *Heart & Lung: The Journal of Acute and Critical Care, 25,* 169–171.

Index